Michael Emmans Dean
The Trials of Homeopathy

edition forschung
Herausgegeben von der Karl und Veronica Carstens-Stiftung

Hans Walz Preisschrift

The Trials of Homeopathy

Origins, Structure and Development

Michael Emmans Dean

gefördert von der Robert Bosch Stiftung, Stuttgart

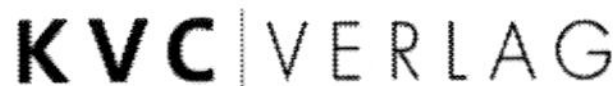

Karl und Veronica Carstens-Stiftung
im Stifterverband für die Deutsche Wissenschaft
Am Deimelsberg 36
45276 Essen
Tel.: 0201/56305-0
Fax: 0201/56305-30
www.kvc-verlag.de

Dean, Michael Emmans
The Trials of Homeopathy – Origins, Structure and Development

edition forschung
Herausgegeben von der Karl und Veronica Carstens-Stiftung

ISBN 3-933351-40-5

Umschlaggestaltung: eye-d Designbüro, Essen
Druck: Union Betriebs-GmbH, Rheinbach

Foreword

It is with great pleasure that, in conjunction with the Karl and Veronica Carstens Foundation, we present the winning entry of the first Hans Walz Prize. Working in close partnership with the Foundation's publishing arm, we have been able to publish this in an unusually short time following the awarding of the prize, on 30 October 2003 at the Robert Bosch House in Stuttgart, Germany.

Hans Walz (1873–1974) was Robert Bosch Senior's right-hand man. For many years he was Chairman of Robert Bosch GmbH and on the board of the Stuttgart Homeopathic Hospital. He had a lifelong professional and personal commitment to homeopathy.

The aim of this prize is to promote research in the history of homeopathy outside the Robert Bosch Foundation's Institute for the History of Medicine. Works eligible for the prize (e.g. undergraduate or Master's dissertations, PhD theses, monographs or extended essays) must be either unpublished, or published no more than one year before submission. They may be in German, English or French. The prize will be awarded on a biennial basis.

The response to the first call for entries, in 2002, was most gratifying. We received works from Germany, and also from Britain and the USA. The jury (consisting of Dr K.H. Gebhardt, Karlsruhe; Dr I. Wünning, Robert Bosch Foundation; Prof. Dr M. Dinges and Prof. Dr R. Jütte) awarded the prize to M.E. Dean's University of York PhD thesis, the original title of which was 'The Trials of Homeopathy. A critical-historical account of the origins, structure and development of Hahnemann's scientific therapeutics, and two systematic reviews of homeopathic clinical trials, 1821–1953 and 1940–1998.'

This is the first systematic review of all clinical trials of homeopathy, predominantly in Europe and North America, from its beginnings to the present day. Dean shows that homeopathy has a long history of scientifically conducted trials that have not received the recognition they deserve. At a time when the place of homeopathy in a changing health landscape is under discussion, this work provides a valuable historical context. The current debate about the merits of different therapies is informed increasingly by trial evidence. The rediscovery of homeopathy's clinical research tradition is, therefore, of particular importance.

We hope this book will be widely read.

Prof. Dr R. Jütte
Head of the Institute for the History of Medicine

Prof. Dr M. Dinges
Head of the Homeopathy Archive

der derzeitigen Diskussion um die Neupositionierung der Homöopathie in einem sich verändernden Umfeld gibt dieser Text historische Orientierung: In einer immer stärker durch wissenschaftliche Forschung geprägten Auseinandersetzung um den Wert bestimmter Heilweisen ist die Wiederentdeckung der klinischen Tradition der Homöopathie bedeutungsvoll.

Wir wünschen dem Buch eine große Leserschaft.

Prof. Dr. R. Jütte
Institutleiter

Prof. Dr. M. Dinges
Leiter des Homöopathie-Archivs

Vorwort

Wir freuen uns, gemeinsam mit der Karl und Veronica Carstens-Stiftung die erste Hans-Walz-Preisschrift der Öffentlichkeit übergeben zu können. Durch die hervorragende Kooperation mit dem Verlag dieser Stiftung gelang dies innerhalb einer ungewöhnlich kurzen Frist nach der Preisverleihung am 30. Oktober 2003 im Robert Bosch Haus, Stuttgart.

Hans Walz (1873–1974) war enger Mitarbeiter von Robert Bosch d. Ä. und langjähriger Vorsitzender der Geschäftsführung der Robert Bosch GmbH sowie Aufsichtsratsmitglied der Stuttgarter Homöopathischen Krankenhaus GmbH. Er hat sich zeitlebens beruflich und persönlich für die Homöopathie eingesetzt.

Ziel des Preises ist es, die homöopathiegeschichtliche Forschung auch außerhalb des Instituts für Geschichte der Medizin der Robert Bosch Stiftung zu fördern. Das Preisgeld wird für eine erst ein Jahr vor der Bewerbung oder noch nicht veröffentlichte Arbeit (Staatsexamens-, Diplom- oder Magisterarbeit, Dissertation oder Monographie, umfangreicheres Aufsatzmanuskript) in deutscher, englischer oder französischer Sprache ausgesetzt. Der Preis wird in zweijährlichem Rhythmus ausgelobt.

Das Echo auf den 2002 erstmals veröffentlichten Preisaufruf war sehr erfreulich. So wurden neben deutschen auch Arbeiten aus Großbritannien und den USA eingereicht. Die Jury (Dr. K.H. Gebhardt, Karlsruhe; Dr. I. Wünning, Robert Bosch Stiftung; Prof. Dr. M. Dinges und Prof. Dr. R. Jütte) entschied sich für die von Dr. M. E. Dean (Universität York) eingereichte Dissertation mit dem ursprünglichen Titel. „The Trials of Homeopathy. A critical-historical account of the origins, structure and development of Hahnemann's scientific therapeutics, and two systematic reviews of homeopathic clinical trials, 1821–1953 and 1940–1998".

Es handelt sich um die erste systematische Untersuchung sämtlicher klinischer Versuche zur Homöopathie, überwiegend in Europa und Nordamerika, von ihren Anfängen bis in die Gegenwart. Dean zeigt, dass die Homöopathie eine lange Geschichte dieser wissenschaftlichen Versuche aufweist, die bisher völlig unzureichend zur Kenntnis genommen wurde. Gerade in

Acknowledgements

First thanks go to Professor Ian Russell, my supervisor, for his original suggestion that I undertake a review of homeopathy's effectiveness, and his subsequent encouragement and support as systematic review began to resemble an archeological dig. Thanks also to the other members of my research advisory group, Dr David Reilly and Dr Kim Jobst, for sparing time from their clinical and teaching duties to share their valuable insights. I think it is fair to say that, in his own way, each of these researchers is interested more in the quality of patient care than in healing technologies per se, and I have tried to retain this emphasis throughout.

For various types of assistance, including the retrieval or translation of some primary documents reviewed here, I should like to thank: Henning Albrecht, Jean Jacques Aulas, Zelda di Blasi, Diana Fernando, Mary Gooch, the late Gustav Hildebrandt, Lois Hoffer, Alexander Kotok, Colin Lessell, Klaus Linde, Corine Mure, Francis Treuherz and Hegge Urdahl.

The library staff at the following institutions also deserve thanks: Allegheny University of Health Sciences, USA; British Homeopathic Library, Glasgow; British Homoeopathic Association, London; British Library, London and Boston Spa; (former) Goethe Institut, York; Halle Universität; Homoeopathic Trust, London; Robert Bosch Stiftung, Stuttgart; Wellcome Institute for the History of Medicine, London; York Minster; J.B. Morrell Library, University of York.

I would like to record a special debt of gratitude to Anneliese, my wife, who aided and abetted by translating from six languages, by suggestions that improved the clarity of my writing, and by meticulous proofreading. Any errors that remain are mine alone. I cannot thank her enough for her support and patience during this project.

York, July 2001 M. E. Dean

Abstract

The controversial discipline of homeopathy is examined from three original perspectives.

Conceptual background: The structure and presentation of Hahnemann's research programme is contrasted with philosophical assumptions about medical science and emerging theoretical structures in German academic medicine circa 1800, and the subsequent rift between homeopathy and allopathy is explained at this level. The sources of homeopathic theory and method are located in mainstream eighteenth-century experiment. Alleged relationships to alchemical medicine are discounted, with the exception of certain pharmacy techniques introduced after 1816. Divergent schools and approaches within homeopathy are traced to their sources, and mapped onto a unified therapeutic field.

Historical importance: A systematic review of prospective clinical evaluations of homeopathy, 1821–1953, contends that these played an important but neglected part in the evolution of the clinical trial. Placebo-controlled trials by sceptics most probably originated in prior Hahnemannian use of within-patient placebo controls. Pragmatic trials of homeopathy versus allopathy in the mid nineteenth century show that judgements of homeopathic inefficacy made by influential nineteenth-century opponents, which have coloured debate ever since, were not evidence-based. Early twentieth-century clinical trials by homeopaths were methodologically in advance of biomedical trials in some respects.

Clinical relevance: A systematic review of 205 prospective controlled clinical trials published since 1940 found evidence of homeopathy's safety, and specific and global efficacy in trials of high internal validity. Implications for clinical research and practice are considered, founded on analysis of intra-homeopathic differences and trends. On the basis of trial evidence, the relative merits of placebo-controlled and pragmatic evaluations of homeopathy are discussed. Clinical relevance was found particularly in areas that pose problems for biomedicine, and proposals for pragmatic trials of homeopathy versus standard treatment are made in the following conditions: unexplained female infertility; postviral fatigue syndrome; influenza; atopy.

Contents

Part IV: Conclusion

1. Introduction

1.1. Rationale

Public demand for alternative and complementary medicine has never been greater, and homeopathy is high on the list of sought-after therapies (House of Lords 2000). Commissioners looking for evidence to justify funding naturally turn to published reports of clinical trials or reviews of those trials. At this point several problems emerge.

Accessibility of information: Because of homeopathy's isolation from mainstream medicine, most homeopathic trials have been published in grey literature, inaccessible through Medline, Embase or other standard databases.

Representativeness of contemporary trials: Many homeopaths claim theirs is a general therapy, applicable and successful in a wide range of conditions. Situated outside orthodox medicine, homeopathy has been starved of funds for research – Albrecht (1999) estimated spending no higher than $1.5 million annually worldwide for all types of homeopathy. As a consequence, there are few contemporary clinical trials overall (fewer than 300 were found in the comprehensive literature search conducted for this thesis). Of these trials, the majority have used standardized treatments, on the lines of a conventional drug trial, even though the majority of homeopaths practise a therapy where treatments are tailored to the individual, particularly in chronic disease. Some conditions, such as bronchial asthma, for which homeopaths claim their therapy works particularly well, are very underrepresented in the trial record.

Homeopathy's controversiality: Like some other complementary therapies, homeopathy is regarded as a placebo therapy by many scientists, regardless of evidence of efficacy from clinical trials (Vandenbroucke 1997). Unlike most other complementary therapies, however, homeopathy began as part of orthodox western medicine, at the beginning of the nineteenth century. Its controversiality and present fringe status stem from judgements made about it in the nineteenth century by powerful opponents in orthodox medicine (e.g. Académie de Médecine 1835a; Holmes 1842; House of Commons 1854–55). Whether or not those judgements were scientifically valid, they still inform current debate (Ernst 1995b; Crellin 1997).

Relevance of existing reviews: Traditional review articles in homeopathy, as is the case in most fields, have generally been unsystematic and written by opponents or proponents of the therapy as a whole (or even of one approach within it). Monographs and textbooks containing reviews, which might be regarded as sources, are highly selective in their choice of examples (e.g. Aulas, Bordelay, Royer 1991; Meyer 1996). Well-conducted recent systematic reviews (with protocols) have used wide-ranging literature search strategies to answer the scientific question 'Is homeopathy any more than a placebo effect?' (e.g. Boissel, Cucherat, Haugh et al. 1996; Linde, Clausius, Ramirez et al. 1997). Because of the question posed, however, these reviews have tended to leave out study designs which might inform health services research and provision.

Exclusion of historical evidence: The widespread use of homeopathy in the nineteenth century has been acknowledged by medical historians (e.g. Kaufmann 1971; Nicholls 1988), but only rarely evaluated for evidence of effectiveness (e.g. Leary 1994). Since homeopathy tends to add to rather than replace its clinical treatments, and since the numbers involved in nineteenth-century trials were many times greater than the sum of all contemporary trial participants, exclusion of the historical record may also misrepresent the therapy.

For these reasons, a historical approach to the evaluation of homeopathy is proposed, one which connects the discipline to its past, and to that of orthodox medicine. In one sense this thesis contains two concise histories of important aspects of homeopathy: Part I accounts for the origins, characteristics and development of the content and methods of the therapy from before 1800 to the present day, while Part II examines evidence from clinical trials of homeopathy from the early nineteenth century up until the middle of the twentieth century. Part III is not historically oriented, but contains a systematic review of clinical trials from 1940 to the end of 1998, looking at issues of current concern including safety and clinical relevance.

Questions concerning the nature of highly diluted homeopathic medicines and the manner in which they are biologically active fall outside the scope of this thesis.

1.2. Overview

1.2.1. Homeopathy's place in the history of therapeutics

The historiography of homeopathy has tended to come from inside the profession. Where different evolutionary streams in homeopathy have been discussed, the treatment usually reflects the allegiances of the author, and tends to be antagonistic towards competing schools of thought (e.g. Coulter 1977; Demarque 1981). More recently, following trends within the 'new' non-medical academic historiography of medicine, the field has enlarged to include accounts and analysis from outside homeopathy: for example, studies of specific historical moments, regional microhistories, sociological analysis of casebooks of well-known homeopaths, and accounts of political and economic conflict between homeopathy and orthodox medicine. But, as in social constructionism generally, little attention has been paid to the content or theoretical and practical adequacy of homeopathy (e.g. Berliner 1982). Therefore, Part I (Chs 2–4) explores the discipline by means of explanatory coverage of its historical origins, conceptual foundation, pharmacological techniques and internal development, without any attempt to impose norms based on what is currently acceptable within any one area of the discipline.

Ch. 2 contrasts the structure of Hahnemann's research programme with emerging structures in German academic medicine around 1800, and is also innovative in attempting to account for Hahnemann's formal presentation of homeopathy by detailing his rhetorical use of academic conventions in his bid to overthrow them. Ch. 3 examines the generally assumed irrationality of homeopathic theory and method by a thorough exploration of Hahnemann's allegedly covert debt to alchemy. Ideas from alchemical medicine that are frequently presumed to survive in homeopathy – such as the doctrine of signatures (e.g. Flaherty 1995) – are shown to have been decisively rejected, yet an acknowledged but overlooked borrowing from Islamic alchemical pharmacy is shown to have transformed the preparation of homeopathic medicines after 1818. The probable origins of Hahnemann's avant-garde miasmatic and germ theory in a forgotten eighteenth-century treatise are also explored, again possibly for the first time. Ch. 4 recounts the post-Hahnemannian development of the principal schools and approaches within homeopathy, and is innovative in showing that allegedly irreconcileable theoretical and practical differences can be mapped and understood as a unified therapeutic field – one which is systematically traversed by many therapists in the present day.

1.2.2. Homeopathy and the development of clinical evaluation

Part II (Chs 5–9) consists of a comprehensive and systematic review of prospective historical trials, 1821–1953. Ch. 5 presents the background against which such a review must take place, namely the neglect of the clinical trial in orthodox medical historiography, compounded by the even greater neglect of homeopathy's clinical record.

The great majority of historical trials found in the literature search fall neatly into three methodological groups corresponding to three chronological phases in the evaluation of homeopathy (and perhaps medicine generally): open observation, pragmatic comparison, and explanatory trial. Ch. 6 reviews mainly prospective case series from the period 1821–35, and the significance of the cut-off date will be apparent when it is remembered that 1835 was the year in which the Académie de Médecine issued its ostensibly evidence-based pronouncement against homeopathy, and the therapy's journey from centre to fringe began in earnest. Ch. 7 reviews mainly pragmatic comparisons with allopathy from the period 1844–86, some of which were clearly an embarrassment to the increasingly powerful medical establishment, as evidenced by attempts to prevent trials and comparisons from being carried out, or to suppress the results once completed. Ch. 9 looks at the increasing adoption of the orthodox explanatory research model in the years 1914–53, at a time when homeopathy had been almost entirely displaced by biomedicine. The evidence found in each chapter is reviewed along with the reception of the trials where found, and then synthesized in relation to the judgements made on homeopathy at the time.

A fourth group of historical trials is reviewed in Ch. 8. These are trials in which placebo controls were used in the period 1829–1903. Such a disparate group – only 2 placebo-controlled therapeutic trials, plus 5 placebo-controlled pathogenetic drug tests and 3 trials of placebo alone regarded as the rhetorical equivalent of homeopathy – deserves separate treatment from the therapeutic trials in Chs 6 and 7. This is in view of the importance accorded to the introduction of masked evaluation, including placebo controls, in the history of clinical evaluation, and again the evidence is synthesized in relationship to nineteenth-century (and current) opinion. All the reviews in Part II are innovative, but Ch. 8 particularly so. It contains the first detailed account of within-patient placebo controls in everyday homeopathic practice as used throughout the nineteenth and twentieth centuries. Evidence that this internal usage was imitated in the first external placebo-controlled evaluations of homeopathy is presented, in complete contrast to the normative view that homeopaths adopted placebo controls in trials as early as they did because of external prompting.

1.2.3. Is homeopathy clinically relevant?

In view of the problems of accessibility mentioned in 1.1 above, the development of a comprehensive database of controlled trials was paramount. This has been based on a search for every prospective controlled homeopathic clinical trial published between 1940 and the end of 1998, with controls including orthodox treatment or no treatment as well as placebo, as in an earlier systematic review (Kleijnen, Knipschild, ter Riet 1991). Part III (Chs 10–13) constitutes a systematic review of the contemporary trials found, split into chapters for convenience: Ch. 10 Rationale, Ch. 11 Methods, Ch. 12 Results, Ch. 13 Discussion. Exploratory rather than hypothesis-based, it is innovative in its inclusion of:

- more trials than any previous review;
- analysis of intrahomeopathic differences and trends;
- an evaluation of homeopathy's safety;
- the evaluation of a generic methodological quality assessment tool designed to allow meaningful inclusion and comparative evaluation of prospective controlled trials other than randomized placebo-controlled ones – as well as allowing other nonexperimental designs to be evaluated and added to the database at a later time;
- discussion of homeopathy's clinical relevance;
- identification of areas that appear to hold most clinical relevance and warrant further research.

1.2.4. Retrospect and prospect

The conclusions drawn in the thesis as a whole are summarized and extended in Ch. 14. These relate to empirical evidence concerning the origins of homeopathy's epistemology, pharmacognosy and theories of disease transmission; and to empirical evidence of its efficacy drawn from nearly two centuries of clinical trials.

Part I: Homeopathy's Place in the History of Therapeutics

2. Homeopathy and 'the progress of science'

Material in this chapter appeared in: Dean M.E. (2001). Homeopathy and "the progress of science". *History of Science*. 39: 255–283.

Background: Eighteenth-century medical practice became increasingly irreconcilable with Enlightenment principles. The 1790s saw French attempts to reconstitute medicine based on observation, leading to better insight into the results of pathological processes. This coincided with German attempts to create a scientific medicine on deductive rational principles aimed at the hypothesized cause of disease. A different response, homeopathy, emerged at the same time.

Questions: How did the conceptual foundation of homeopathy differ from prevailing approaches to the creation of a new medical science? Can differences at this level explain its later exclusion from biomedicine?

Argument: Hahnemann shared the aspirations of those contemporaries who wished to create a medicine to match the real achievements of the sciences. He borrowed the rhetorical structures of German academic medicine, while advancing an approach to healing fundamentally opposed to rationalist assumptions. Further examination of the epistemological basis of homeopathy shows he adopted a procedure of global hypothesis formation and testing, which allowed him to believe homeopathy answered the call for a Kantian medical 'science'. Homeopathy's attention to the person diverged strongly from contemporary trends, and may have contributed in large part to its rejection by orthodoxy.

2.1. Introduction

In 1790, after he had turned his back on medicine and looked to translation to earn a living, a German doctor summarized the state of therapeutics in an annotation to the *Treatise of Materia Medica* of William Cullen (1710–90), the eminent Edinburgh physician (Cullen 1789; Cullen 1790):

> Blood-letting, fever remedies, tepid baths, lowering drinks, weakening diet, blood cleansing and everlasting aperients and clysters [enemas] form the circle in which the ordinary German physician turns round unceasingly. (cited in Haehl 1927, i: 35)

Cullen's despairing translator and annotator was Friedrich Christian Samuel Hahnemann (1755–1843). Born in Meissen, he became a physician, chemist and linguist, studying medicine in Leipzig and Vienna, and finally graduating from Erlangen in 1779. After 1790, for the remaining five decades of his long life, he mounted a sustained attack on blood-letting, purging, blistering, polypharmacy, massive doses and the abusive treatment of the mentally ill, that aligned him with Roger Bacon, Paracelsus, J.B. Van Helmont and G.E. Stahl, who had all addressed the same issues, frequently in the same terms. Before involving himself with therapeutic reform, he had achieved prominence and respect from his peers in each of his chosen professional fields. Christoph Hufeland (1762–1836) is often described as the greatest German clinician of the late eighteenth century (e.g. Habrich 1991), and he described Hahnemann as 'one of the most distinguished of German physicians ... a practical physician of matured experience and reflection' in his preface to Hahnemann (1801a). A quantitative survey of peer citations found in Lorenz Crell's *Chemische Annalen* in the years 1784–89 ranks Hahnemann in the first 15 German chemists (Hufbauer 1982: 91). Translations of scientific, medical, and literary works into German from English, French, Latin and Italian were highly regarded enough to earn him awards and many commissions for further translations and also original textbooks. His translation of the influential *Wholesale Manufacture of Chemicals* by J.F. Demachy (1784) was considered by the reviewer in *Chemische Annalen*, ii (1785): 77 (cited in Haehl 1927, i: 28) to be an improvement on the French original, because of Hahnemann's many critical annotations and amplifications. His own *Apotheker Lexikon* (Hahnemann 1793–99) treated every aspect of best practice in pharmacy so definitively and comprehensively that it constituted a major reform, superseding its competitors in the opinion of three reviewers also cited by Haehl (1927, i: 49).

At the same time, he advocated positive public health measures as progressive as anything to be found in Rickmann (1771) or Frank (1779–1819), though without the latter's statist intentions: his programme encompassed improved diet and housing for the working people, reform of prisons, strict control of trades such as rag-picking and papermaking that harboured and spread contagious disease, and compulsory isolation of infectious patients (Hahnemann 1792/1795). Developing from this, in the two decades after 1790, Hahnemann created a new pharmacotherapeutic system he believed to be more humane and effective than any known before that time, and which he eventually named homeopathy. In spite of a seemingly secure polymathic foundation, Hahnemann was vilified like his iconoclastic predecessors, and his proposed solution to the therapeutic anarchy of the day earned him even more notoriety than his critique. Typically, he was portrayed as a quack unable to earn a living from orthodox medicine (Holmes 1842), dishonest or insane (Guy 1860), and, in a dismissal extending to all who followed his precepts, as 'too weak mentally to practise medicine or even to take care of himself' (Spooner 1882).

Here I make no attempt to give more than the briefest mention of the philosophical and scientific basis of Hahnemann's attack on traditional therapeutics, or of the sources and precursors Hahnemann drew on in designing his system (for which see Ch. 3), or of his influence on nineteenth-century therapeutics and pharmacology. I would like simply to examine some of the ways in which Hahnemann tried to position homeopathy in German medical life at the beginning of the nineteenth century, and some of the difficulties inherent in his rhetorical and practical engagement with a theoretical academic discourse which started with a fundamentally different assumption from his about the place of therapeutics in medicine, a discourse which at its most extreme led to the abandonment of therapeutics in the interests of science. I try to show that homeopathy's eventual exclusion from biomedicine may be more plausibly accounted for at this level, rather than by the notorious infinitesimal doses usually advanced as the self-evident explanation.

2.2. Philosophy, medicine and the *Aufklärung*

Hahnemann was not alone in his dissatisfaction with medicine's failure to fulfil the ideals of the German Enlightenment or *Aufklärung*. During the 1790s many German physicians supported the call for a reconstituted medicine, based on the critical philosophy of Immanuel Kant (1724–1804), to match the certainties of the physical sciences. In 1784 a Berlin journal had asked several leading thinkers to contribute an answer to the question, What is Enlightenment? Kant's essay famously opens:

> *Enlightenment is man's emergence from his self-incurred immaturity.* (Kant 1784, original emphases)

And in 1798 the doctor Johann Karl Osterhausen paid direct homage to Kant in an essay 'On medical enlightenment', which he defined as:

> Man's emergence from his dependence in matters concerning his physical wellbeing. (quoted in Gay 1970: 17)

The conceptual gulf separating the lowly craft of medicine from the established sciences was spelled out by Kant in a letter of 1799: doctors were currently fighting symptoms, whereas in Brown's system 'the disease was like an X equation' (quoted in Risse 1972). Kant was promoting his doctrine that scientific knowledge was necessarily quantitative by referring to the system of John Brown (1735–88), the Scottish student of Cullen who had reduced all disease to a single fundamental category: variation in 'excitement', or degree of vitality (Brown 1780). The health of any organism consisted of maintaining a balance between its 'excitability', or predisposition to excitement, and internal and external 'stimuli' – food, drugs, emotions, for example – which constantly impinged on excitability: increase in excitement led to 'sthenic' disease, and decrease to 'asthenic' disease. Conventional disease labels, such as 'jaundice', 'dropsy' or 'fever', were assigned points between two extremes on a graduated scale similar to that of a thermometer, and treatment was correspondingly simple:

> The indication for the cure of sthenic diathesis is to diminish, that for the cure of asthenic diathesis is to encrease the excitement, and to continue to encrease it. (Brown 1791 cited in Conner 1966)

In practice, debilitating treatments such as blood-letting or opium, and stimulants such as alcohol answered every clinical need. Brown's revival of early Greek Methodism is the best-known and most influential example of the rationalist trend in late eighteenth-century medicine. German interest in the Brunonian system, as it was called, was such that medical students and faculty fought in the streets of Göttingen in 1802 for several days to decide the truth of the doctrine, until the cavalry were sent in (Hegel 1970, iii: 379). In complete contrast to the better known French attempts to reconstitute medicine as an inductive science based on Linnaean nosological categories and the search for the lesion, the German task was to look for first principles which would underlie nosology and therapeutics, and so elevate rationalism to new heights.

Andreas Roeschlaub (1768–1835), professor of medicine at Bamberg University, was one of the initiators of the German trend. As the leading German Brunonian, Roeschlaub had developed Brown's simple irritation 'equation' by adding a vital principle with which irritation came into conflict. In touch with the latest developments in other fields, he also attempted to reconcile Brunonianism with Lavoisierian chemistry and accounted for the disease polarities in terms of oxidation and disoxidation (ibid.). His interest in chemical explanations of disease was paralleled elsewhere. For instance, J.-B.-T. Baumes (1756–1828), professor at Montpellier, proposed a division of diseases based on deficiencies of hydrogen, azoth (nitrogen), caloric (Lavoisier's elastic fluid from which heat derived), phosphorus or oxygen (Baumes 1798; 1801–02). Roeschlaub's main ambition though was to provide the conceptual illumination for a formal deductive science of medicine, and in an important article of 1799 he constructed a hierarchical framework to support the practice and teaching of such a system (Roeschlaub 1799).

The preliminary phase of the operation required the creation of a standard terminology to allow unambiguous description of theory and practice. Among other things, this involved clarification of the terms *Heilkunde* and *Heilkunst*, about which it seems there had been some confusion. Etymologically, both are based on the root *Heil* – cure, heal. The suffix *-kunde* indicates knowledge and theory, and turns an entity or activity into a subject or discipline: *Heilkunde* is medicine in the same way that *Erdkunde* is geography. The noun *Kunst* means art or skill, and was added to many terms during the eighteenth century to indicate a craft or professional activity employing an organized body of knowledge or *Wissenschaft*. According to Roeschlaub, *Medizin* – medicine – contains two fundamental divisions: *Heilkunde* – theoretical, scientific – and *Heilkunst* – technical, practical. It is important to realize that *Heilkunde* is concerned solely with ridding patients of diseases. It does not include background fields such as chemistry, anatomy and physiology, nor does it encroach on the areas occupied by hygiene and health maintenance. *Heilkunde* is further subdivided into general and applied sections, dealing with the laws of health and disease, their manifestations in pathology and classified nosology, and pharmacology. *Heilkunst* meanwhile consists of what doctors do in practice to realize this theoretical knowledge, and includes diagnostics, prognostics and therapeutics. The word was in fact the eighteenth-century German equivalent of the Hippocratic *techne iatrike* (Latin *ars medendi*), and a down-to-earth definition from 1803 helps to clarify its essentially practical objective: *Heilkunst* could be 'implemented internally in various forms, or externally, as with salves' (cited in Grimm & Grimm 1862).

Roeschlaub was explicit that his variant of Brunonianism sat at the apex of the new Kantian medical science, and would provide the a priori guidelines for successful therapeutics. His ideas were highly influential, and stimulated the philosopher Friedrich Schelling (1775–1854) – whose medical degree from Landshut (1802) was purely honorary – to articulate an even more ambitious programme for the realization of a medical science that would transcend Brunonianism and embody the highest ideals of post-Kantian *Naturphilosophie*. Man was coincident with the universe, but had lost touch with this essential oneness. Not until he had learned to understand external nature, through contemplation of his own innermost reality, could he hope to formulate laws of existence. From this certain knowledge would come insight into health and disease, thus allowing a rational therapeutics to be deduced from metaphysical principles without the need for empirical testing (Schelling 1797; 1799).

Nevertheless, German attempts to create a deductive medico-philosophic science and the better-known French attempts to reformulate medicine on inductive clinical lines were therapeutically unproductive, in the lifetime of their patients at least. By the end of the nineteenth century, in spite of enormous advances in descriptive pathology, normal and abnormal physiology, surgery, and public health, the internal medicine of the end of the eighteenth century had advanced scarcely at all:

> Blood-letting gradually lost favour, but … the pharmacopoeia was a bag of blanks … the few medicines that were effective included mercury for syphilis and ringworm, digitalis to strengthen the heart, amyl nitrite to dilate the arteries in angina, quinine for malaria, colchicum for gout – and little else … (Porter 1997: 674)

If safety had been a criterion of use as well as efficacy, the list would have been even shorter.

2.3. Conceptual foundation of homeopathy

Praktische Arzneykunde was another expression for *Heilkunst*, at a time when German technical terminology was in state of creative flux, and Christoph Hufeland's *Journal* of that name was programmatically opposed to the theoretical turn in academic medicine. It was there that Hahnemann (1796b; 1852b) chose to announce his 'new principle for ascertaining the curative powers of drugs'. Treatment under the new system differed from current medical practice in consisting of single pure drugs that had been subject to thorough experimental testing on healthy volunteers (in moderately small doses) before being given in smaller, and hence safer, doses to the sick. These pathogenetic trials (*Prüfungen*, tests, anglicized as provings) indicated the therapeutic sphere of influence of each drug, according to the similia principle – *similia similibus curentur*, let likes be cured with likes. Hahnemann later published his first experiments with greatly attenuated therapeutic doses in 1801 in Hufeland's *Journal*, and several important critical and homeopathic articles followed, which invariably appealed to clinically validated experience as the arbiter of therapeutic efficacy, not theory or tradition (Hahnemann 1801a; 1801b; 1801c; 1801d; 1805c; 1806; 1807).[1]

[1] All except the last two can be found in the collections *Kleine medicinische Schriften* (Hahnemann 1829) and *The Lesser Writings* (Hahnemann 1852b).

It is probably on this account that homeopathy has been dismissed as pure empiricism – that is, lacking any explanatory theory (e.g. House of Commons 1854–55) – as often as it has been dismissed as a survival of eighteenth-century rationalism – that is, theory unconnected with experimental confirmation (e.g. Shryock 1948: 138). It is often pointed out that since Hippocrates official medicine had tended to oscillate between empirical and rationalist poles (Faber 1921; Temkin 1963). It is also true that Hahnemann favoured the biographical natural-history-of-disease approach of the empirical school, exemplified by Hippocrates and Sydenham, over the ontological claim of rationalists such as Galen and Brown to know the essential nature of disease:

> We were never nearer the discovery of the science of medicine than in the time of Hippocrates. This attentive, unsophisticated observer sought nature in nature. He saw and described the diseases before him accurately, without addition, without speculation (Hahnemann 1805c; 1852b).

Because of this, recent historians have tended to see homeopathy as an empirical discipline, in conflict with Brunonianism (e.g. Schwanitz 1983), or even as empiricism's final answer to 1500 years of Galenic rationalism (Coulter 1977). Admittedly, Hahnemann (1801a) demolished Brown's *Elements of Medicine*, regardless of Roeschlaub's advocacy; and early in the history of *Naturphilosophie*, Hahnemann (1808c) was wondering whether satire or elegy would be the most appropriate vehicle to commemorate the self-spun 'gossamer' fabrications of Schelling and his emulators. Even chemical nosologies such as Roeschlaub's and Baumes's were new flasks for some very old ideas (Albury 1977), and Hahnemann (Hahnemann 1801c; 1852b), the chemist, believed rudimentary chemistry was being used as a medical figleaf. However, recalling Bacon's (1620, i: §95) observation that empirical ants were no more effective than rationalist spiders, Hahnemann (1801c) also made searching criticisms of empirical treatments aimed at ill-defined 'diseases' that were hardly more than a vague symptom or two – such as 'rheumatism' and 'dropsy' – and not just the sorts of cause that rationalism claimed to know. He pointed out that the empiricists had known how to observe but not how to cure, hence their reliance on diet and the 'healing power of nature' above all. In 'Examination of the sources of the ordinary materia medica' he also criticized the random nature of testing one substance after another in each disease: the tiny number of known specifics – scarcely more than mercury for syphilis, cinchona bark for malaria and sulphur for skin eruptions in the 1500 years since Galen – had been discovered by the empiricists as if by chance, or appropriated from folk medicine (Hahnemann 1817; 1852b). And he was not alone in wondering how the specifics worked. As Kant's successor G.W.F. Hegel (1770–1831) pointed out contemporaneously in his review of biology and medicine:

> The *materia medica* has not yet uttered a single rational word on the connection between a disease and its remedy; experience alone is supposed to decide the matter. Experience with chicken droppings is therefore as valuable as that with the various officinal plants, for human urine and the droppings of chickens and peacocks were formerly used medicinally, in order to produce nausea. (Hegel 1970, iii: 206)

Homeopathy's resistance to simple binary classification was addressed to some extent by Guttentag (1940), who developed the rational-empirical oscillation further in the time dimension by representing medical history since Hippocrates as a spiral. He located Hahnemann at a cusp point midway between the two poles of the spiral, along with other late eighteenth-century figures such as Withering and Jenner. Guttentag did not analyse further the scientific basis of homeopathy, except to say that it was an empirical clinical discipline, not an explanatory biological hypothesis.

In fact, the technical term with the closest epistemological fit for Hahnemann's conceptual innovation is abduction (or retroduction), introduced at the end of the nineteenth century by the philosopher C.S. Peirce. This was his translation of *apagoge*, Aristotle's third form of inference – along with induction and deduction – which had hitherto been translated as reduction (and is often referred to now as 'inference to best explanation'):

> The form of inference, therefore, is this: The surprising fact, C, is observed; But if A were true, C would be a matter of course. Hence, there is reason to suspect that A is true. Thus, A cannot be abductively inferred, or if you prefer the expression, cannot be abductively conjectured until its entire content is already present in the premiss, 'If A were true, C would follow as a matter of course.' (Peirce 1935 vi, 522–528)

According to Hanson (1958: 70ff), abduction is not synonymous with the better-known hypothetico-deductive model, associated with the theorists Whewell and Popper, although Hanson's main example of abduction – Kepler's reconceptualization of the Copernican circular planetary orbits – has for some reason left many unconvinced that the two forms of inference can be distinguished. Hahnemann's 'surprising facts' were the inexplicable empirical specifics, long an embarrassment to rationalism, such as cinchona, mercury and sulphur. He had seen many cases of malarial fever while practising in Transylvania in 1777–79 (Cullen 1790, ii: 114). The mercurial disease was often confused with syphilis, sulphur workers produced itching rashes, so, suspecting a hitherto unnoticed relationship between the medicinal action and toxicological symptoms of cinchona, Hahnemann's footnote to Cullen (ibid. ii: 108) describes how he took in 1790,

> by way of experiment, for several days 3 drachms of good bark twice a day. My feet, finger-ends, &c., first became cold, and I felt tired and sleepy, then my heart began to beat, and my pulse became hard and quick; I got an insufferable feeling of uneasiness, a trembling (but without rigor). A weariness in all my limbs; then a beating in my head, redness of the cheeks, thirst, – in short, all the old symptoms with which I was familiar in ague [malaria] appeared one after another, yet without any actual chill or rigor. In brief, even those particularly characteristic symptoms which I was wont to observe in agues – obtuseness of the senses, a kind of rigidity in limbs, but especially that numb disagreeable feeling which seems to have its seat in the periosteum of all the bones of the body – all put in an appearance. This paroxysm lasted each time 2 or 3 hours, and came on afresh whenever I repeated the dose, but not otherwise. I left off, and was quite well.

Hahnemann, it turns out, illustrates Hanson's distinction as well as Kepler. Aristotelian abduction originated as a logical description and justification of the process of inference from disparate biological species to the genera which contain them. In other words it seeks higher level ontological groupings which subsume lower level data – synthetic a priori insights, in Kantian terms. The specifics were doubly surprising, because they showed a paradoxical ability to produce the very symptoms they were reputed to cure. Hahnemann's explanatory hypothesis and conceptual definition was the similia principle, or homeopathicity, which subsumed known treatments of vastly different appearance and qualities for diseases that were themselves unrelated.

And as Atran (1990: 89ff) points out, *apagoge* has not only this dual function for Aristotle – to provide an intuitive hypothesis and then a concept or definition which figures as the major premiss in syllogistic demonstration – but most importantly is required to 'factor out … the truly essential from the natural incidents of the common-sense type.' The similia hypothesis allowed Hahnemann to reject the plausible explanations of his contemporaries, such as Cullen's (1790, ii: 108) entirely orthodox claim that cinchona cured malaria because its bitter taste had a tonic effect on the stomach. Fulfilling Peirce's requirement that the abductive hypothesis be subject to experimental validation, Hahnemann's tests from 1790 onwards involved making careful records of what happened when he gave different drugs first to himself and then to other healthy volunteers, and what happened when he treated the sick with drugs capable of producing the same symptoms (Hahnemann 1805b).

2.4. The appearance of the *Organon*

Hahnemann's textbook of homeopathy, first published in 1810, provides theoretical and practical instructions for the new approach to therapy he had created in the previous 20 years, and integrates his similia hypothesis with a Hippocratic natural-history approach to nosology, Stahl's homeostatic vitalism, Plenciz's germ theory, John Hunter's theory of medicinal counter-irritants, placebo controls and many other disparate and previously unrelated influences (Hahnemann 1810; Hahnemann 1913; Hahnemann 2000). It went through five editions in his lifetime, and has been in print continuously since then in many languages. Before examining the internal structure of his programme as laid out in the book, it is worth trying to estimate the impact Hahnemann wished the book to have, judging by the way he presented it.

Although the bones of the system had first been presented in Hufeland's *Journal* under the title *Heilkunde der Erfahrung* (*The Medicine of Experience*) in 1805, the change of title to the more imposing *Organon der rationellen Heilkunde* indicates that Hahnemann believed that appeals to experience were unlikely to sway a medical establishment wedded to a priori theories of disease and how medical knowledge was to be structured. The term *Organon*, which can be a conceptual tool, systematic treatise or physical instrument, echoes the collective title traditionally given to Aristotle's treatises on logic, and Francis Bacon's *Novum Organum* of 1620. Apart from Aristotle's and Bacon's, there had been remarkably few *Organons* before Hahnemann, although the word had achieved some currency in Germany following the appearance of J.H. Lambert's (1764) *Neues Organon*. Hahnemann might conceivably have read this epistemological treatise – which contains the first use of the word phenomenology – by the most important German philosopher of the generation immediately before Kant.

The meaning of the rest of Hahnemann's title has become obscure, because the implications of *Heilkunde* at this date – medical theory – are unfamiliar in modern German. *Heilkunde* now inclusively means medicine, or medical science in the broadest sense, in which theory and practice are held to be integrated, or therapeutics. And unsurprisingly, the Terminology Office of the European Commission in Luxembourg defines *Heilkunst* – ID Number 3102196 in the Medicine Collection (RLM76) – as just 'another word for *Heilkunde*'. The *rationell* of the first edition is equally remote. *Rationell*, signifying 'technical', 'scientific', 'validated by empirical reason', had been introduced in 1798 by Goethe from French. It was distinct from the existing but rarely used *rational,* a term with traditional philosophical overtones, and filled an important gap left unoccupied by *Wissenschaft*. Hahnemann's employment of the term in a medical context seems intended to occupy a rhetorical high ground similar to that enjoyed by 'evidence-based' in present-day clinical discourse, while prefiguring Jakob Henle's (1846) later use of *rationell* in a book title to draw a line between his empirical research and the speculative physiology that *Naturphilosophie* was famous for. Once again, the word's original sense has faded, leaving an identifiable gap: Rudolf Carnap, Karl Popper and others complained that psychoanalysis and Marxism did not deserve their self-descriptions as scientific – *wissenschaftlich*. The disappearance of the original meaning of *rationell* might even have been a factor in the foregrounding of the demarcation problem by the Vienna Circle. Nowadays it simply means rational, although a secondary meaning of 'economically efficient' was introduced in the 1930s (equivalent to one of the meanings of 'rationalized' in English) reconnecting the word to its 'empirically-proven' origin. Nevertheless, the original title called attention to itself as constituting the architectonic 'science' the Kantians, Brunonians and *Naturphilosophen* aspired towards.

The title page was adorned with C.F. Gellert's (1715–69) quintessentially Enlightenment verse:

> The truth we humans need | Us blest to make and keep,
> A wise hand lightly covered o'er | But did not bury deep.[2]

We may guess from this that the book will not advance any theory of the occult essence or origins of disease. This is confirmed by the preface which informs us that 'no occupation is more unanimously declared to be a conjectural art than medicine', but that the author's researches had led him 'very far from the common highway of medical routine ... away from the old edifice, which, being built up of opinions, was only maintained by opinions.'

Interestingly, the term homeopathy is absent from the title page. An unpaginated half title, between the Introduction and the main text, is a partial exception: *Organon der rationellen Heilkunde nach homöopathischen Gesetzen* is found in the first edition, but not in any of the five later editions Hahnemann prepared for the press. A legitimate translation would be: 'Treatise of scientific medical theory according to homeopathic laws'. Hahnemann had coined *Homöopathie* (Greek *homoios*, similar + *pathos*, suffering) together with the pejorative *Allöopathie* to describe unsystematic treatment (*alloios*, other, dissimilar) in 1807 in a scholarly literature review that became the Intro-

[2] Die Wahrheit, die wir alle nöthig haben, | Die uns als Menschen glücklich macht, | Ward von der weisen Hand, die sie uns zugedacht, | Nur leicht verdeckt, nicht tief vergraben. I have adjusted thc translation in Hahnemann (1893: 155).

duction to the *Organon* (Hahnemann 1807; 1833a: 48–101). It contains nearly 250 examples of the mostly unconscious use of the similia principle by 440 named physicians, past and present, as evidence for the method elaborated in the rest of the book.

The main body of the *Organon* is laid out as 271 numbered sections containing propositions and arguments, grouped thematically, like the aphorisms of the *Novum Organum*, emphasizing the book's critical philosophical intent. They vary in length from single sentences to extensively footnoted paragraphs spanning several pages. The first two aphorisms set the tone:

> The physician has no higher aim than to make sick people well, to heal as it is known.
> The highest ideal of cure is the speedy, gentle and enduring restoration of health, or the removal and annihilation of disease in its entirety, by the quickest, most trustworthy, and least harmful way, according to *principles* that can be readily understood.

2.5. The structure of the *Organon*

To understand the structure of Hahnemann's medical programme as formalized for the first time, Roeschlaub makes a convenient point of reference. As noted, the *Organon* was ostensibly concerned with *rationelle Heilkunde*, which to a Roeschlaub implied a priori knowledge of the causes of disease. Hahnemann (e.g. 1801c; 1808c) believed history had shown this was an unprofitable line of inquiry, but a hierarchic presentation of his therapeutic posed difficulties because the similia principle ran counter to the causal model required by Western science. In the essay that was expanded to become the *Organon*, Hahnemann (1805c; 1852b) had written:

> Medicine is a science of experience; its object is to eradicate diseases by means of remedies. The knowledge of diseases, the knowledge of remedies, and the knowledge of their employment constitute medicine.

This tripartite division lacks any overarching theory of disease causation, and, although Hahnemann was a contagionist, and the influence of Plenciz's (1762) germ theory can be found in his writings from 1801 onwards (see Ch. 3), he recognized that most diseases could not be so easily explained. The components of the homeopathic method differ radically from its rationalist (not to mention empiricist) counterparts, and Hahnemann was obliged to create a theoretical justification to give the appearance that the rest of the book had been deduced a priori. Accordingly, the similia principle is placed at the apex of the system, and incorporated into the Roeschlaubian hierarchy as far as possible by dividing the *Organon* proper into four sections dealing successively with:

1. disease as response to disturbance of homeostasis; theory of specific medicinal counter-forces, i.e. the similia principle;
2. individual case-taking;
3. conduct of collective pathogeneses;
4. practicalities of medicine selection, case-management and pharmacy.

Table 2.1 Correspondence of the internal structure of Hahnemann's *Organon* (1810) to Roeschlaub's (1799) deductive schema

	Roeschlaub		**Hahnemann**
1. *Heilkunde* or Theoretical medicine	General	Disease concept and causation	Disease concept; theory of cure by similars (§§ 1–38)
	Applied	Pathology Nosology Pharmacology	i. Case-taking (§§ 39–82) ii. Pathogeneses (§§ 83–125)
2. *Heilkunst* or Technical medicine		Diagnostics Prognostics Therapeutics	iii. Medicine selection (§§ 126–99), dosage, case-management (§§ 200–71)

Hahnemann's original tripartite division corresponds to sections 2–4, and the way in which it can be superimposed (numbered i–iii, as in the *Organon* § 38) on Roeschlaub's categories is shown in Table 2.1. In complete contrast to the determinist chain of cause, classified nosologies, their attached treatments, and pigeon-holed patients, Hahnemann's system is essentially circular, despite the superficial resemblance in the way the material is ordered. Its justification – the similia principle – lies at its heart, not at its head. The impression of seamless continuity is reinforced by the absence of conventional section headings or chapters: the paragraphs run uninterruptedly, and sections i–iii are mentioned only in the text.

In contrast to systems emerging to take the place of humoralism, such as the chemical nosologies of Roeschlaub and Baumes, or the diathesis construct (Ackerknecht 1982a), disease is not to be viewed as purely idiopathic or essential. Yet, although disease is occasioned by external causes, and there are even 'fixed' contagious diseases, these causes have no independent disease-existence apart from their effects on the organism:

> The invisible disease-producing alteration in the inward man together with the visible alteration in health (the sum of the symptoms) make up that which is called disease; both together actually constitute the disease. (Hahnemann 1913 § 6)

Virus, miasms, poisons and drugs all have the ability to alter health, for better or worse, and the homeopathic principle demands that their pathogenetic capacity be correlated with the symptoms of the patient:

> a few berries of belladonna are just as much disease-producing forces as inoculated vaccine-matter, or a viper-bite, or a great shock, and every one of these influences, just because it has the power to produce disease, can become a remedy and a force to counteract disease, as soon as it is opposed to a similar disorder already existing in the body. (ibid. § 32)

Disease, nevertheless, must be viewed holistically, since

> the oneness of life forbids the idea that any bodily disease can remain completely and absolutely local so long as it is not confined to a part of the body entirely shut off from all the rest. The remainder of the system simultaneously suffers more or less, and betrays its suffering in this or that symptom. (ibid. § 43)

Moreover, diagnosis does not involve matching patients to the static nosologies of Sydenham, Cullen and Pinel, which

> even if it could be accomplished with tolerable accuracy and completeness, would serve the physician only as a natural historian, in the way that the classification of other natural phenomena and natural objects is of value in general natural history. In other words, it would aid his historical perception by means of a tabulated and ordered survey. But for the physician as a practitioner of the art of medicine it would be of no value whatever, (ibid. § 45)

because each disease, properly examined, has never been seen before.

Pathology (subdivision i) therefore must be discovered in a process of unbiased phenomenological inquiry, in which the patient's experience is not merely a pointer to an explanatory or reductive diagnosis. The therapist notes the observable manifestations of illness and records the account of physical and psychological suffering related by the patient and his carers, 'using their exact expressions' without translation into transient medical codes, and paying particular attention to qualities, modalities and concomitants of symptoms, as well as general disturbances of function (ibid. §§ 62–69). The extensive and detailed anamnesis does not provide a mere collection of symptoms, however, but must be integrated in the therapist's mind as a unified *Symptomeninbegriff*. This is a term of art for Hahnemann, who exploits *Inbegriff*'s dual meanings of totality and epitome. The same procedure is adopted in collective diseases, such as epidemics: a symptom-complex is built up from the partial manifestations of the disease seen in each individual, allowing a valid collective remedy to be synthesized (ibid. §§ 79–81).

A similar form of meticulous case-taking is used in the pathogenetic drug tests which constitute homeopathy's nosology (subdivision ii). This spans the *Organon*, where the detailed instructions for conducting provings are given, and the materia medica where the results of systematic drug tests are listed – again using the provers' own expressions (Hahnemann 1805b; 1811–21; 1822–27; 1828–30; 1833–37).[3] The aim was the creation of a materia medica in which nothing was 'conjectured, asserted without proof, imagined, invented; but all is the pure reply of Nature to careful questioning', (Hahnemann 1913 § 121).

> In the investigation of these drug-symptoms all suggestion must be as rigidly avoided as in the examination of the symptoms of disease. The greater part of what is recorded as the genuine result of experiment must be the voluntary statements of the prover; nothing must be conjectural, nothing guessed at, and as little as possible should consist of answers to formal questions; least of all should the record contain expressions relating to sensations with which the prover has previously been prompted, or the results of questions that suggest the answers 'Yes' or 'No'. (ibid. § 115)

In a footnote to § 122, Hahnemann called on others to carry forward his investigations of the previous 20 years:

> When thousands of exact and tireless observers, instead of one as hitherto, have laboured at the discovery of these first elements of a scientific Materia Medica, what will it not be possible to effect in the whole extent of the endless kingdom of disease! Then the art of medicine will no longer be mocked as an art of conjecture lacking all foundation.

The practical details of prescription, case-management and pharmacy (subdivision iii) correspond to *Heilkunst*, therapeutics, where many instructions are given for the selection of the remedy in individual cases. The defining aspect of homeopathic diagnosis–prescription is an individualization based on the unique, as opposed to common, aspects of the patient's symptoms:

> In this search for a specific homoeopathic remedy, that is, in this comparison of the totality of the symptoms of the natural disease with the symptom-lists of

---

[3] For tabulated analysis of the development and publication history of Hahnemann's materia medica, see Hughes (1893: 17–39).

> available medicines, the more striking and unusual of the characteristic symptoms of the disease should especially be kept in view; for it is precisely to these symptoms that analogues must be found among the disease-symptoms of the drug which is to be the most suitable remedy. On the other hand the general signs, like loss of appetite, weariness, discomfort, disturbed sleep, and so forth, are of little significance when unaccompanied by more precise indications, because they are found in the symptomatology of most drugs as of most diseases. (ibid. § 129)

In other words, the subtle variations of symptoms experienced in relation to time, position, temperature, weather and so on – the so-called modalities – are of greater importance than the same undifferentiated symptoms or nosological category. It is also here, rather than under nosology, that the usual distinction made between mental and physical illness is declared to be purely conventional:

> Indeed, [mental diseases] are in no wise really an exceptional class of disease, though often sharply separated off from others in classification. For in every other kind of disease the condition of the mind and of the disposition is invariably altered in some way, and the disposition and mental characteristics of the patient form symptoms of prime importance in all cases which the physician has to treat. (ibid. § 186)
> We shall, therefore, never learn to cure scientifically or homeopathically, unless we consider in every case of disease these alterations in mind and disposition, and choose as a counter-force the remedy which is capable of causing similar alterations. (ibid. § 189)

In practical terms:

> *Aconite* will never bring about a speedy or lasting cure in a patient of quiet, equable disposition; *Nux vomica* is as little serviceable to gentle phlegmatic patients, *Pulsatilla* as little to the gay and happy, *Ignatia* as little to those who are imperturbable and disinclined either to fear or to vexation,

since each of those had shown itself capable of producing the opposite disturbances of mind in the healthy.

The *Organon* does not contain worked examples of the method, but these were published soon after as 'Cases illustrative of homoeopathic practice' (Hahnemann 1817; 1852b). For instance, to illustrate the process of conceptualizing the symptoms and matching them with the materia medica, Hahnemann presents the simple case of Frau Sch—, a middle-aged laundress with a troublesome condition that had kept her from work for 3 weeks. The unique symptoms she presented with on 1 September 1815 were:

> (1) Any movement, especially on stepping, and worst on making a false step, leads to shooting pain in the epigastric region coming every time from the left side. (2) Complete relief on lying down, no pain anywhere, neither in the side nor in the epigastrium. (3) Sleepless after 3 a.m. (4) Enjoys her food, but feels nauseous after eating only a little. (5) This leads to increased salivation which runs from her mouth, like water-brash. (6) Frequent empty eructations after each meal. (7) Passionate temper, disposed to anger. —Covered in perspiration when the pain is severe.—Menses normal two weeks earlier.

Hahnemann details how each symptom of Frau Sch—'s ailment can be found in the pathogeneses contained in the materia medica, and distinguishes between several medicines for each symptom on the basis of the modalities. To give only his working out of the first symptom:

> *Belladonna*, *China* and *Rhus toxicodendron* cause shootings in the epigastrium, but none of them *only on motion*, as is the case here. *Pulsatilla* certainly causes shootings in the epigastrium on making a false step, but only as a rare alternating action, and has neither the same digestive derangements as occur here at (4) compared with (5) and (6), nor the same mental state. *Bryonia* alone has among its chief alternating actions, as the whole list of its symptoms demonstrates, pains *from movement* and especially shooting pains, as also stitches beneath the sternum (in the epigastrium) on raising the arm, and on making a false step it causes shooting in other parts. (ibid.)

The other symptoms are dealt with in the same way, each being compared with medicines which produce the general symptom, then distinguished on the basis of the individualizing modalities. For instance, nausea after eating was common to eight drug pathogeneses, but none so constantly or associated with such enjoyment of food as *Bryonia*. Frau Sch—'s psychological state was an important factor in differentiation, and again *Bryonia* was preeminent.[4]

Hahnemann points out that the individualization of simple cases is carried out as a rapid mental operation once the materia medica is memorized or the practitioner knows where to find the symptoms, but giving all the reasons for

---

4 The follow-up to this case is interesting. Hahnemann prescribed a drop of (undiluted) *Bryonia* tincture in the customary single dose and asked Frau Sch— to see him in 48 hours, telling a colleague present at the time that she would be better the next day. She never returned, and when the colleague sought her out later from curiosity, she replied: 'What was the use of going back? The very next day I was quite well, and could start my washing again. I am extremely obliged to the doctor, but the likes of us have no time to leave off our work. For three weeks previously my illness prevented me from earning anything.' (ibid.)

and against each stage of the process in writing leads to 'tedious prolixity'. Since each disease is a unique process, not a fixed entity, case-taking merges with prescription and case-management:

> Now we can neither enumerate all possible aggregates of symptoms of all concrete cases of disease, nor indicate *a priori* the homeopathic medicines for these (*a priori* undefinable) possibilities. For every individual given case (and every case is an individuality, differing from all others) the homeopathist must himself find them. (ibid.)

And because the treatment is a unique analogue of the patient's symptom-complex, the distinction between theory and therapeutics is blurred and circles back to the similia principle, or general *Heilkunde*.

2.6. Hahnemann and the academy

Homeopathy might have been the product of a controversial iconoclast, but it was regarded as part of orthodox medicine at first, as Hegel's (1970, iii: 205) account of its pharmacological mechanism shows. Nevertheless, it was not aimed at hypothesized proximate or ultimate causes, as in rationalist or symptomatic medicine. Still less did its explicitly holistic individualization of disease states hand doctors a bagful of easy-to-remember empirical specifics, to which more or less plausible justifications could be attached; even the 'fixed' contagious diseases seen in epidemics required different remedies to be calibrated at each outbreak (Hahnemann 1810 § 79). The *Organon* pointed in a different direction from its German and French contemporaries, yet it appeared at a time when Hahnemann wished to acquire a secure academic base from which to promote homeopathy and transform therapeutics, and the detailed critique of existing practices, for which its author had become notorious, is notably absent. It would be surprising therefore if it were the sole example of his rhetorical deployment of terminology and structures corresponding to the mindset of German academic medicine. Two years after the appearance of the *Organon*, he presented his habilitation thesis at Leipzig University, where university regulations allowed anyone capable of successfully defending a thesis to lecture as an unsalaried *Privatdozent* (Hahnemann 1812; 1852b). His demonstration that the 'hellebore' used in Classical Greece, Rome and Islam was none other than the plant known to the moderns as *Veratrum album*, cites more than 500 sources from Greek, Roman, Arabic, English, French and Italian authors in the original languages, up to the year 1200. An idea of the aloofness of the work can be got from Hahnemann's disdainful prefatory note that he would 'leave it to others to give an account of the use of hellebore in modern times'. Medical and linguistic historiography that combined 'fearsome erudition and minute scholarship, quite divorced from any practical problems in medical practice' (King 1958: 173) was an unusual departure for Hahnemann, given his outspoken rejection of unvalidated historical authority and philosophical theorizing in medicine, and seems to call for explanation absent from the text.

In a discussion of the pecking orders that scientific and scholarly communities create for different disciplines, Jardine (1991: 111ff) points out that they are important when we want to find out which disciplines serve as models of procedure and presentation for others. For example, in Renaissance Italian medical training physicians nearly always gained doctorates in philosophy as well as medicine, as part of a process of professional legitimation aimed at raising the status of mere empirics. Jardine cites von Seemen (1926) who described a similar situation in German medical teaching in the first decades of the nineteenth century, and casts much light on Hahnemann's remarkable thesis. As the limitations of Brunonianism became more apparent, medical textbooks became increasingly obsessed with historical precedent, even to the exclusion of current theory and practice. This 'history craze' became as characteristic of the Romantic movement in German medicine as *Naturphilosphie*, and led its followers to worship the 'record of the manifestations of the original ideas which underlie all sound medical theory and practice.'

A reinterpretation of his thesis in this light suggests that, in order to gain the right to lecture at Leipzig, Hahnemann abandoned the well-known practical urgency that enlivens the rest of his considerable output and instead presented the authorities with an academic performance designed to flatter – or flatten – their judgement at that moment in 1812. The strategy worked. His opponents had anticipated a field day demolishing a homeopathic thesis, but in the event Hahnemann was unopposed and obtained his platform.

2.7. The transformations of the *Organon*

This historiographical display had been anticipated in the Introduction to the 1810 *Organon*, albeit grounded in the demands of day-to-day therapy. The German academic world was not won over on its own terms, however, and vitriolic attacks on Hahnemann by Hecker and others followed (see Haehl 1927, i: 89ff). At the same time, the attractions of *Naturphilosophie* were beginning to prove irresistible for many. The professor of pathology at Jena, published a medical system (Kieser 1817–19) in which less than a fifth of the section on diagnosis mentioned practical observation, the bulk being devoted to speculation about the meaning of various symptoms in relation to Schelling's theories of male-female polarities and positive and negative electrical charges (cited in Schenk 1966: 180). In the same year Hahnemann reaffirmed his traditional practical stance in 'Nota bene for my reviewers', declaring that homeopathy stood or fell on the evidence of validly conducted clinical experiments (Hahnemann 1817; 1852b).[5]

The difficulty of fitting a unified acausal methodology into deductive hierarchies such as Roeschlaub's and Kieser's no doubt explains another important change in the second and subsequent editions: a new title, *Organon der Heilkunst*, acknowledged that, in its essential form, homeopathy began and ended in therapeutics. Moreover, for Hahnemann, it was the only therapeutics worth the name. At the same time, Gellert's verse was replaced with a new motto: the Horatian challenge *aude sapere*, dare to know (*Epodes* I, 2, 40). This could be seen as forming yet another connexion with Kant, whose essay 'What is Enlightenment?' continues:

> The motto of enlightenment is therefore: *sapere aude!* Have courage to use your *own* understanding! (Kant 1784, original emphasis)

Yet Hahnemann was a child of the Enlightenment – literally, after his father had brought him up according to Rousseau's principles (which Hahnemann later translated: Rousseau 1796) – and scarcely needed lessons from Kant. Also in 1784, Hahnemann had written in one of his earliest publications that the true physician

> rejects nothing not investigated by himself, nor takes the word of another, and has the courage to think for himself and to treat accordingly. (Hahnemann 1784: 179)

The *Organon*'s brief first aphorism acquired a lengthy footnote, burning any academic bridges that might have been under construction. It attacks 'learned reveries' about the essence of life and origin of disease, identification of disease with its cause, 'unintelligible and pompous expressions' designed to impress, and chairs of 'theoretical medicine', and ended with another call to arms:

[5] Perhaps it was a sign of the times, or just of his normal impatience, that he pushed the historical review to the end of the *Organon*'s Introduction in the second edition, and preceded it with an equally lengthy recension of his medical critique. The history of homeopathy's precursors was later reduced to a handful of examples in the fifth edition of 1833. Hahnemann's extensive annotations and revisions to the 5th edition were not published until much later (Hahnemann 1921).

> It is high time that all those who call themselves physicians should cease to deceive suffering humanity with words that have no meaning, and begin to act – that is to say, to afford relief, and cure the sick in reality. (Hahnemann 1819a; 1833a)

However, in spite of Hahnemann's efforts to reform therapeutics, many conceptual, scientific, economic, sociological and psychological obstacles stood in his way. Fashions in medical jargon may also have played a small part in homeopathy's struggle for recognition. *Heilkunst* – the working-out at the individual level of medical theory – was being replaced as a term, even in the early 1800s, by *praktische Heilkunde*, and later by *Therapie*. By the mid nineteenth century, outside of internal homeopathic literature, *Heilkunst* had been pushed to the margins in terms such as *Wasserheilkunst*, hydrotherapy – in other words, those fields rapidly being shed by the growing body of biomedicine.[6] The Viennese 'therapeutic nihilist' Joseph Dietl complained (1845) that the physician had been for too long a mere *Heilkünstler* – therapist – and should strive to become a *Naturforscher* – scientific researcher (cited in Lachmund 1998). *Heilkunde* itself began to be affected by the same process of semantic displacement and decline: Jütte (1998) points out that in the 1880s dissident therapies were dismissed as *Naturheilkunde*, nature-cure, by the practitioners of scientific *Schulmedizin*.[7] Yet Hahnemann maintained he was advancing a scientific therapeutics till the end, as shown by the references to *rationelle Heilkunst* in the later editions of the *Organon*. Increasingly, the expression is used as an ironic reproach to the followers of different medical gods, either those who perpetuated the old abuses, or such as Dietl, whose calls for a new *rationelle Therapie* (cited by Lachmund 1998) unconsciously echoed Hahnemann's rhetorical claim of 30 years before.

Readers of translations not based on historical German usage faced further problems. For instance, the only English translation of the first edition – usefully clear in most respects – conflated the titles of the first and second editions, distorting the German terms at the same time: *rationelle Heilkunde* – scientific medical theory – and *Heilkunst* – therapeutics – became 'rational healing art' (Hahnemann 1913). Since all doctors believe they act rationally

[6] I am grateful to an anonymous reviewer for *History of Science* who drew my attention to the historiographical survival of the term in *Die Apologie der Heilkunst: eine griechische Sophistenrede des fünften vorchristlichen Jahrhunderts*, transl., ed. and annotated by Theodor Gomperz (Leipzig, 1890).

[7] *Naturheilkunde* survives as naturopathy; see Wiesenauer (1992) for evidence that it might even be *rationell*, in the modern sense of economically efficient.

and practise the 'healing art', they could be forgiven for asking what Hahnemann meant.

2.8. The grounds for rejection

The tendency of sceptical opponents of homeopathy to base their entire critique on the a priori impossibility of infinitesimal doses while ignoring more fundamental components of the therapy, such as drug tests, the similia principle and individualization of prescriptions, was noted by August Bier (1925), the influential Berlin surgeon who critically investigated the subject. Hahnemann is still excluded from accounts of early pharmacological investigation of the pure effects of drugs in humans, despite the priority and scale of his work (between 1805 and 1837, he published provings of 100 drugs that he had personally conducted or directed), and the sometimes explicit indebtedness of canonical pioneers such as Magendie, Orfila and Purkyne to his methods, because homeopathy is held to 'contradict the most elementary scientific knowledge' (Weatherall 1994). Nevertheless, infinitesimal doses were not part of the homeopathic hypothesis, were rarely used in drug tests, and were only gradually introduced into treatment as Hahnemann's experience with the method increased.[8] They were a refinement and not a requirement of the system. Even though Hahnemann (1833b; 1852a) repeatedly claimed that chemistry was as inappropriate to the analysis of his triturated and succussed medicines as it was to detecting the difference between plain and magnetized iron, the fact that infinitesimal doses have always been open to clinical testing, regardless of prior beliefs about their plausibility, suggests that explanations of homeopathy's comprehensive rejection by official medicine should be sought elsewhere.

Philosophy and medicine were explicitly connected in German intellectual life in the period 1790–1840 in a manner not countenanced elsewhere. Later, Romantic medicine came to be seen as a blind alley in the onward march of medical progress, disavowed nowhere more strongly than in Germany, and the era's coincidence with Hahnemann's working life ensured he was tarred with the same brush. Shryock's (1948: 138) claim that homeopathy

> was established in Germany during the last days of the *Naturphilosophie*, and was characterized … by a monistic pathology and therapeutics

[8] See: Hughes (1893: 930-939) for a chronological review of Hahnemann's posology.

is typical of its period in its inaccuracies of date, intellectual relationships, nosology and treatments. Yet it remains true that the reorientation of medical and scientific historiography in the second half of the twentieth century away from intra-professional triumphalism and 'great men' towards socially-oriented reflexivity has generally left homeopathy's content and methods on one side, in favour of regional studies of its clientele or its political and economic battles with allopathy.[9]

Much therefore remains to be explored in the relationships of homeopathic science to the intellectual environment of its birthplace, and the parallel formation of biomedicine in the nineteenth century. Hahnemann came from a similar Pictist background to Kant, and the enactment of the categorical imperative in a medical context underlay his life's work, long after he had left Pietism behind. Nonetheless, he was not bound to accept Kant's confidence in Brunonian theory. He was just as critical of visionary hyper-Brunonianism such as Schelling's (Hahnemann 1808c), and maintained – rightly it would appear – that a fallacious association with *Naturphilosophie* and Romantic medicine had retarded the acceptance of homeopathy (Haehl 1927, ii: 287). Yet, ironically for a philosophy that seems to have had such an influence on Hahnemann's critical outlook, it was a Kantian pronouncement about the legitimate domains of scientific inquiry that hastened the marginalization of homeopathy, more subtly but possibly even more thoroughly than the 'infinitesimal' doses that proclaimed a self-evident absurdity.

As noted, Hahnemann emphasized the individuality of each sick person, and the crucial importance of emotional and cognitive states in determining the simillimum – the most similar and thus most suitable medicine:

> It is not too much to say that the mental symptoms of a patient often form the determining factor in the choice of the medicinal counter-force. They are the characteristics which the observant physician can least of all afford to overlook. (Hahnemann 1810; 1913 § 187)

Kant had said that the contents of the mind could not be studied scientifically, on the interesting grounds that they exist in time but not in space, and are hence unamenable to mathematical description. This orientation helped to underwrite the tendency towards identification of disease processes with their lesional endstates that came to characterize 'hospital' and 'laboratory' definitions of illness, the assumption being that the classification and diagnosis of

---

[9] For recent social historiography of homeopathy, see: Faure (1992b), Jütte (1998). Notable content-based exceptions are: Schmidt (1990) and Dellmour (1997).

any disease should indicate essential organic and biochemical characteristics common to all patients who present with it, and that any symptomatic or causal treatment ought ideally to be valid at all times, in all places, for everybody (Foucault 1963; Ackerknecht 1967; Jewson 1976; Maulitz 1987). The search for the single apodictic answer to each species of disease came to the fore in the milieux that proclaimed their devotion to empirical fact most loudly; but was linked, not just with the now-familiar disappearance of the patient narrative but, moreover, with an explicit and institutionalized disbelief in what the patient or experimental 'subject' might have to report (Lachmund 1998). Since that time, many trained in what became the dominant medical model, including the practical majority who were uninterested in nosology, have had difficulty comprehending a therapy that side-stepped causation and elevated the individual's 'claims' to subjective experience above her common mammalian reactions. For example, the idea of compiled personal reactivities clearly mystified an otherwise sympathetic commentator (Berkowitz 1994) on a recent successful randomized placebo-controlled trial of infinitesimal doses for childhood diarrhea (Jacobs, Jiménez, Gloyd, et al. 1994).

Another objection to homeopathy's acausal descriptive personalism was the unfalsifiability of its prescription–analogues.[10] Hahnemann rejected the relevance of the Kantian a priori to the understanding of disease, but the quest for the simillimum invoked another kind of Kantian a priori, one that functions as an ideal exemplar or paradigm (in the traditional, Aristotelian sense of *paradeigma*, pattern). Kant (1787: 384) discusses this under the heading 'Of the regulative employment of the ideas of pure reason', using geometrical and physical illustrations such as the circle or vacuum:

> The most remarkable circumstance connected with these principles is, that they seem to be transcendental, and, although only containing ideas for the guidance of the empirical exercise of reason, and although this empirical employment stands in an asymptotic relation alone … that is, continually approximate, without ever being able to attain them, they possess, notwithstanding, as *a priori* synthetical propositions, objective though undetermined validity, and are available as rules for possible experience. In the elaboration of our experience, they may also be employed with great advantage, as heuristic principles.

Many drugs might produce similar symptoms to the patient's, but only the one offering the closest fit to the symptom-complex was chosen. It follows that the

[10] Popper's criterion was applied to homeopathy in falsificationism's heyday (Cioffi 1970; Campbell 1978; Schwanitz 1983: 177).

simillimum remains as an ideal of treatment that can only be approximated in any case of illness, albeit using a teachable heuristic involving an equation of analogous qualities, as in the case of Frau Sch—. Falsifying such an hypothesis poses considerable difficulties, given the astonishing number of variables at play in symptom collection and matching, not to mention evaluation of the clinical results. Are the difficulties therefore evidence of homeopathy's lack of scientific plausibility? Hahnemann believed not, but his warning that valid appraisals had to follow his method of individualizing were usually ignored. And even Hahnemann's care in case-taking could also be held against him: it might have been 'in line with the best modern teaching and considerably in advance of the average *practice*' (original emphasis) of the next century even, but it was clear that the undeniable therapeutic benefits of homeopathy were a non-specific effect due to patient–practitioner interaction (Suttie 1936: 130ff).

The theory's predictive power in the face of new diseases such as cholera or old ones such as pneumonia that defied orthodox treatment might reasonably have been considered a better test of its plausibility (see e.g. Tessier 1850; Eidherr 1862; Lasveaux 1988; Leary 1994), but even its clinical successes could be held against it, most notoriously in Britain, where the behaviour of the Medical Council, set up by the President of the Board of Health, Sir Benjamin Hall, to compare results of different treatments in the 1854 London cholera epidemic, exemplifies the difficulties that impartial clinical evaluation of competing therapies posed for the profession at this date. The historic importance of this large-scale trial was apparent to its participants at the time, and has been emphasized more recently as a defining moment in the evolution of the clinical trial (Lilienfeld 1982). When asked by Hall to explain the suppression of the returns from the London Homoeopathic Hospital, Golden Square, Soho (at the epicentre of the epidemic), the Council tacitly acknowledged the dramatic superiority of the independently evaluated homeopathic results, but agreed unanimously that:

> by introducing the returns of homoeopathic practitioners, they would not only compromise the value and utility of their averages of cure, as deduced from the operation of known remedies, but they would give an unjustifiable sanction to an empirical practice alike opposed to the maintenance of truth and to the progress of science. (House of Commons 1854–55: 194)

Rudolf Virchow believed the possibility of an explanation was not a scientific criterion (cited in Guttentag 1966), but it was probably more realistic to say that

> Western knowledge is a form of having … If knowledge is a form of possession, it follows that one possesses only what one understands. For what is not

> understood cannot truly be called a possession. Pragmatism is a disinherited offshoot of the true idea of Western knowledge because it is satisfied with the fruition of what it does not possess by comprehension. (Haas 1956: 182)

When that celebrated ironist Jean Paul (1826–28, ii: 292) exclaimed:

> *Hahnemann, double-headed prodigy of philosophy and learning* – whose system spelled the final ruin of the prescription-mongers, but was nevertheless little taken up by practitioners, and is more reviled than investigated,

he may not have guessed his judgement would stand for nearly another two centuries before it could be gainsaid.

3. Origins of Hahnemann's pharmacognosy and miasmatic theory

Material in this chapter appeared as: Dean M.E. (2000). Homeopathy and alchemy: (1) A pharmacological gold standard. *The Homeopath* (79): 22–27; Dean M.E. (2001). Homeopathy and alchemy: (2) Contagion from miasms. *The Homeopath* (80): 26–33.

Background: Critics traditionally object that homeopathy involves not natural phenomena and scientifically grounded method but manufactured or irrational techniques and ideas. Many homeopaths and occultists claim that Hahnemann was mainly inspired by alchemy, a debt which he concealed.

Questions: Were the essential elements of homeopathic theory and practice inventions of Hahnemann? What connexion if any do they have with pre-scientific alchemical theory and practice?

Argument: The main elements of Hahnemannian theory and practice – such as the similia principle, drug tests, theory of infectious miasms, and even small doses – had emerged in orthodox medical debate in the decades immediately before he wrote. Serial dilution and potentization appear to be the only elements derived from medieval alchemical medicine, but Hahnemann only accepted them into homeopathy after empirical testing. He is best seen as an experimentalist and systematizer of much that was previously unexplained and uncoordinated.

3.1. The main objections

By 1805 the essential groundwork had been accomplished, and Hahnemann began to formalize his system. As noted in Ch. 2, homeopathy was initially regarded as part of orthodox medicine. However, Hahnemann's dilution of doses beyond the point where Avogadro's hypothesis (contemporaneously announced in 1810) stated that no molecule of the original substance could remain, proved to be the most visible single stumbling block to the therapy's acceptance, and prevented consideration of almost everything else. Then as now, virtually all critique of homeopathy ignored its clinical method and the evaluation of its efficacy. Rejection came on a priori grounds: homeopathic medicines are sometimes diluted beyond the Avogadro number N_A, so any effects of homeopathy must be placebo effects. Despite the fact that attenuation is a secondary development of and subordinate to the similia principle, and even though many homeopathic medicines are not diluted beyond N_A, critics have continually based their rejection of homeopathy solely on its so-called 'infinitesimal' doses. The criticism has been expressed in much the same terms during two centuries:

> The waters of the whole world would require the addition only of 1.32603 grains to make the dilution such that each drop should contain but the quadrillionth of a grain; ... The belief, therefore, that anything so small could have any effect on disease is too ridiculous to require comment. (Routh 1852: 8)
>
> The laws of physics and chemistry are the same in Bangkok, Bristol and Buenos Aires, and homeopathy is just as much nonsense in one part of the world as in another. (Fisken 1996)

Even when formal clinical evaluation is involved, the situation is little different. A recent meta-analysis of 89 randomized placebo-controlled trials of homeopathy included 51 trials in which at least one group received medicines not diluted beyond N_A (Linde, Clausius, Ramirez et al. 1997). Yet one of the two hostile editorials commissioned to accompany the publication of the meta-analysis rejected its largely positive findings on the basis of homeopathy's 'infinitesimal doses' (Vandenbroucke 1997).

In contrast, the criticism of homeopathy made by the epidemiologist P.C.A. Louis at a meeting of the Académie de Médecine in 1835 is more thoughtful: he said that 'Homeopathy shows many signs of being invented rather than discovered' (Académie de Médecine 1835a). His implication was that there was no scientific research tradition leading up to homeopathy, and that the similia principle, serial dilution and potentization were arbitrary inventions not grounded in empirical observation of nature. In keeping with the prevailing therapeutic nihilism of the French school, Louis was pessimistic about the value of any treatments available at that time, orthodox or dissident, and his criticism of homeopathy is less vitiated by self-interest or chauvinism than was the norm (see Ch. 6). The well-known American doctor O.W. Holmes (1809–94) took up Louis's strain in his polemic *Homeópathy* [sic] *and its Kindred Delusions* (1842), an essay still revered today as a humiliating demolition of Hahnemann (King 1958: 157; Ernst 1995b; Crellin 1997). As if it were not incredible that Hahnemann had discovered something of such importance as the similia principle, was it not completely implausible that he had discovered the potentization of medicines, not to mention the miasmatic origin of disease? One major discovery can be allowed to any scientist, but three undermine his credibility. Holmes's sarcasm was obvious: Hahnemann was not a scientist, and he had not 'discovered' anything, but simply made it all up.

It should be clear from the account in Ch. 2 that Hahnemann did not conjure the similia principle, but formed and tested a hypothesis to unify the 'surprising facts' of empirical specifics known to him, and supported it with hundreds of examples of paradoxical cures found in the literature. Nevertheless, Louis and Holmes aimed at the techniques of homeopathy as much as the epistemological foundation. The issue is complicated by the fact that Hahnemann also received criticism in the early positivist period for allegedly deriving his entire method from alchemy, more specifically from the great Swiss dissident alchemist physician Paracelsus (c.1491–1541) (Schultz 1831). Academic historians still claim today that Hahnemann proposed a 'modified form of Paracelsianism' (Brock 1992: 38), and based his therapy on the doctrine of signatures (Flaherty 1995). The therapy was not merely invented, but was a relic of the superstition and witchcraft that preceded the scientific revolution, completely undermining Hahnemann's claims to scientificity and rationality. This charge is even more grave than Louis's, and merits investigation.

3.2. Hahnemann and alchemy

It has to be acknowledged that the question of direct alchemical influence on Hahnemann's development of homeopathy remains open, in spite of his denials of any connexion with Paracelsus. Proponents of the theory of personal esoteric involvement point out, for instance, that Hahnemann's father painted plates in the Meissen factory set up after the alchemist Johann Böttger (1682–1719) had stumbled on the secret of Chinese porcelain while trying (unsuccessfully) to manufacture gold (Fernando 1998). Moreover, during his period in Vienna Hahnemann was introduced by his mentor and tutor, the Freemason Joseph von Quarin (1733–1814), to an influential fellow Mason, Baron Samuel von Brukenthal, who invited Hahnemann to his estate in Hermannstadt (now named Sibiu, in Romania). Hahnemann was admitted to the craft almost immediately on arrival in Hermannstadt in 1777, and spent two happy years practising medicine in the locality, as well as cataloguing von Brukenthal's collections of coins and early medical and alchemical texts (Haehl 1927). Since many of the Viennese lodges, in the higher degrees, adhered to a synthetic ritual that contained Masonic, alchemical and Rosicrucian elements (Palou 1966) the origins of homeopathy can surely be found in the heady atmosphere of late eighteenth-century Austrian Freemasonry, so the argument goes. Moreover, Burnett studied the information that was available in the late Victorian period and concluded that Hahnemann had failed to give Paracelsus his due (Clarke 1923), and Oosterhuis (1937) later published an impressive catalogue of parallels between the two reformers – which tends to suggest that Hahnemann might indeed have had something to hide.

On the sceptical side, within homeopathy, an interpretation has emerged which seeks to minimize alchemical connexions, while promoting Hahnemann's undoubted empiricist and scientific credentials (e.g. Coulter 1977; Demarque 1981). After all, Hahnemann was one of the 15 most cited chemists in Lorenz Crell's *Chemische Annalen* in the years 1784–89, a journal which above all others laid the foundations for the German chemical community's preeminence in the coming century (Hufbauer 1982: 91). Why should such a prominent experimentalist have had recourse to discredited superstitions like the doctrine of signatures? Hahnemann claimed in 1825 to be unaware of the similarities between his and Paracelsus' medical systems, and when Schultz (1831) published what he regarded as evidence of direct influence, Hahnemann then dismissed the Paracelsan writings as incomprehensible (Haehl 1927, ii: 274). This is hardly surprising in view of the fact that it has taken lifetimes of scholarship to unravel the contradictory opinions, obscure jargon, proto-science and occultism found in the Paracelsan corpus (e.g. Pagel 1982b) – lifetimes that were unavailable to Hahnemann, who was busy with his own task.

Attempts to absolve Hahnemann of alchemical sympathies are as understandable as the interest in his possible esotericism. How then should such conflicting claims be evaluated? Hahnemann's vitalist ideas, which appeared comparatively late in his career, can be plausibly traced to Paracelsan and ultimately Oriental theories, but they were often held by other eighteenth-century European medical thinkers. For instance, Georg Ernst Stahl (1660–1734) opposed the advance of Cartesian dualism, which was rapidly leading to the relegation of mind to the bottom of the medical hierarchy of systems, and reintroduced the idea of an *anima*, or 'biomedical soul', arguing essentially that

> medicine is the science of life … and physicians repudiate medicine when they refuse to ask what life is … many diseases are remedied by the spontaneous 'autocracy' of some sort of vital guide or direction. We must study the mode of action of this guide, and base our therapeutic method on seconding its operations. (Hall 1975. i: 352)

Stahl's influence was noticeable in German medicine throughout the eighteenth century, and his term *autocratie* is used by Hahnemann – who had previously rejected the idea in 'The value of the speculative systems of medicine' (Hahnemann 1808c; 1852b) – as a synonym for *Lebenskraft* and *dynamis* in the

1833 *Organon*. Similar observations can be made about holistic features of Hahnemann's system, such as the protective nature of symptoms: recent research has shown that the threat of metastasis was commonly used by eighteenth-century physicians as a means of ensuring loyalty and compliance with instructions among their patients (Nicolson 1988).

Because aspects of vitalism and holism were still reasonably widespread at the beginning of the nineteenth century, especially in Germany, the characteristics of homeopathy which it seems most fruitful to investigate for evidence of a unique debt to alchemy are its research methods and pharmacological techniques. In other words, the similia principle, drug tests, pharmacopeia, dilutions, trituration and potentization. Hahnemann's theories of infectious disease causation – the acute and chronic miasm concepts – also deserve a closer look in this context, since they went against most current trends.

By way of definition, 'alchemy' is broadly treated here as the complex of magical and metallurgical lore, herbal and mineral therapies, spiritual practices and metaphysics which: surfaced in turn in China, Hellenistic Egypt and under Islam; took an increasingly medical form in Islam; came to medieval Europe courtesy of Islamic conquests and contacts; were especially associated with Paracelsus and the iatrochemists who followed him; and which continued to affect medicine during the Scientific Revolution, while being gradually replaced by chemistry. Prominent in this tradition at different times were transmutation of elements, and the attempt to produce the – real or metaphorical – philosophers' stone. According to your heart's desire, the object was the attainment of illumination, immortality, longevity, health or simply gold.

3.3. Pharmacology

3.3.1. Similars and signatures

Hahnemann insisted that the similia principle had been used in medicine, consciously or otherwise, long before him. He found traces of the doctrine as far apart as the Hippocratic writings – quoted in 'The medicine of experience' (Hahnemann 1805c; 1852b) – and the suggestion by Quarin's Viennese colleague Anton von Störck (1731–1803) that stramonium should be tried in some mental disorders because it can induce dissociation, mania and hallucinations (Störck 1762). Hahnemann claimed only to have hypothesized and validated the principle, via provings of known specifics such as cinchona, and systematized it as a means of discovering the sphere of action of new medicines.

What relationship if any is there between the similia principle and alchemy? As a guide to pharmacology, Paracelsus taught not symptom similarity but the doctrine of signatures. This identified medicines for illnesses from their shared appearances or qualities. These so-called correspondences could function at various semiotic levels. As Hahnemann (1817; 1880) indicates in 'Examination of the sources of the common materia medica', doctors gave

> the testicle-shaped orchis-root in order to restore manly vigour; the *phallus impudicus*, to strengthen weak erections; ascribed to the yellow turmeric the power of curing jaundice, and considered *hypericum perforatum*, whose yellow flowers on being crushed yield a red juice (*St John's blood*), useful in haemorrhages and wounds.

It is easy to see that such a doctrine may plausibly have originated in preliterate societies as an aide-memoire for reputed cures which happened to bear a resemblance to their target illness, but it had been turned into a magical dogma by the Renaissance. Some Paracelsan notions of signatures are imaginative to say the least: mercury was named for the god of the marketplace, where the French disease – syphilis – could be picked up cheaply.

Signatures, and the astrological lore attached to them, were rejected in the strongest terms by Paracelsus' follower J.B. Van Helmont (1579–1644) in spite of his immersion in alchemical medicine (Pagel 1982a). Hahnemann expresses similar contempt for the doctrine in the essay just quoted, continuing that he would 'refrain from taunting' his medical contemporaries with the traces of the absurd superstition which could still be found in the most recent materia medicas – presumably because he had already taunted them in 'The value of the speculative systems of medicine' (Hahnemann 1808c), where many examples of the survival of the doctrine are enumerated. In his article on *Chelidonium* – whose bitter yellow juice bore the signature of bile, and hence all hepatic disease – he elaborated that it was impossible to use even those remedies which appeared to verify the doctrine because: (a) the alleged clinical indications were so imprecise; and (b) the plants had generally been compounded with many other ingredients in those cases where they were reputedly effective (Hahnemann 1811–21; 1880). He attacked the 'criminal frivolity' of those who were satisfied with such guesswork:

> Only that which the drugs themselves unequivocally reveal of their peculiar powers in their effects on the healthy human body – that is to say, only their pure symptoms – can teach us loudly and clearly when they can be advantageously used with certainty; and this is when they are administered in morbid states very similar to those they are able to produce on the healthy body.

3.3.2. Drug tests

There is no doubt that Hahnemann's systematic investigation of materia medica gave a major impetus to the establishment of scientific drug testing and hence clinical pharmacology. Are there any Paracelsan or alchemical precedents? Apparently not. Or simply a link with earlier times? The Persian philosopher and physician Ibn Sina (Avicenna, 980–1037) is famous for his *Kitab al-Qanun* (Canon of medicine) which was still required reading in European medical schools centuries after it was written (e.g. Avicenna 1473; 1564). It contains seven precepts for the scientific evaluation of drugs on humans, some of which derive from Galen. The principles include the idea, revolutionary for the time, of controlled tests of uncompounded single drugs on the sick (Crombie 1953). Hahnemann was well aware of Ibn Sina's central contribution to medicine, and even quotes – in Arabic – from Book ii of the *Canon*, on simples, in the thesis of 1812 that gained him the right to lecture at Leipzig University (see Ch. 2). This early call for a rational pharmacology was not for pathogenetic trials (provings) but empirical tests of possible curative agents. Even though it sought to avoid the time-honoured errors due to polypharmacy, it was a precursor of the random Baconian inductivism that Hahnemann rejected:

> Either a single drug must be tried in all diseases … or all drugs must be tried in a particular disease … Thus, after thousands upon thousands of blind trials with innumerable substances upon, perhaps, millions of individuals, the suitable, the specific remedy is at last discovered *by accident*. (Hahnemann 1811–21; 1880)

A more probable origin for Hahnemannian provings can be found much closer to his time. He applauded Albrecht von Haller (1708–77), who had conducted physiological experiments on healthy animals and recommended their extension to humans. In fact, the first recorded test on a healthy human seems to have been made somewhat earlier by Van Helmont (1648), who noted the strange alterations in his perception after putting a piece of aconite root on his tongue, but this seems to have been an isolated instance before more systematic programmes emerged in the next century. Richard Mead (1673–1754), society physician and advocate of smallpox inoculation, tried a few poisonous substances on himself, including viper venom and opium, but from the standpoint of a contagionist who wished to find how epidemics were transmitted (Mead 1745). More therapeutically oriented were Störck's tests in which he tried one or two poisonous plants on himself before experimentally treating patients with them. Störck's work was so well known throughout eighteenth-century Europe that his self-test of *Colchicum autumnale* appeared in English in the popular *Gentleman's Magazine* (Störck 1764). From different starting points, Mead and Störck appear to have started a trend: others who tested drugs on themselves after this date include the Dublin doctor Alexander (1768), and Monro (1788) and Crumpe (1793) of the Edinburgh school.

Yet there was another fundamental difference between Hahnemann's experiments and those of his immediate predecessors. Alexander set out to see whether common drugs such as castor and camphor did to him in a state of health what they were supposed to do in sickness; because castor was reputed to combat fever but didn't reduce his normal healthy temperature, he concluded it was valueless. Alexander may have been right about its efficacy in fever, but his method was hardly the way to find out. And as Hahnemann (1811–21; 1880) points out in his article on *Camphora*, earlier researchers had neglected the all important personal element, concentrating on rudimentary quantitative measures such as pulse and temperature:

> the pure effects of it, observed by Alexander, are very meagre and confined to mere general expressions.

Hahnemann's orientation towards pure symptoms uninfluenced by *a priori* theories of drug action, and his emphasis on the existential subjectivity of illness states, differed completely from earlier investigations of the effects of drugs in the healthy. Still, he did not hide his debt, as claimed recently (Oliver 1999): experimental symptoms discovered by Van Helmont, Mead, Störck, Alexander, Monro, Crumpe and many others were included and correctly referenced (along with a much greater number of alleged side-effects observed during Old School treatment of sick patients) under the appropriate drugs in his materia medica, and in the historical survey of 1807 that later served as the first introduction to the *Organon*.

3.3.3. Therapeutic poisons and the minimum dose

Hahnemann was well aware of the historical precedents for using highly poisonous plants in therapy – his Leipzig thesis, discussed in Ch. 2, concerned the use of hellebore in Classical Greece, Rome and Islam. Although Paracelsus had used such plants, and Hahnemann included Van Helmont's symptoms of self-poisoning with aconite in his materia medica, a far more likely initial stimulus for Hahnemann's interest again lay much closer to home, since it was a corollary of the proving idea. As mentioned, Störck (1760) was one of the first to envisage the systematic reintroduction of highly toxic plants to the official materia medica. This triggered widespread interest in the plants' therapeutic potential in the 1760s – for instance, Quarin (1761) published a monograph on cicuta at this time – but enthusiasm quickly waned because of the unacceptable number of fatalities that occurred. Poisonous plants then re-emerged in medicine – in parallel with Hahnemann's first homeopathic experiments – in suitably reduced doses. William Withering (1741–99) isolated digitalis from a folk remedy for dropsy containing many less useful plants (1785) and in 1789 wrote:

> Poisons in small doses are the best medicine; and useful medicines in too large doses are poisonous.

Hahnemann's pre-homeopathic 'Description of Klockenbring during his insanity' (Hahnemann 1796a; 1852b) mentions a prescription of 2 grains of stramonium seed for mania made in 1792. The prescription is more remarkable for being the patient's own instruction to Hahnemann during a relatively lucid interval. Klockenbring was not a doctor, but an author and intellectual who had presumably become acquainted with Störck's conjecture, and Hahnemann comments favourably on the suitability of the medicine and the dose. Also in the early 1790s, John Alderson (1758–1829) was cultivating *Rhus toxicodendron* at the Hull General Infirmary, and used small doses in the treatment of various forms of paralysis. He mentions the novelty of giving such a toxic plant as medicine, and the trepidation felt by some of his patients (Alderson 1811). He reports some astonishing successes with longstanding well-attested paralyses, and symptoms from his monograph were included in the homeopathic materia medica (Hahnemann 1811–21).

After announcing the similia principle in 1796, Hahnemann continued to use doses similar to those of his more cautious and scientifically minded contemporaries, and only after 1800 did he begin to reduce them gradually towards the levels that eventually made homeopathy notorious, as seen in 'Cure and prevention of scarlet fever' (Hahnemann 1801b; 1852b). For instance, a letter to Stapf, dated 3 September 1813, shows provers were expected to take 1 oz of a simple dilution of helleborus niger containing the equivalent of 1/160 grain (= 0.0004 g), every two hours, as long as they were 'not too severely affected' (Hahnemann 1889). This was a small dose, but certainly not 'infinitesimal'. In fact, ultra-small doses seem to have been reserved for treatments at this time, simply because patients were more sensitive than provers, not because smaller doses were more powerful. Paracelsus is well-known for his claim that small doses of poisons were the most effective medicines, but it is unnecessary to invoke his influence on their use by Withering, Alderson, Hahnemann or other late eighteenth-century experimentalists.

3.3.4. Drug preparation

Hahnemann's pharmacopeia was mainly herbal in the first two decades of homeopathy, and prepared solely from liquid tinctures. Juices were expressed from fresh plants, dried plants were steeped in alcohol for several hours, and in one or two cases metallic salts of various degrees of solubility, such as *Causticum*, were used to make a 'tincture' which could then be further diluted as needed (Hahnemann 1805b). He modified the process of simple dilution with succussion as a more efficient means of mixing the material with the diluent, but there is no suggestion at this time that he had discovered processes which not only made the medicines safer – the original motivation for dilutions – but also released a hidden medicinal power. Dilutions were standardized in 1816, on a metric (centesimal) scale quite dissimilar to the traditional apothecaries' measures used in homeopathy until then. Two years later Hahnemann claimed that even substances declared to be biologically inert because of their insolubility were capable of pathogenetic and therapeutic action, after lengthy trituration with lactose, and he now began to call the process 'dynamization' and the attenuations 'potencies'.

Plausible influences from alchemy are much easier to find here than with the similia principle, provings or poisonous plants. The call for common alchemical processes such as serial dilution to be used in the preparation of medicines was frequently heard in Europe from the time of Ramon Lull (c.1232–1315, but the works fathered on him belong to more than one author, like the Hippocratic, Jabirian and Paracelsan writings) and the experimentalist philosopher Roger Bacon (c.1214–92) onwards. Instructions for alchemical projection – the final process of transmuting base metal with the philosophers' stone to produce gold – demand accurately measured serial dilutions, typically of one part in 100 (Lully 1330). And, of course, the more times the process was repeated the more powerful it became, as the cynical but well-informed Ben Jonson observed in 1610[11]:

> For look, how oft I iterate the work,
> So many times, I add unto his virtue.
> As, if at first one ounce convert a hundred,

[11] *The Alchemist* II. iii. 106–14.

> After his second loose, he'll turn a thousand;
> His third solution, ten; his fourth, a hundred.
> After his fifth, a thousand thousand ounces
> Of any imperfect metal, into pure
> Silver or gold, in all examinations
> As good as any of the natural mine.

Trituration of insoluble substances was another of alchemy's many processes, and in his article of 1818 on *Aurum foliatum* Hahnemann records how he came to adopt the practice only after reading its history in early medico-alchemical texts:

> I was delighted to find a number of Arabian physicians unanimously testifying to the medicinal powers of gold in a finely pulverized form, particularly in some serious morbid conditions, in some of which the solution of gold [tri-chloride] had already been of great use to me. (Hahnemann 1818; 1880)

The alchemists' legendary *aurum potabile* (drinkable gold) had of course disappeared from European medicine by the late eighteenth century, dismissed by nearly all Hahnemann's contemporaries as a primitive superstition. He recounts the history of gold therapy in Islamic and European medical alchemy, quoting Geber's celebrated phrase *materia laetificans et in juventute corpus preservans* (a substance that gladdens and preserves the youthfulness of the body) that he had found in *De alchemia*, in the edition of 1598 brought out by Lazarus Zetzner, a leading publisher of alchemical works (Geber 1598). The book was attributed to Jabir ibn-Hayyan (c.721–c.815), the 'father' of Islamic alchemy, until the twentieth century, when it was shown that it belongs to the thirteenth century and was probably written in Europe (Newman 1991). Nevertheless, the author of the *Summa perfectionis*, as it is usually called, had an intimate knowledge of Arabic alchemy, and the book has always been accepted as the fountainhead of the European alchemical tradition. Interestingly, this emergence of the 'gold as elixir of life' theme in Europe in the thirteenth century ties the practice ultimately to Taoist alchemy, rather than Hellenistic Egypt as previously thought: the Chinese took the immortality theme literally, unlike the Greek alchemists, and it was transmitted to Europe via the Middle East (Needham 1974).

Hahnemann then cites Serapion the younger (c.900) and Ibn Sina for their use of gold in various conditions including cardiac disease and depression, showing his knowledge of Arabic in the process. One of the conditions Ibn Sina treated with gold could be 'talking to oneself' or 'dyspnea', depending on the diacritical mark: Hahnemann claims that his proving demonstrated it was the latter, and respiratory distress is certainly accepted now as an aspect of gold toxicology. The early methods of making pure gold biologically available are then detailed: Abu'l-Qasim al-Zahrawi (Abulcasis, 936–1013) first showed how to prepare gold powder by rubbing it on a rough linen cloth in a basin filled with water, and Zacutus, the Portuguese, later rubbed gold on a grindstone. Hahnemann cites over 20 more recent alchemical and medical texts that recommend gold powder – including Francis Bacon's *Historia vitae et mortis* (1623) – and decided the idea was worth testing empirically:

> But leaving these authorities out of the question, I thought I might attach more value to the testimony of the Arabians as to the curative powers of finely powdered gold than to the theoretical unfounded doubts of the moderns.

Accordingly, trituration with lactose was introduced for the first time into homeopathic pharmacy, though it was a common technique elsewhere. Here for example are Störck's (1762) instructions for preparing aconite:

> Take extract of Blue Monkshood, two grains; white sugar, two drachms; mix and grind them together for a long time in a marble mortar, to the finest powder.

Hahnemann's innovation combined an existing technique for preparing dried plant materials – previously unused by him, because he preferred to steep them in alcohol – with an alchemical technique that had been eclipsed:

> I triturated the finest gold leaf (its fineness is 23 carats, 6 grains) with 100 parts of milk-sugar for a full hour, for internal medicinal use. (Hahnemann 1880)

His provers took substantial quantities of triturate:

> 100 grains of this powder (containing one grain of gold), and on others, 200 grains (containing two grains of gold), dissolved in water, sufficed to excite very great alterations in the health and morbid symptoms.

The results satisfied him that

> the assertions of the Arabians are not without foundation, as even small doses of this metal given in the form mentioned caused even in healthy adults morbid states very similar to those cured (in unconscious *homeopathic* manner) by those Orientals, who deserve credit for their discovery of remedies.

Prior to 1818, metals had been available to homeopathy only as solutions of their salts such as copper sulphate, mercury sulphides and iron acetate (introduced respectively in 1805, 1811 and 1816). This seems to have been true of post-Paracelsan iatrochemistry generally: in spite of the example of gold powder, only the nitrate of silver had been used in Europe, notably by Robert Boyle (1627–91) whose renowned diuretic pills Hahnemann criticized for their large doses and antipathic action in his *Argentum* article (1811–21). Could Hahnemann have known of J.A. Chrestien's (1758–1840) successful revival of gold powder in the treatment of syphilis (Chrestien 1811)? Burnett (1879) thought Hahnemann probably did, while Hughes (1893) took the opposite view. Whether or not Hahnemann was aware of contemporary allopathic experimentation is less important than the use made of the discovery in the two schools: gold powder therapy did not function as an exemplar in allopathy and soon fell out of fashion, whereas the homeopathic materia medica was transformed following the successful experiment in 1818. Pure metals such as silver and tin and insoluble minerals and plant materials were submitted to the trituration process for the first time. Many of the post-1818 medicines are reputed to be the deepest-acting, in spite of their innocuous appearance before trituration: these include *Silica*, *Carbo animalis* and *Carbo vegetabilis*, and the notable triad of *Calcarea*, *Lycopodium*, *Sulphur*.

Hahnemann did not record whether he adopted centesimal dilutions from alchemical sources – and he need not have as the metric scale was being used increasingly by scientists – but the date justifies the conjecture and his bibliographic references show he cannot have been unaware of the precedents.

3.4. Disease theory

3.4.1. Acute 'miasms'

Hahnemann was orientated towards successful therapeutics, and his writings betray a comparative lack of interest in the causes of disease. This was a reaction to the theorizing about the ultimate nature of disease that had dictated treatments since Galen, and an admission of how little could be known with certainty at this date. Even when causes could be found, they were not to be confused with diseases – which were the response of the organism to the disease-provocation and knowable only by their symptomatic manifestations.

> It may be granted that every disease must depend upon an alteration in the inner working of the human organism. This disease can only be mentally conceived through its outward signs and all that these signs reveal; *in no way whatever can the disease itself be recognized.*
> The invisible disease producing alteration in the inward man together with the visible alteration in health (the sum of the symptoms) make up that which is called disease; both together actually constitute the disease. (Hahnemann 1810; 1913 §§ 5, 6)

This idea corresponds to modern notions of disease as a response to disturbance of homeostasis, and Stahl is the most obvious precursor of this aspect of Hahnemann's thought. Nevertheless, in our quest for alchemical sources, it is worth tracing the evolution of Hahnemann's theories about disease transmission and causation in the period 1790–1830.

Following the decline of humouralism in official medicine, external causes for disease were sought. In the period 1700–1860 diseases that we now class as infectious were generally believed to result from miasmata – nonspecific noxious atmospheres or effluvia (Greek *miasma*, pl. *–ata*, bad air). Hahnemann (1792 / 1795) begins conventionally enough, for a late eighteenth-century doctor: epidemic diseases were the results of these miasmata, according to *The Friend of Health*.

However, venereal disease was an obvious exception to the general nonspecific rule of disease transmission, since it was only contracted after intercourse with someone already infected. In *Instructions for Surgeons respecting Venereal Disease*, Hahnemann (1789; 1852b) states that gonorrhea and syphilis are primary and secondary manifestations of the same disease, and ascribable to contagion. Ironically the two diseases had been clearly distinguished in the sixteenth century by Jean Fernel (c.1497–1558) and others. However, Paracelsus claimed they were the same and his error was believed and perpetuated until after Hahnemann's time. Most famously, John Hunter (1728–93), the Scottish surgeon, had inoculated himself with matter taken from a gonorrheal patient in order to demonstrate that it was the same as syphilis (Hunter 1786). He thought the symptoms he produced had proved his point – unaware that the donor also had syphilis. Hunter's reputation ensured that his confounding of the two diseases was taken as definitive for many decades, as was his rejection of the possibility of inherited syphilis or extra-genital transmission. Hahnemann followed Hunter's teaching about venereal disease in many respects, and the explanation of the action of homeopathic medicines he put forward later was particularly influenced by Hunter's theory that mercury provoked a medicinal disease which acted as a counter-irritant to the infection. Nevertheless, Hahnemann was independent enough to observe the existence of congenital syphilis at this date.

In his early homeopathic writings, such as 'Observations on the three current methods of treatment' (1801c; 1852b), Hahnemann thought disease was knowable purely by its symptomatology, and maintained that removal of the symptoms in toto was the radical cure. However, it is also at this date that he began – confusingly, and against contemporary usage – to restrict his use of the term 'miasm' to describe a transmissible principle that lay behind a specific contagious disease. (The quote marks are intended to distinguish Hahnemann's use of the term from orthodox miasmatic theory.) 'Cure and prevention of scarlet fever' (1801b; 1852b) refers to the causal mechanism of a transmissible scarlatina 'miasm', or 'virus'. (The quote marks distinguish 'virus' from the modern concept: from the eighteenth century to the mid twentieth, 'virus' meant morbid disease matter that could be inoculated thus passing on a disease and conferring immunity against future attacks.) The concept of a transmissible 'virus' was based on smallpox inoculation which had been introduced into European folk medicine from China and the Middle East in the sixteenth century. It was taken up by the medical profession in the early eighteenth century before the emergence of the much safer cowpox vaccination at the end of the century. Even more remarkably for the era, one section of Hahnemann's article – 'Prevention of scarlet fever in its first germs' (*Keimen*) – suggests the 'virus' contains or originates in a microscopic disease principle.

The theory is generalized to a variety of specific diseases in 'The medicine of experience', where 'miasmatic' is employed as the equivalent of what we would now call 'infectious':

> We observe a few diseases that always arise from *one and the same* cause, e.g. the miasmatic maladies; hydrophobia, the venereal disease, the plague of the Levant, yellow fever, small-pox, cow-pox, the measles and some others, which bear upon them the distinctive mark of always remaining diseases of a *peculiar* [particular] *character*; and because they arise from a contagious principle that always remains the same, they always retain the same character and pursue the same course, excepting as regards some accidental concomitant circumstances, which however do not alter their essential character. (Hahnemann 1805c; 1852b)

In Hahnemann's hands the concept of contagion was only applicable to a 'few diseases' but nonetheless allowed him to grant them a specific name *and* treatment (when discovered). And it was more than a precursor of the germ theory of specific diseases, which came to dominate medicine. The similia principle is based on the equivalence of diseases, poisons and medicines – they are capable of producing similar states. In his letter on the 'regeneration of medicine' he pointed out that

> the little of a positive character to be found amid the enormous mass *of* medical writings, consists in the accidentally discovered mode of cure of two or three diseases which always arise from identical miasmata; these are, the autumnal marsh ague [malaria], the lues venerea [syphilis], and the itch of workers in wool; to these must be added that most fortunate discovery, the protec-

> tion from variola [smallpox] by means of vaccination. And these three or four cures take place only according to my principle *similia similibus*. (Hahnemann 1808a; 1852b)

By the time of the first edition of the *Organon*, Hahnemann is talking about the difficulty of using specific diseases in provings:

> The invisible influences whereby the ordinary diseases of mankind are produced are all too little known, and are all *too* little under our command, for us to use them for the production of diseases at our will, and thus as remedies against diseases of longer standing. (Hahnemann 1810; 1913 § 34)

Using 'miasm' in his now familiar restricted sense of communicable disease matter, he continues, generalizing from smallpox vaccination to immunization against other diseases:

> Even the miasms, which might conceivably be inoculated for the removal of certain diseases, are too few in number to be used even to a limited extent as remedies. (ibid. § 35)

'On the venereal disease and its ordinary improper treatment' (Hahnemann 1816; 1852b) develops the thesis further, on the basis of observation: acute infectious diseases with fever and skin rash, such as smallpox, cowpox, measles, gonorrhea–syphilis and others are systemic poisons. Nothing can prevent the rapid spread of the inoculated 'virus' through the body, as evidenced by hydrophobia which develops even after immediate excision of the bite wound.

In 'Examination of the sources of the common materia medica' (Hahnemann 1817; 1852b), the distinction between Hahnemannian 'miasms' and conventional miasmata could not be clearer. Specific remedies only exist for those diseases

> of a *constant character* … some are *produced by a miasm which continues the same* through all generations, such as the venereal disease; others have *the same exciting causes*, as the ague of marshy districts …

In other words, he withholds the term 'miasm' from malaria, the very disease which appeared to confirm his contemporaries' theory of effluvial miasmata.

In a better-known passage from 'The mode of propagation of the Asiatic cholera', Hahnemann (1831; 1852b) returns to the microscopic origins of infectious disease hinted at in 1801. He claims that the cholera pandemic was not 'epidemically atmospheric-telluric' – i.e. not caused by a miasma – as his contemporaries continued to think for many decades, but was probably transmitted by

> a swarm of infinitely small, invisible living organisms, which are so murderously hostile to human life, and which most probably form the infectious matter of cholera.

Hahnemann was wrong in believing the bacteria multiplied in vapour rather than water, but correct in identifying human contact as an important vector. He warned that handling of patients by medical attendants without careful hygiene could spread the disease, and proposed preventive measures, such as sterilization of clothing and bedding, that would undoubtedly have been helpful if they had been followed. It is often forgotten that he recommended spirits of camphor to be used externally as an antiseptic, as well as diluted with water and taken orally, because of its homeopathicity to cholera symptomatology.

3.4.2. Sources of acute 'miasm' theory

Although theories of contagion had been advanced in Europe in the sixteenth century, in the wake of the great plague epidemics and the recent introduction of syphilis, the opposing effluvial theory had gained the upper hand by the eighteenth century and was dominant in the first half of the nineteenth century. In spite of being an incorrect theory, the value of the public health measures it inspired is undeniable. For instance, Edwin Chadwick (1801–90), the great instigator of Victorian sanitary reform, was a convinced effluvialist and anticontagionist, as was Charles Creighton whose important late nineteenth-century work on epidemiology was motivated by a desire to refute germ theory (Creighton 1891–94).

It seems unlikely therefore that Hahnemann could have been influenced by his contemporaries at a time when germ theories were almost totally unknown, so could there be an alchemical influence on homeopathic acute 'miasm' theory?

Traditional Hippocratic and Galenic medicine believed disease was due to an internally-generated – idiopathic – imbalance of the four humours: bilious, choleric, phlegmatic and sanguine. No surviving Greek text mentions contagion; even in epidemics, treatments were not aimed at protecting the community but at restoring the lost balance of the individual. Before 600 AD Chinese medicine held similar dyscrasic theories, but between then and 1600 it began to conceptualize diseases as separate entities which could be attacked with specific treatments that were valid at the population level (Unschuld 1998). Tellingly, the Chinese pictogram for cure includes the image of an arrow in a quiver – conceptually related to Erlich's specific chemotherapy or 'magic bullets' from the end of the nineteenth century. The idea of specific disease entities requiring specific treatments began to be reflected in Islamic sources in the ninth century, completely contradicting the stereotypical dismissal of Arabic medicine as a passive conduit for Galenism. For instance, in Book I of the *Canon*, Ibn Sina lists three main categories of specific diseases that can be passed on, either by infection, or by family or racial inheritance. Group 1 includes scabies, leprosy, smallpox and phthisis; groups 2 and 3 include gout, phthisis, and endemic goitre. This concept of intrinsic disease entities only began to surface in European medicine during the Renaissance. Alchemical sources were among the first to reflect the shift of emphasis, and alchemical illustrations of the body as a castle, repelling invasion by different diseases from the four quarters, survive from the seventeenth century.

This covert trend against the Galenism of the medical schools was made public by Paracelsus, who rejected humoural theory and replaced it with what he termed the *archeus*. *Archeus* is a Latinized Greek root, connoting rulership (-archy, in modern English) and fundamental principles (arche- or archi- in modern English). It is generally translated as life-force (although the theosophist Rudolf Steiner (1948) characteristically claimed that Paracelsus meant the etheric body). Paracelsus also believed that each disease has its own *archeus*, marking a clear break with the earlier theory of internal dyscrasias and imbalance, although he retained more primitive beliefs in attributing epidemics to the stars or the imagination. Moreover, the introduction of specifics for diseases in Europe, as against general treatments for imbalance, is also associated with Paracelsus: *Spezifikum* is in fact another Paracelsan coinage that quickly became common currency.

Van Helmont, Paracelsus' most prominent successor, believed that disease came about because of the struggle between the host's vital force and the vital force of the disease factor, and elaborated his idea of the effects of the invasion of the body by alien spiritual beings (*archei*):

> Once they had established a foothold he supposed that they took over the vital processes of the host for their own benefit, producing waste products that were poisonous to the victim. (Harré 1983: 97f)

Anachronistically viewed, this struggle between host and invader seems to prefigure modern germ theory. Unfortunately for what seems to promise an alchemical influence, in 'The value of the speculative systems of medicine' Hahnemann (1808c; 1852b) had dismissed the Paracelsan and Helmontian *archeus* – in its sense of an externally imposed rulership of the body – as an example of the error of attributing an ontological essence to disease. He does not seem to have been aware of the theory of independent disease *archei*, so any connexion remains highly conjectural.

Are there any more likely sources? Contemporaneously with the essentially dynamic ideas of Paracelsus, the idea of infections as due to *seminae* or seeds is associated with Girolamo Fracastoro (1478–1553), possibly influenced by the atomism of Democritus and the philosophical poem *De rerum naturae* by Lucretius (Fracastoro 1546). Fracastoro is sometimes cited as the originator of European contagionism, but his 'seeds' seem to have been as dematerialized as Van Helmont's. In any case, the idea was lost during the ascendancy of effluvial theory. However, it is possible to find an influence on Hahnemann's contagionism much closer in time and place than Paracelsus, Fracastoro or Van Helmont, one as plausible and immediate as Störck's anticipation of homeopathic pharmacology and method.

Marcus Antonius Plenciz (1705–86) belonged to the generation immediately before Quarin and Störck. He practised successfully in Vienna from 1735, and summarized his theories about disease in *Opera medico-physica*, published in 1762 at the same time as his younger contemporaries' monographs on therapeutic poisons (see 3.3 above). Plenciz (1762) seems to have been almost the sole voice of contagionism in the eighteenth century. His ideas have an extraordinarily modern ring because by continuing Anton van Leeuwenhoek's (1632–1723) investigations of microscopic lifeforms Plenciz became the first to realize the relevance of *animalculae* to disease transmission. He groups diseases according to whether they are epidemic, contagious or both. Infectious diseases are the results of specific causes, analogously with plants that only emerge from a seed of the same species. Noxious atmospheres do not satisfy this requirement, so disease transmission can only be explained by hypothesizing specific airborne disease germs that flourish under favourable conditions. Several terms are used for the means of infection, such as *miasma animatum, miasma verminosum*, and *seminia animatum*. These 'minute worm-like living germs' possess the capacity to multiply rapidly once they have gained access to the host. Inoculation against smallpox supports the theory, since a minute amount of inoculated 'virus' can cause disease, and also demonstrates the way that evolutionary modification of the original germ can confer immunity. Plenciz even had a modern-sounding explanation for the action of the well-known specific drugs, mercury and cinchona: these were capable of killing the germs of syphilis and malaria respectively. Generally, he recommended that therapy should be directed at predatory microorganisms, and favoured investigation of the antibiotic properties of heavy metals. His book contains two further essays – on smallpox and scarlet fever – to illustrate the theory.

These prophetic ideas were forgotten, except by the biologist-historian Kurt Sprengel (1821–28) who derided them. Brettoneau (1778–1862) is remembered for identifying diphtheria as a specific illness in 1826, but his suggestion – made only in a personal letter – of bacterial infection as the causal agent came twenty years after Hahnemann's cholera publications of 1831. The discovery in 1835 by Agostino Bassi (1773–1856) that the silkworm disease muscarine was probably due to a microscopic fungus is sometimes mentioned (Bassi 1835–36), but the revival of germ theory is usually dated from 1840 when the pathologist Jakob Henle (1809–85) claimed – against great opposition – that infectious diseases were probably caused by living parasites (Henle 1840).

Could Hahnemann's remarkably avant-garde contagionist ideas – which were only confirmed by the empirical discoveries of Pasteur and Koch in the second half of the nineteenth century – be connected with Plenciz's theories? The circumstantial evidence is strong. In his two main publications on scarlet fever, Hahnemann (1801b; 1808b; 1852b) acknowledges his reliance on the symptomatology in *Opera medico-physica*; and Plenciz's observational accuracy gained him the rare honour of Hahnemann's published approval (*Organon* edns 5 & 6, § 38) – which he accorded to Hippocrates, Sydenham, Haller and very few others. Scarlet fever seems to have been pivotal, not only for the greatly reduced doses introduced around 1800 to treat it, but also for the development of Hahnemann's contagionism.

3.4.3. Chronic disease theory

A standard mid twentieth-century medical dictionary defined homeopathy *inter alia* as a system that holds: 'that eruptive diseases of the skin must be allowed to come out, and should not be driven in' (Jones, Hoerr, Osol 1949). Although related to his general rejection of symptom suppression, this is particularly pertinent to Hahnemann's theory of chronic diseases which he developed in the 1820s, and which has been the most problematic part of his system, for homeopaths as well as critics.

After his semi-retirement to Cöthen, Hahnemann's patients were mainly those who travelled from many parts of the world to consult him with non-urgent longstanding illnesses that had defied conventional treatments. It was at this time that he found that the acausal 'general' model of homeopathy that had been so effective in acutes was not always successful in chronic disease. The theory of chronic miasms he put forward in *Chronic Diseases* (Hahnemann 1828–30; 1896) combined the ideas of infection and susceptibility: the sequelae of infectious episodes and other incidents gave rise to slowly developing conditions, leading to layered states of ill-health and susceptibilities to many other forms of illness. These all constituted blockages to cure using the 'general' model, and required sequential treatment.

His three examples of primary causal infections are 'itch', syphilis and gonorrhea, which were rife if not endemic at the time, and led to the chronic miasms of 'psora', 'syphilis' and 'sycosis' respectively. 'Itch' has usually been identified with scabies, which was later found to be a parasitic infection requiring external treatment with parasiticides, but it also traditionally covered a larger category of eruptive, and often contagious, skin diseases (Jones, Hoerr, Osol 1949), and it is clear that Hahnemann included leprosy and psoriasis among many others in his classification. These eruptions had traditionally been suppressed by external means such as ointments, and driven inwards with repercussions for general health, according to his theory of the protective nature of symptoms.

The possible origin of such a highly unusual theory has given rise to much speculation. *Chronic Diseases* was published two years after the appearance of an important article on homeopathy by Hufeland (1826). Although Hufeland's review was mainly favourable, especially regarding the benefits for patients of single pure drugs (see 3.5 below), he was critical of Hahnemann's apparent neglect of the causes of disease. The period 1800–50 saw widespread attempts in the orthodox medical world to provide explanations for disease after the decline of humouralism. Effluvialism has already been mentioned in connexion with epidemics, but at same time the notion of diathesis was revived, and became enormously popular because it seemed to account for chronic disease. We succumb to particular illnesses because we are predisposed to them: cancer occurs because of a cancerous diathesis, tuberculosis because of a tubercular diathesis, to name just two that crop up repeatedly in the many different systems and lists of diatheses published by orthodox nineteenth-century doctors. Hufeland named 12 'dyscrasias' in 1836, and Ackernecht (1982a) pointed out in his important review of the concept that eight of them had previously appeared in the list of diatheses in the *Dictionnaire des sciences medicales* of 1818. The 'explanation' is circular, however, and reminiscent of Molière's doctors who believed opium's tendency to induce sleep was the result of its 'dormitive virtue'. So, although external pressure and example might have been influential in provoking Hahnemann into announcing a causal theory when he did, it does not help to explain the theory's content.

There is some question over whether Hahnemann plagiarized Autenrieth's discussion of psora from 20 years earlier, or Wenzel's theories about syphilis–gonorrhea published in 1825 (Wood 2000: 69). Autenrieth (1807–08) had said that external suppression of psora led to metastasis, and severe illness such as asthma, but Hahnemann rejected the influence, claiming that Autenrieth's treatment was unknown to him at the time. This seems reasonable since Hahnemann had already cited Juncker (1750) as a much earlier source of ideas about the consequences of suppressed psora, supported by scores of references from the literature. Hahnemann also used an analytic approach to symptomatology to differentiate syphilis and gonorrhea, unlike Wenzel. The question of whether syphilis and gonorrhea were one or two diseases was frequently debated between 1750 and 1850. As late as 1853, the erudite and highly qualified homeopath Robert Ellis Dudgeon (1820–1904) was able to dispute Hahnemann's opinion on this issue (Dudgeon 1853: 300f). Phillipe Ricord (1800–89) is still given priority in histories of medicine for the correction of Hunter's mistake in 1838, a decade after Hahnemann – and 45 years after Benjamin Bell (1749–1806), who seems to have been the first into print (Bell 1793; Ricord 1838). Yet Hahnemann's ideas on the source of chronic disease can be seen taking shape in 'On the venereal disease and its ordinary improper treatment' (1816; 1852b), where the disastrous results of external suppression of contagious disease are detailed. The discussion includes psora and the venereal disease, i.e. gonorrhea–syphilis, which he still thought of as a single entity at the time, and confirms Hahnemann's claim that he developed the theory in the decade before Wenzel published.

However, we are no nearer understanding why these three contagious diseases, and these three only, assumed such importance for Hahnemann. Could there be an alchemical origin? One of the alchemists' most pervasive doctrines was the sulphur-mercury theory of metallic composition. Although the development preceded him, Paracelsus is usually credited with the expansion of the sulphur-mercury doctrine into the *tria prima*, three universal principles of 'sulphur', 'mercury' and 'salt', which underlay the material universe. These metaphorical principles should not be confused with the chemical substances of the same name, since the quality of 'mercury', for instance, could be found in many other substances. In *De natura rerum* Paracelsus provided an esoteric interpretation as well:

> Mercury is the spirit, sulphur is the soul and salt is the body. (cited in Crosland 1962, i: 14)

It has been claimed that when 'sulphur', 'salt' and 'mercury' are translated back into Arabic, it is easy to hear their alliterative equivalence to the terms for human qualities that initiates cultivated in order to bring about personal transformation; only later was this esoteric psychological code exteriorized as part of the well-known search for metallic gold (Shah 1964: 194f).

A resemblance between the chronic 'miasms' and the Paracelsan trinity has been pointed out many times (e.g. Voorhoeve 1936; Coulter 1977; Zissu 1977–78). Hahnemann's diseases, it is claimed, must be related to the *tria prima* pharmacologically by homeopathic analogy: if 'sulphur', 'mercury' and 'salt' are fundamental principles, then the diseases for which their eponymous material elements are homeopathic – itch, syphilis and sycosis – must be fundamental conditions. Unfortunately, this only works for psora–*Sulphur* and syphilis–*Mercurius*; and proponents of the theory of Paracelsan influence have not offered to explain the connexion between 'salt' and *Thuja*. However, there is a way of saving appearances that involves recalling that *Nitricum acidum* was regarded as even more fundamental than *Thuja* by Hahnemann (1828–30), since he used it to complete the treatment of the sycotic 'miasm'. It may be objected that nitric acid is not a salt, but in metallurgical alchemy it was assumed that because acids precipitate salts they were merely salts in solution, and so 'salt' carried the quality of acidity: *aqua fortis* (nitric acid) was a prime 'salt' (Boas 1958: 84). Surely, then, there can be no coincidence that the remedies associated by Hahnemann with the chronic 'miasms' happen to be identical in name with such fundamental alchemical terms and principles?

The plausibility of such a relationship has to be measured against Hahnemann's opinion of the *tria prima* in 'The value of the speculative systems of medicine' (1808c):

> the Alchemists forced the infinite multiplicity of chemical substances into the triangle, salt, sulphur, mercury. What cared they for the numerous varieties of metals? They prided themselves on dictatorially fixing the number of metals at seven, and these they falsely and boldly referred to a single original substance, the metal-seed.

It seems unlikely therefore that alchemy or numerology was involved, especially as Hahnemann believed that psora was responsible for by far the greatest proportion of chronic disease, syphilis and sycosis playing minor roles. Sulphur for skin conditions and infestation and mercury for syphilis just happened to be two widely used specifics of the day. *Thuja* and *Nitricum acidum* for sycosis seem to have been Hahnemann's own discoveries.

3.5. Discussion

At this point it is useful to outline the key stages in the development of Hahnemann's new medical orientation and therapeutics.

1789–	abandonment and critique of traditional medical practice (Hahnemann 1805a);
1790–	systematic pharmacological research with single pure drugs on healthy humans (Cullen 1790);
1792	establishment of a humane asylum for the mentally ill (Hahnemann 1796a);
1796	announcement of a 'new principle for determining the curative power of drugs' which is acausal and analogical (Hahnemann 1796b);
1800	drastic reduction of doses used in treatment (Hahnemann 1801d);
1801–	introduction of theory of infectious microorganisms; coupled with a dynamic theory of health and disease: symptoms are an expression of disease, which should not be confused with its immediate cause;
1805–	publication of a new pure materia medica, based on signs and symptoms expressed in the 'language of the patient' (Hahnemann 1805b; 1811–21; 1828–30); establishment of a new method for careful examination and treatment of patients in their semiotic, psychological, social and ecological totality (Hahnemann 1805c; 1810);
1816–	development of the potentization principle: biologically inert substances used as drugs after serial trituration and agitated dilution (Hahnemann 1818);
1821–	theory that chronic disease originates from infections and other acute episodes (Hahnemann 1828–30).

Most of the distinctive elements of homeopathy – provings, poisons as medicines, small doses, similars, miasms – had surfaced in rudimentary form in orthodox medicine in the three or four decades before Hahnemann began to synthesize his system, and it is easy to rule out alchemical or Paracelsan influence. Nonetheless, there is a documented direct link from alchemy to at least one important aspect of Hahnemann's technique: trituration of pure gold was a turning point in the evolution of homeopathic pharmacy and pharmacology, and its origin in authentic, pre-Paracelsan alchemical medicine is perfectly transparent. It led to the expansion of the pharmacopeia in a direction unimaginable to his immediate predecessors, and seems to have been the stimulus for the announcement of the dynamization principle.

Can Hahnemann therefore be identified as an occultist, rather than an exceptionally open-minded scientist? Leaving aside the accusations of critics such as Schultz (1831), the entry into homeopathy, after Hahnemann's death in 1843, of Paracelsan ideas from several sources has undoubtedly muddied the water. To mention only two streams (discussed in Ch. 4), there were organ remedies based on signatures (Rademacher 1841; Steiner 1948), and versions of Swedenborgian emanationism, itself traceable to the archetypal correspondences of Böhme and Paracelsus (Wilkinson 1857b; Kent 1900). Given such pervasive occult influences it is unsurprising to find the signatures doctrine misattributed to Hahnemann, not merely by anti-homeopathic positivists and homeopathic occultists, but also by historians of ideas (Flaherty 1995). It is nonetheless important to distinguish those trends from Hahnemann's own writings, where not a trace of them can be found.

Yet the possibility of a personal involvement with esotericism has continued to fascinate some of Hahnemann's later followers – perhaps anxious to attribute their own beliefs to their hero – who support their claims with circumstantial evidence such as the plate factory and the Hermannstadt episode. It must be admitted though that the evidence is thin. Böttger was long dead; and Hahnemann was admitted only to the first Masonic degree while in Hermannstadt, advancing no further for many years. Moreover, Austrian Freemasonry, as in France, was not under Papal interdiction – and was close to being an alternative state religion, centred on Enlightenment ideals of free intelligence, generosity and social progress (Kuéss-Scheichelbauer 1959). Lodges were one of the few places where people from different strata of society could meet on an equal footing, and many radicals and scientists like Hahnemann became Freemasons – along with many in the Austrian Catholic church hierarchy. In any case, it is easy to overestimate the authenticity of the esoteric teaching available. Freemasonry was a recently constituted movement, trying hard to invent a distinguished lineage for itself. The bogus Orientalism of Giuseppe Balsamo – or Count Cagliostro as he styled himself – was welcomed with open arms; and the *Sethos* novel by the hoaxer Terrasson was accepted as a genuine firsthand account of hermetic initiation in ancient Egypt well into the nineteenth century. Accounts of the rituals in many Viennese lodges of the day show they were fabricated even when they managed to avoid actual silliness (Palou 1966). And North German Freemasonry, which Hahnemann belonged to after his brief stay in Austro-Hungary, was far less exciting. It was primarily a devout non-denominational ethical movement heavily coloured by the Protestant Pietism that Hahnemann had been born into, a branch of Lutheranism which sought the inner light through self-examination in a manner analogous to Quakerism.

However, although Hahnemann's strong objections to 'magic, incantations and divinations' agree with this interpretation – if his Leipzig thesis and disavowal of the Paracelsan writings are to be believed – and although he seems to have been entirely free of Pietist emotionalism – as evidenced by his preference for Confucius over Jesus – those determined to find a personal occult connexion bring forward a final unanswerable argument: Hahnemann hid his involvement, perhaps because he had been sworn to silence. This was true to some extent of Boyle, whose anti-Paracelsan pronouncements in the *Sceptical Chymist* have long been regarded as foundational for the Scientific Revolution, but actually concealed an immersion in alchemy as great as Newton's (Newman 1994; Principe 1998). Boyle's case allows a further twist to the argument, one that has so far not been advanced: Could Hahnemann have belonged to an anti-Paracelsan stream *within* an esoteric framework? Only recently has external scholarship penetrated far enough behind the deliberate mystifications of alchemical literature to realize that not all alchemists thought alike, allowing an explanation of the apparent contradictions between Boyle's and Van Helmont's alchemical interests and their highly selective approach to Paracelsan ideas. And there is a different kind of precedent in the example of the anti-Jesuit Bavarian Illuminist cult of 1785–90 (which was politically neutralized by absorption into Austrian Freemasonry after 1788): there the initiation into each degree involved repudiation of the revelations of the preceding level. Tempting though it might seem to impute both an esoteric vow of silence and anti-Paracelsanism to Hahnemann, once again the evidence is flimsy. His use of authentic alchemical documentation to justify his gold experiment makes it an improbable combination, especially when Chrestien's example would have provided the perfect mask.

The two facets of homeopathy which particularly exercised critics such as Louis and Holmes, the similia principle and serial dilution, seem to have been part of a long-submerged tradition which they cannot have been aware of. However, Hahnemann acknowledged the new direction that alchemy had given to his researches as openly as one could wish for. Conceivably, the initial seed of his interest in some aspects of Islamic medicine – derived as we now know from Taoist alchemy – might have been planted in the pseudo-Oriental atmosphere of Austrian Freemasonry, although his own professorial knowledge of pharmacological history seems more likely to have been ultimately responsible. What reveals most about his real source of inspiration is the fact that he did not simply take the archaic elixir at face value, however central a feature of alchemical medicine it might have been. Instead, he submitted the substance and the manufacturing process to empirical testing within the research programme he was creating out of the scattered hints and speculations of other scientists.

The aspect of Hahnemann's thought and practice which Holmes said wasn't worth the effort of refuting – infectious and chronic miasms – still causes much scorn (e.g. Vickers 2000). However, it was an early manifestation of the germ theory that swept all before it in the 1880s, and demonstrates the progressive nature and complexity of Hahnemann's thought, and the difficulties that created for many of his contemporaries. Although Hahnemann did not accept Plenciz's bactericidal explanation of the pharmacological action of specifics such as mercury and cinchona – preferring Hunter's counter irritation theory – the parallels between Hahnemann's and Plenciz's notions of specific contagious diseases transmitted by microorganisms are obvious, and clearly distinguishable from Hunter's much more orthodox ideas.

The development of acute 'miasms' into the source of chronic disease is further evidence that Hahnemann's ideas need to be seen in the context of eighteenth- and nineteenth-century medical debate rather than the hidden esoteric sources that later followers wished for. As suggested here, Hahnemann may well have responded to external pressure from critics such as Hufeland in announcing his theory of chronic disease when he did. Nevertheless, there is an important difference between Hahnemann's chronic diseases and the diatheses of nineteenth-century allopathy. Hahnemann believed the chronic 'miasms' were the superimposed sequelae of suppressed contagious disease, not essential characteristics or typologies. Moreover, he believed they could be treated and removed, quite unlike diatheses. The crucial distinction was obscured by later homeopaths such as Grauvogl, who refashioned Hahnemann's chronic diseases into conventional diatheses, opening a door to the introduction of Galenic humours and magical typologies into homeopathy (discussed in Ch. 4).

There is little in Hahnemann that seems irrational or evidence of charlatanry or weak-mindedness once it is accurately described and some attempt made to understand its origins. A classical scholar and student of philosophy as well as chemist and physician, he was uniquely qualified to synthesize many factors into a coherent humane therapeutics. Hufeland (1826) listed the advantages and disadvantages of the system impartially. He faulted Hahnemann for lack of interest in the ultimate causation of disease, and seems to have regarded ultra-small doses as often no more than a placebo. He also felt reliance on drugs could sometimes prevent patients from receiving valid treatments such as blood-letting. Nevertheless, Hufeland concluded that if the system were generally adopted it would:

- prohibit large doses
- simplify prescriptions
- encourage accurate testing of drugs on humans (which he acknowledged had already begun to some extent following Hahnemann's example)
- encourage better attention to drug preparation, and stricter supervision of druggists
- prevent actual harm
- allow the sick more time to recuperate quietly and naturally; and
- reduce drug costs remarkably.

Revolutionary for their time, these points are all now regarded as desiderata of any scientific pharmacopraxy, and are a further indication of the rationality of the Hahnemannian contribution to medical science.

4. Homeopathy after Hahnemann

Background: Hahnemannian homeopathy represents a distinct medical focus within the early history of biomedicine. However, present-day homeopathy contains a number of different approaches or schools, leading to dissension within the field and confusion for those outside.

Questions: What are the different approaches and schools? Are there real conflicts between them?

Argument: The evolution of the major streams in post-Hahnemannian homeopathy is outlined. A schema for the conceptualization of different homeopathic approaches is proposed, allowing them to be seen not as irreconcilable schools, but as foci within a coherent field of therapeutic information and action. Homeopaths frequently move freely within this therapeutic field treating individual patients on many levels, diachronically as well as synchronically.

4.1. The division

> 200 years later, however, far from being a unified therapeutic approach, 'homeopathy' is probably best understood as an outlook with many interpretations, which sometimes contradict each other. (Kleijnen, Knipschild, ter Riet 1991)

The principal division that Kleijnen and colleagues allude to is that between individualized and standardized treatments, both of which exist in more-or-less pure forms, as well as in many intermediate mixed grades. Both approaches stem directly from Hahnemann: his normal procedure was to individualize, but he looked for collective medicines in epidemics or common traumas, for example.

The later years of Hahnemann saw many refinements of these two heuristics, and the years after his death saw a trend towards polarization among his followers. The purists, such as Hering and Kent, based treatment almost entirely on symptomatology, usually weighting the diagnosis towards mind symptoms. They were at the opposite end of the spectrum from the more scientifically orientated homeopaths such as Griesselich in Germany and Hughes in England who were interested in correlating homeopathy with developments in orthodox physiology and pathology.

The two groups were popularly called the 'highs' and the 'lows' respectively, because of a tendency to favour potencies above or below N_A, and they also insulted each other as 'metaphysical' or 'pathological' prescribers from time to time, but these terms caricature what was a complex debate about the direction homeopathy ought to take.

The British homeopath J.H. Clarke (1840–1921) combined both streams in his own work and publications; he described the purist approach as 'classical', and the other as 'clinical' (Clarke 1911). The names he chose are memorable, descriptive and nonpejorative, and are used here.

4.2. Symptomatic classical homeopathy

Immediately after Hahnemann, the most influential figures in this stream are Constantin Hering (1800–80) and Clemens von Bönninghausen (1785–1864), followed much later by James Tyler Kent (1849–1916). Each made many contributions to homeopathic theory and practice, but only the principal theoretical innovations from each will be discussed here because of their significance in present-day homeopathy.

4.2.1. Directions of cure

Hahnemann had introduced the idea of chronic miasms which posed blockages to cure in *Die chronischen Krankheiten* (1828–30) (see Ch. 3). The miasms preceded the patient's current state and their persistence was believed to prevent the simillimum from acting, requiring antimiasmatic drugs to antidote them. In the foreword to the first translation into English of the *Chronic Diseases*, his close associate Hering observed that:

> Every homoeopathic physician must have observed that the improvement in pain takes place from above downward; and in disease, from within outward. … The thorough cure of a chronic disease is indicated by the most important organs being first relieved; the disease passes off in the order in which the organs had been affected, the more important being relieved first, the less important next, and the skin last. (Hahnemann 1845)

This became formalized as a set of rules for evaluating the progress of treatment in any chronic case. Cure was supposed to proceed:

- from within outward
- from the most important organs to the least important organs
- in the reverse order that symptoms had first appeared.

These observations became known as 'Hering's laws of cure', naturally enough, in an era that unselfconsciously believed in 'laws' of nature, and clearly relate to Hahnemann's theory of the protective nature of symptoms. They underpin a strong directional tradition in homeopathic case analysis, associated later in the nineteenth century with James Compton Burnett (1840–1901), in which cases are seen as layered histories, requiring sequential treatment to unblock and remove each layer before cure can be said to have happened.[12]

4.2.2. Repertories and keynotes

Hahnemann (1805b, ii) provided an index to his first materia medica, allowing the pathogeneses to be searched by symptom. Hahnemann (1811–21) does not develop the idea, but his materia medica was limited to a few score medicines which were thoroughly known to him and the early homeopaths who compiled them. However, the expansion of the materia medica which began towards the end of Hahnemann's life, and continued unabated throughout the nineteenth century, posed an increasing strain on the practitioner's memory. The need for a comprehensive symptom-based index to the materia medica was recognized, and Hahnemann wrote the foreword to one of the first (Bönninghausen 1832).

Bönninghausen's repertories were highly analytic: symptom complexes that had been found in provings were broken down into their components and listed in separate regional sections. For instance, Frau Sch—'s first symptom (see Ch. 2), 'Any movement, especially on stepping, and worst on making a false step, leads to shooting pain in the epigastrium, coming every time from the left side', might have occurred as a complete proving symptom. Bönninghausen could then have generalized from it to 'pain on movement', 'pain on stepping', 'shooting pain in the epigastrium' and so on, if these modalities were found in enough provers and cured patients.

This was seen as an advantage by some, allowing a new case to be covered by rubrics derived from medicines that had not shown the presenting symptom

[12] This idea of therapeutics as archeology later became an integral part of the psychoanalytic worldview. Freud's apostate disciple Wilhelm Reich (1897–1957) then exteriorized the psychoanalytic process from the mind to the body, and originated the concept of 'character armour', where the patient's musculature is held to retain memories of psychological conflict and physical traumas (Reich 1942). Following Reich, various forms of deep massage were developed which were believed to allow the armour (or equivalent concepts) to be removed (Rolf 1977). Such therapies formed an important component of the personal growth movement associated with Esalen, California in the 1960s (Murphy 1993).

complex in any single prover, but generalization from fragmented symptoms has always been controversial. Bönninghausen seems to have answered this in part by laying greater stress on concomitant symptoms in subsequent editions of his repertory. However, Hughes (1886–91) in particular objected that the repertorial approach per se ignored the prover's records of the sequence of the pathogenesis – important, presumably, if the sequence of development of chronic illness was a factor.

Combinatorial symptomatology went hand in hand with Bönninghausen's analytic approach to case-taking. It may have been his previous training as a lawyer which led him to amplify Hahnemann's approach to case-taking and symptom evaluation along classical juristic investigative lines: who?, what?, where?, accompanied by what?, why?, modified by what?, when?, derived from a Latin hexameter belonging to the medieval scholastics: '*Quis? quid? ubi? quibus auxiliis? cur? quomodo? quando?*' (Bönninghausen 1908). Since his time it has been standard practice to use these questions to obtain a full description of each patient in terms of personality, sensation, location, concomitants, immediate aetiology, modalities and times of occurrence.

Bönninghausen also began the process, still in use, of weighting medicines relative to each other in the repertory rubrics according to the prominence and frequency with which their component symptoms had appeared in provings and clinical responses. This early attempt at quantification (analogous to confidence intervals) led indirectly to the development of 'keynote' materia medicas and prescribing. For instance, T.F. Allen (1837–1902), compiler of an encyclopaedic 11-volume materia medica, also produced a single-volume primer, and there have been many others (Allen 1874–80; 1936). Authors such as Allen always caution that their keynote handbooks are aide-memoires for the experienced, and a way into the subject for the student, and are not intended as a substitute for careful comparison of the patient's symptoms with the full materia medica. Nevertheless, 'keynote' prescribing developed, almost inevitably, in response to the pressures of busy clinics.

4.2.3. Constitutional types

Throughout the nineteenth century, repertories continued to be compiled from different theoretical positions. Kent is famous for the one most frequently used today (Kent 1945). He did not favour the combinatorial method, and his repertory is based on complete symptoms, although it includes in fact fewer concomitants than Bönninghausen's later repertories. Kent addressed the shortcomings of the repertorial method in a different manner. He used a retelling of the materia medica to lay the foundations for one of the strongest traditions in present-day classical homeopathy: the so-called 'constitutional types' and 'drug pictures'. As noted in Ch. 2, Hahnemann stressed the importance of mental symptoms in individualizing, and left rudimentary examples of how character states can be used to distinguish one medicine from another. This seems to be the germ from which an entire philosophy of prescribing grew.

Kent (1912a) is on record as deprecating 'constitution' as a basis for prescribing, but he was probably referring to contemporary developments in German and French homeopathy (see 4.4.3 below). What is currently termed constitutional prescribing has its origins in the vivid descriptions of 'remedy types' that formed the subject of his lectures on materia medica (Kent 1911). The fastidious and highly-strung dandy needing *Arsenicum* is worlds apart from the physically slothful but intellectually active 'ragged philosopher' needing *Sulphur*, though both might present with eczema. Kent's students and followers have continued and developed his tendency to conflate states with traits. In Tyler's *Drug Pictures* (1952) the indications for medicines become minor 'characters' from Victorian novels. Coulter (1986) turns the process round in her *Portraits of Homeopathic Medicines*, and diagnoses and prescribes for historical characters from life and literature, analogous to the procedure once popular in the psychoanalytic movement. Current theories of 'essence' prescribing, where a unifying theme is sought in all the patient's symptoms – physical, psychological and situational – also derive from Kent. This rhetorically-worded summary of the *Aurum* picture by a mid twentieth-century American homeopath is fairly typical:

> Heaviness runs through the whole picture. Heavy build, a heavy gait, heaviness of heart, a heavy mind. Darkness is the main color of this picture, a dark complexion, darkening of vision, dreams of darkness, a dark mind. Destruction is its meaning, slow destruction of the body, of the big glands, of the bones, finally destruction of the self through suicide. (Gutman 1978: 82)

As with keynotes, what started as an aide-memoire took on a life of its own.

4.3. Nosological and pathological homeopathy

The 1830s saw the emergence of a movement within homeopathy which challenged many of Hahnemann's later ideas, such as miasm theory and exclusive use of high potencies (Gross 1837; Wolf 1837; Griesselich 1848). Known at the time as the 'critical'[13] homeopaths, they encouraged a sceptical scientific attitude, leading to the systematic reevaluation of the materia medica, and comparative tests of potencies above Avogadro's number with molecular low potencies (see also Chs 7 & 8).

4.3.1. Clinical

The 'clinical' nosological perspective was a natural development of Hahnemann's epidemic remedies, which were found by seeking the central common symptoms from many cases of the same illness and comparing these with the symptoms in the materia medica. Hahnemann (1814) published evidence of the efficacy of this approach in treatment of a typhus epidemic in 1813 (see Ch. 8). Most famously, he was able to calibrate treatments for cholera from case reports sent to him by colleagues in Russia, before the disease reached Germany (see Ch. 2). Empirical confirmations of the efficacy of medicines in particular clinical conditions, even when proving data was missing or incomplete, were incorporated later, by Griesselich (1848) and others who started a trend away from the predominantly psychological tendencies of classicists such as Bönninghausen and Hering, moving instead towards a materia medica of etiological and nosological 'specifics'. Later still began the correlation of the materia medica with the increasingly well-defined pathological descriptions and categories of orthodox medicine. For example, the critical British homeopath Richard Hughes (1836–1902), made an extensive study of paralytic disease and was able to point to the similarity between the symptoms of progressive muscular atrophy and lead poisoning. (Hughes 1869; Hughes 1893: 752) It was this trend, marrying homeopathy with advances in pathology, but without introducing treatments aimed at hypothesized causes, that led Hughes's contemporary, Compton Burnett, to write:

> The pathologic simillimum is the furthest point yet reached in drug therapeutics, and embodies a very great and fertile idea. (Burnett 1896: 78)

Clinical homeopathy seems to have been most influential in Germany. The classical model was superseded there during the nineteenth century, only to resurface after translations of Kent began to appear in 1945. Before then it had been usual to make a conventional diagnosis and differentiate on the basis of

---

[13] In his essay *Bentham*, first published in 1838, John Stuart Mill contemporaneously explained that the equivalent English term for the continental 'critical' philosophy was 'subversive' (Mill 1867, 1: 334).

etiology or lesional factors. As Leeser (1936: 369f) made clear, the use of *Sulphur* in every case of furunculosis was inappropriate, not because of neglect of mind symptoms or the total symptom-complex, but because:

> only if the furunculosis stands on the soil of such skin and metabolic alterations which lie in the sulphur trend, will the homeopathic physician select sulphur. It might be that he would select arsenicum if there were a diabetic basis, or again arnica if there were a pyemic state in the degenerative condition of issue and skin, and a tendency to ecchymosis spoke particularly for it.

Another reason for the emergence of the critical perspective was the doubt raised about the validity of many of Hahnemann's later provings, which seem to have been conducted on patients rather than healthy provers (Hahnemann 1828–30). This led to cured symptoms being substituted for pathogenetic symptoms, as well as to the mistaken inclusion of symptoms of prior disease, and there were also many who were equally sceptical of provings based only on high potencies (Griesselich 1848; Dudgeon 1853; Kleinert 1863) (see Ch. 8).

4.3.2. Complex

Griesselich (1848: 146) summarized the task facing orthodox classical homeopaths. They were required to select a single medicine to cover:

- the patient's whole individuality, constitution, predisposition
- the symptoms, from their first appearance to their present state, including modalities and concomitants
- the originating cause of the disturbance.

The simultaneous use of more than one medicine as a response to the difficulties of selecting a single medicine for this entirety began during Hahnemann's lifetime. K.J. Aegidi (b. 1795) reported that he had found numerous combinations more effective than single medicines, and Bönninghausen and Hahnemann both welcomed this development (Aegidi 1834). Hahnemann wrote a new section endorsing the approach for the fifth edition of the *Organon*, but was persuaded by colleagues that such an inclusion would be misinterpreted by the allopaths as conceding the principle of polypharmacy – one of the main objections that he had always raised against traditional therapeutics (Haehl 1927, ii: 253). Aegidi later repudiated double remedies (ibid. ii: 86), no doubt for similar reasons. Arthur Lutze (1813–70) published an unauthorized edition of the *Organon* including the omitted § 274b (Hahnemann 1865), and his own case histories show the approach that he learned personally from Bönninghausen to have been worth following up (Lutze 1874). Majority opinion was against him, and an interesting development was thus nearly stifled at birth for political rather than scientific reasons. Research into complexes only re-emerged at the end of the nineteenth century. British homeopaths have often used low-potency combinations of 2 or 3 medicines – such as SSC (*Sulphur*, *Silica*, *Carbo-veg*), for acne – but the principle was expanded greatly in Germany and France, where complexes of 10 or more components have been formulated since the 1900s. Recent pathogenetic investigations suggest that complexes may have beneficial synergistic effects, not necessarily predictable from the individual components (Vakil & King 1997). They certainly form a researchable area in homeopathy.

4.3.3. Isopathy and nosodes

Treatment and prevention of diseases with their own morbid products, or snake bites with venoms, were widespread practices in folk medicine, but only gradually accepted by the medical profession in Europe after smallpox vaccination naturalized the concept. It has always been a controversial area in homeopathy, because the similia principle is believed by many to contradict the aequalia principle of isopathy.

Against this, Hahnemann's case-records show he occasionally experimented with potentized isopathic preparations towards the end of his career, in a difficult tubercular case for instance, 60 years before Koch's experiments (Handley 1997: 102). Hering had been the first to potentize and prove nosodes (his coinage from the Greek *nosos* disease), derived from disease matter such as infectious pus and sputum.[14] He even suggested treating rabies with *Lyssin*, potentized saliva from a rabid dog, which seems to be the first instance of isopathy within homeopathy. The veterinarian Johann Lux (b. 1776) then began the systematic use of isopathic nosodes in the early 1830s (Lux 1833). Hahnemann was following their precedent.

The history of nosodes is closely bound up with isopathy for obvious reasons, and many homeopaths since Hahnemann's time who object to isopathy have nevertheless used the same medicines as individualized prescriptions. They have based this on proving data where available, and materia medicas of

[14] He was one of the most innovative in the search for new materia medica from many sources, testing snake venoms, amyl nitrite, lithium carbonate and many others, well before their adoption by official medicine. His encyclopedia of materia medica is comparable with T.F. Allen's mentioned above (Hering 1879–91).

these provings eventually appeared (Swan 1888; Allen 1910). Ironically the nosodes etiologically connected with the chronic infectious miasms were widely used to treat the sequelae of the same miasms – but not the acute phase of the disease – in addition to the conventional anti-miasmatics. As a pragmatic complement to individualized prescribing, this and other sorts of isopathy have been fairly widespread, particularly in preventive homeopathy.

Some classical homeopaths, however, believe isopathy is heretical, alleging that Hahnemann never used it, and disapproved of it. In the face of evidence that he did, it is even suggested that if it worked it couldn't have been isopathy, but must have been homeopathy: the causal agent was in some way transmuted into something else during the potentization process. It is true that Hahnemann spoke out against isopathy, but it seems to have been against early enthusiasts who were trying to replace homeopathy with isopathy (Haehl 1927, 2: 292). As in the case of complex homeopathy, it is important to remember that many of Hahnemann's public pronouncements in the 1830s were political rather than scientific.

Isopathy is an area of homeopathy closer than most others to orthodox immunology, and has been used not just for its clinical results, but as a convenient model to to test the efficacy of ultramolecular dilutions per se. In 1892 Behring, who discovered antitoxin prophylaxis of diphtheria and tetanus, demonstrated immunity produced by infinitesimal doses of tetanus antitoxin (Behring 1905; Coulter 1994). Later, Paterson and Boyd used potentized diphtheria toxoid and *Diphtherinum* C201 to alter positive Schick tests to negative (Paterson & Boyd 1941).

The English homeopath Charles Blackley (d. 1900) was the first (a) to offer empirical tests showing that hayfever could be attributable to pollen sensitivity (1873), and isopathic treatment with potentized pollen soon followed. Research to replicate this model was again undertaken to test the reality of biological activity of ultramolecular medicines, and its widely reported success has been influential in establishing the fact in recent times (Reilly, Taylor, Beattie et al. 1994).

A related isopathic approach is termed tautopathy – potencies of chemical substances, especially conventional drugs and vaccines, used to antidote adverse effects and sequelae (see 4.5.2 below).

4.4. Parahomeopathic concepts and homeopathic neorationalism

During the nineteenth century several variants or simplifications of homeopathy emerged, in parallel with the miasm and keynote concepts. These often tried to tie homeopathy in with aspects of scientific physiology, and influenced mainstream homeopathy to a greater or lesser extent, and in some culture areas more than others. Some are still extant. At the same time occult etiological theories proliferated in areas of classical homeopathy. Both these trends had a rationalist basis, in that they tried to identify and treat causal factors in illness, material on the one hand, spiritual on the other.

4.4.1. Organ remedies

Johann Gottfried Rademacher (1772–1850) was a younger contemporary of Hahnemann who explicitly revived Paracelsan ideas, and associated remedies with specific internal organs. He seems to have practised quietly as a country doctor, and published only one book on his method late in life (Rademacher 1841).

Hahnemann made a German abstract of a treatise on dysentery by Rademacher from Latin in 1810, and a few drug symptoms observed by Rademacher found their way into Hahnemann's materia medica, but it is not clear whether he knew of the younger man's medical system. Rademacher certainly knew of Hahnemann, and seems to have felt overshadowed by him (Rückle 1942). He was not a homeopath, and his ideas were derived from a close study of Paracelsus, with treatments based on the doctrine of signatures and the phases of the planets. Rademacher's system involved a fundamental tripartite categorization of disease with an associated Paracelsan 'universal' for each: copper, sodium nitrate and iron. He also employed many other more specific 'organ remedies', again following Paracelsus and the doctrine of signatures. These subsequently became popular in French homeopathy as herbal 'drainage' remedies, and were given to detoxify specific organs and systems before prescribing more powerful potentized homeopathics.

4.4.2. Biochemic tissue salts

Mid nineteenth-century physiology knew of approximately 12 inorganic components of the human body. Wilhelm Heinrich Schüssler (1821–98) devised a simplified therapeutic system based on 12 minerals given in low decimal (D6) potency (Schüssler 1874), in an attempt to reconcile homeopathy with the cellular pathology of Rudolf Virchow (1821–1902). Schüssler later reduced his original 12 medicines to 11, but all 12 have remained in use, possibly due to number mysticism. Some were already part of the homeopathic materia medica but others, such as *Kali phosphoricum*, were absorbed without having been the subject of pathogeneses.

4.4.3. Constitutional biotypes and morphology

The influential German homeopath Eduard von Grauvogl (1811–77) published a chemical–humoural system in the 1860s which echoes the much earlier one of J.B. Baumes, discussed in Ch. 2. Like Baumes, Grauvogl saw disease as attributable to chemical imbalance, but Baumes's five categories are covered by three – oxygenoid, hydrogenoid and carbo-nitrogenoid – possibly because Grauvogl also tried to correlate them with the three chronic miasms of Hahnemann (Grauvogl 1860; 1866).

The French homeopath Antoine Nebel (1870–1954) later developed a tripartite system of constitutional physical types, *carbocalcique*, *phospho-calcique* and *fluoro-calcique*, which overlaps the earlier classification of Grauvogl, and has prompted many modifications, mainly in French homeopathy. These are often correlated with body types, such as the ecto-, endo- and mesomorphic builds of Kretschmer (1926). They are also believed to have different susceptibilities to disease, and are correlated with the chronic miasms.

The fondness for tripartite divisions recalls the *tria prima* of the alchemists, and the relationship of the chronic miasms to alchemical theories of substance has been discussed in Ch. 3. Homeopathic neorationalism seems to have taken at least one of its cues from Hahnemann, even though he was not describing essential types, but the sequelae of infectious episodes. Attempts to fit the components of one or other of these parahomeopathic systems to each other could lead to scholastic absurdities of the sort Hahnemann had rejected so decisively:

> A considerable lack of clarity in the picture of copper arises from the fact that Grauvogl perceived copper as the chief remedy of the carbonitrogenoid constitutional type. He came to this conception by mixing the Rademacherian conception with his idea of the three chronic miasms of Hahnemann. For Rademacher copper was the third of his universals which were given for the two other constitutional types and, indeed, out of [a] natrium nitricum for the sycosis of Hahnemann or the hydrogenoid constitution of Grauvogl and [b] ferrum for syphilis of Hahnemann or the oxygenoid constitution of Grauvogl, only [c]

> copper remained for the psora of Hahnemann which was placed equal to the carbonitrogenoid constitution. (Leeser 1936: 795)

4.4.4. Spiritual neorationalism

Kent, whose qualitative constitutional types were discussed above, is equally well known for his attempt to impose a top-down mentalist hierarchy on the perception and explanation of disease. Like many American homeopaths of the nineteenth century, he belonged to the Church of the New Jerusalem, founded 1787 in London by followers of Emmanuel Swedenborg (1688–1772). This Swedish scientist turned full-time visionary was in many ways far ahead of his time, originating ideas such as: the objective nature of the psyche; psychospiritual individuation; the use of the terms *animus* and *anima* to describe psychological functions; and dream guidance.[15] Swedenborg also revealed a 'doctrine of correspondences', a Paracelsan idea related to the signatures doctrine: every organ of the human body was governed by spirits who dwelt in a corresponding portion of the supersensible mystical body of God – an idea encapsulated many centuries earlier in the hermetic aphorism 'As above, so below'. Swedenborg is equally well-known for his 'doctrine of uses' which provided a heavenly rationale for something close to the Protestant work ethic: souls were graded according to their usefulness to others and the divine plan, and he even claimed that illness and death were the results of sin. It is these darker aspects of Swedenborgianism which underpin Kent's severely hierarchical and judgemental homeopathy, aimed at the spiritual regeneration of fallen humanity:

> Eternal principles, themselves, are authority. The Law of Similars is a Divine Law. So soon as you have accepted the Law of Similars, so soon have you accepted Providence, which is law and order ... Psora is the evolution of the state of man's will, the ultimate of his sin ... Thinking, willing, and doing are the three things in life from which finally proceed the chronic miasms ... The body became corrupt because man's interior will was corrupt. (Kent 1926: 646–70)

The English homeopath and New Church member John Garth Wilkinson (1812–99) was also active in the mid to late nineteenth century. His translations of Swedenborg's treatises on mystical anatomical correspondences be-

[15] Ideas that were later appropriated by Freud's rival Carl Jung (1875–1961). Jung read Swedenborg early in his career but, as Larsen points out, was unwilling to acknowledge the obvious influence (Swedenborg 1984: 16).

came popular in New England transcendentalist circles and were adopted by many American homeopaths such as Kent (Treuherz 1983). His own thought has not received much attention though. Wilkinson's approach to homeopathy was as ultimately Platonic as Kent's but is expressed in much gentler, less direly eschatological terms. He expressed another traditional hermetic idea – emanationism – using a concept that that became better-known from the teachings of Jung:[16]

> There is an image-and-likeness psychology in man himself, for the soul is the archetype of the body as God is the archetype of the soul. (Wilkinson 1890: 16f)

These sorts of beliefs were combined with a notion, attributed to Hahnemann, that the homeopathic materia medica acted 'spiritually'.[17] 'It comes from the mind, and remakes and inspires the nature of drugs', wrote Wilkinson, who claimed Hahnemann had

> established a *materia medica* of mental fineness ... able to enter into relations with the mind in the body, and thereby with the intimate body itself as a mere theatre and extension of the mind. (Wilkinson 1889)

In fact, the mind of the physician was possibly more important for Wilkinson than the tools of the trade. Because most homeopaths are not medical materialists, and inquire into their patients' inward experience,

> patients believe in them, not only for their mode or system, but for themselves. Mind touches mind here as it seldom does in specialism. (ibid.)

---

[16] Jung's unacknowledged Swedenborgian borrowings extend to Wilkinson, who seems to have been an inspiration in more ways than one. Wilkinson (1857a) had advised: 'Let involuntary drawing be introduced then as a normal employment into asylums, and let the class of patients upon whom the spirit-cure is to be tried be those who are functionally deranged, and especially those who are suffering from disappointed affections, and in general mental and affectional causes ... Let each drawing be kept, dated, and numbered, as marking a progress of state'. The link from Wilkinson to Jung, an active proponent of painting as therapy, as well as the notion of psychological archetypes, has been traced via Jung's analysand and student Kristine Mann, another New Church member whose family were friends of Wilkinson (Webb 1976: 392).

[17] Hahnemann's *geistig* and *geistartig* – immaterial, spiritlike – were consistently translated as if he had written *geistlich* – holy, spiritual. It is even claimed that Hahnemann wrote *geistlich* (e.g. Coulter 1977: 343), although neither the electronic version of the sixth edition of the *Organon* nor the index of the variorum *Organon-Synopse* reveal any such usage when searched (Hahnemann 1921; 2000).

Wilkinson is almost forgotten, perhaps unjustly,[18] but his influence via American homeopathy and Kent on the development of twentieth-century homeopathy was considerable. Although Kent himself has been seen as one of the chief culprits behind the accelerating decline and marginalization of homeopathy in the first half of the century (Inglis 1964: 85f), his ideas were a dominant force in its revival in the latter half, when overtly spiritual–mentalist hierarchies were taught as the foundation of a 'science of homeopathy' by some (Vithoulkas 1980; 1991).

The related essentialist notion that homeopathic constitutions represent Jungian archetypes was also taken up enthusiastically (e.g. Gutman 1978; Whitmont 1982). This happened possibly without awareness that some of Jung's most apparently innovative ideas may derive as much from a stream within late nineteenth-century homeopathy (itself deriving from Swedenborg), as from more overtly alchemical and astrological sources (for the latter, see Noll 1992).

It is nevertheless important to separate these trends from Hahnemann's own writings, where hardly a trace of them can be found. Despite his origins in a pietist environment, Hahnemann seems to have been an eighteenth-century deist (borne out by his freemasonry) more in tune with staid Confucian ethics than visionary esoteric Christianity, let alone hellfire American fundamentalism (Haehl 1927, 2: 387f). It is unlikely that his 'dynamic' concept of life, disease and medicinal action is identical with the 'spirituality' of many of his later Swedenborgian and occultist followers.

4.5. The modern synthesis

Many homeopaths have never accepted miasmatic theory, either because they found it implausible (Dudgeon 1853), or because they objected to the reintroduction of causality into a phenomenological discipline (Ledermann, Sutherland, Lunt 1954). Many others have regarded it as a fruitful theory, indispensable for understanding and treating chronic disease. Rau said in 1837 that, in spite of being wrong in details, its importance lay in the acknowledgment of

[18] A Blake scholar as well as translator of Swedenborg, he was friends with many of the great figures of the day, such as Carlyle, Froude, Dickens and Tennyson, according to the *Dictionary of National Biography*. Another friend, the New England transcendentalist Ralph Waldo Emerson (1850), wrote that he 'threw all the contemporary philosophy of England into shade', and possessed a 'vigor of understanding and imagination comparable only to Lord Bacon's.'

the need to account for internal hidden conditions and dyscrasias (Haehl 1927, 2: 163). This opinion has been echoed by several of the most prominent critical homeopaths (for example Wolf 1837; Hughes 1893; Eizayaga 1991). A further linguistic problem lies in Hahnemann's use of the term 'miasm', leaving the misleading impression that he was reliant on an abandoned theory of intangible miasmata, when he was in fact a contagionist and pioneer of germ theory. The historically uninformed retention of 'miasm' in the present day to describe a concept that has moved away from infection towards metabolism, structure and genetic predisposition is particularly unfortunate, and no doubt explains the disappearance of 'miasms' from modern French homeopathic terminology. *Mode réactionel* (reactional mode) has become the preferred term, with collective and individual categories, and subcategories such as acute, constitutional or diathesic (Meriadec 1990).

4.5.1. Layer theory

Homeopaths from Bönninghausen onwards had noticed that during treatment certain drug pictures tended to follow each other in predictable sequences, *Sulphur*, *Calcarea* and *Lycopodium* being the best known. Explicit acknowledgement of these 'zig-zags' and 'ladders of cure' came from Burnett (1887: 53), but they have been developed furthest in French homeopathy (e.g. Zissu 1977–78). This approach has been formalized more recently by Francisco Eizayaga. Eizayaga began as a classicist, but objected to what he saw as antiscientific occultist tendencies in much neo-Kentian homeopathy. Over many years, he developed a rigorous method of analysis in chronic disease, related to the French reactional modes, which involves breaking the case down into three layers, which may require entirely different medicines:

1. lesion, consisting of local, general and mental symptoms of acute phase, plus precipitating factors;
2. fundamental: mental and general symptoms specific to the patient during the disease, which may involve the chronic miasms;
3. constitution: non-pathological general characteristics, correlated with a small number of mineral biotypes.

Eizayaga (1991: 251) states that in 'severe and organic cases, when the remedy for the disease (*similar*) and the remedy for the patient (*simillimum*) are different, one should prescribe the similar first'. He also points out that constitutional treatment will only be successful if the remedy chosen happens (accidentally or not) to include or overlap any lesion, but that starting treatment at the lesional level is frequently so successful as to make subsequent constitutional treatment unnecessary.

He has treated many thousands of cases of serious pathology, including malignant tumours and multiple sclerosis, using this approach. Results of treatment using his system in chronic asthma have also been published (Eizayaga, Eizayaga, Eizayaga 1996).

4.5.2. Sequential therapy

The Swiss Jean Elmiger (1998) also developed a clinical algorithmic approach to chronic disease after experiencing similar disillusionment to Eizayaga with purist neo-Kentianism and the fetish of the single constitutional remedy. In Elmiger's sequential therapy, treatment follows an explicit timeline (reverse chronology) using homeopathic prescriptions for traumas and unresolved acute episodes, intercalated with constitutional prescriptions. In each patient this is followed by antimiasmatic treatment with nosodes. He has claimed particular success with the chronic sequelae of immunizations, antidoted by the potentized vaccine (tautopathy), and has evolved a schedule for pre- and post-treatment of conventional immunization. These potencies are made from the whole vaccine, including the fixatives such as formaldehyde and aluminium phosphate and the preservative thiomersal, a mercury compound. They are claimed to minimize adverse effects and maximize the positive immune response to vaccines.

4.6. Conclusion

Jewson (1976) proposed a sociological explanation for the cosmologies that have dominated Western medicine since the eighteenth century. His theory was that eighteenth-century 'bedside' medical practice was mainly determined by the patronage of well-off patients but was displaced by nineteenth-century medicine aimed at the masses. It is not necessary to accept his thesis to see the usefulness of this categorization in explaining some of the difficulties faced by homeopathy. Table 4.1 shows Jewson's original table, modified only by the introduction of a column containing Hahnemannian homeopathy.

Table 4.1 Western medical cosmologies, 1770–1900, adapted from Jewson (1976)

	Bedside Medicine –1850	**Homeopathy 1790– (Chronic disease 1821–)**	**Hospital Medicine 1790–1900**	**Laboratory Medicine 1870–**
Subject matter of nosology	Total symptom complex	Total symptom- complex (historical symptom-complex)	Internal organic events	Cellular function
Patient-practitioner involvement	Central	Central	Minimal	Peripheral
Focus of pathology	Systemic – dyscrasias	Systemic (miasms, constitution)	Local lesion	Physico-chemical processes
Research methods	Speculation and inference	Provings; Statistically oriented clinical observation and comparison	Statistically oriented clinical observation	Laboratory experiment according to scientific method
Diagnostic technique	Qualitative judgement	Structured anamnesis cf pathogeneses (*timeline*)	Physical examination before and after death	Microscopic examination and chemical tests
Therapy	Heroic and extensive	Optimistic; simillimum in minimum dose	Sceptical (with the exception of surgery)	Nihilistic
Mind–body relation	Integrated: psyche and soma seen as part of the same system of pathology	Integrated: psyche and soma seen as part of the same system of pathology	Differentiated: psychiatry a specialized area of clinical studies	Differentiated: psychology a separate scientific discipline

It is clear that homeopathy shared some of the aspects of bedside medicine, including holistic attention to the individual patient, that were being displaced by a rapidly industrializing medical profession. It is also clear that its extreme precision in differentiating states that are usually lumped together causally or nosologically is radically different from anything before or since. No doubt the acausal diagnosis of these unique illness states in terms of their treatment contributed further to the difficulty faced by allopathy in understanding homeopathy.

Moreover, Jewson's categories are useful in explaining the tensions observable within homeopathy. Paradoxically, at the same time that the individual patient's subjective experience became the central focus of homeopathy, to a far greater extent than in bedside medicine, the same homeopaths were pioneering the investigation and therapeutic use of pathogens derived from morbid matter, and were extending the similia notion to the level of the lesion.
Although the results of classical, clinical, complex and isopathic versions of homeopathy have been categorized and quantified in recent systematic reviews of clinical trials, authors have avoided making qualitative comparisons (Kleijnen, Knipschild, ter Riet 1991; Linde, Clausius, Ramirez et al. 1997). Even within the qualitative literature, detailed comparisons of different homeopathic approaches are rare. The British Jungian psychiatrist and homeopath Anthony Campbell (1984) rearticulated the nineteenth-century distinction made by Hughes concerning the 'two homeopathies': the clinical and the classical, roughly corresponding to Hahnemann's pre- and post-1810 periods respectively (Hughes 1893: 90). Campbell concluded that although the pathological approach might be more acceptable to science, it lacked patient-appeal, which is amply provided for by the metaphysical version, however logically unsustainable the latter.

Van der Steen and Thung (1988) make a similar contrast between two contemporary homeopaths: the neo-Kentian Vithoulkas (1972; 1980), an advocate of homeopathy as 'grand theory'; and Mössinger (1984), who does not accept the similia principle as more than a useful heuristic, or the potentization principle at all, and has investigated empirical disease-based homeopathic specifics in a number of trials (see Part III).

Although our culture favours arguments based on binary oppositions, they tend to oversimplify. Hughes, for instance, has been consistently painted as a sceptical opponent of classical homeopathy and high potencies, but, contrary to received wisdom, was highly sympathetic to the classical viewpoint which took Hahnemann's mature method as its starting point:

> The individualisation of each case … is the only certain method of arriving at the true *simillimum* … The more we generalise, and refer it to a class, the less happy we shall be … Subjective symptoms outweigh objective ones … because they present less of the common than of the peculiar features of a case. They are, moreover, of great value, as being the earliest signs of disorder, before organic change has begun; they constitute the main phenomena of a malady at a stage in which it is still curable. (Hughes 1893: 89)

As for chronic disease theory, he felt that it was of immense benefit in allowing the possible constitutional origin of local and superficial complaints to be treated. Indeed, this was the area classical homeopathy was most suited to, rather than large-scale treatment of acute disease, and was the 'best hope of making certain and speedy cures, whose brilliancy shall recall the earlier days of our history' (ibid.: 91). Again, he easily accepted the pathogenetic effects and therapeutic efficacy of ultramolecular potencies when these were demonstrated in trials of acceptable scientific quality (ibid.: 103, 106).

From the opposite side, Kent devoted some essays to 'pathological' prescribing that make startling reading when compared with the anticlinical and antiepidemiological pronouncements of some of his recent followers (e.g. Vithoulkas 1991). He acknowledged that the study of disease is essential to the study of homeopathy, that semiology is only half the story, the other half being pathology; and went on to say that medicines which could not produce the pathological tissue changes found in any disease could not cure that disease homeopathically (Kent 1885; 1912b). Similarly, Burnett is often presented as a high-potency opponent of Hughes, yet as noted above, Burnett believed the pathological simillimum was a great advance.

Figure 4.1 shows how these allegedly irreconcilable approaches can be mapped straightforwardly onto a graph.

Along the y axis this moves from individual to species, and along the x axis from subjective symptom to external causation. The overlaps and interrelationships between the variants are too complex to indicate visually.

As we have seen, by the 1830s Hahnemann had prescribed across most areas of the field using the individual, epidemic, chronic disease, traumatic and isopathic models. Subsequently, classicists have tended to work in the semiotic–individual area, moving into nosology and pathology only to narrow down the choice of medicines for a patient, or occasionally to treat chronic miasms using nosodes; while some clinical homeopaths have worked from the opposite quadrant, probing symptomatology only to refine a much narrower palette of nosological and pathological specifics.

	Semiology		Nosology	Physiology	Pathology	Etiology
Species		Complexes Heel 1900	Clinical specifics Griesselich 1840	Tissue salts Schüssler 1870	Pathological simillimum Hughes 1880	Isoprophylaxis Hering 1830
Population		Genius epidemicus Hahnemann 1800	Epidemic prophylaxis Hahnemann 1800	Constitutional biotypes Grauvogl 1860		Allergology Blackley 1880
Family	Constitutional psychology Kent 1880	Physical generals Bönninghausen 1830	Chronic miasms Hahnemann 1830		Nosodes Hering 1830	
Individual	Mentals & generals Kent 1880	Symptom-complex Hahnemann 1800	Keynotes e.g. Allen 1880		Isopathy Hering 1830	Tautopathy Hering 1830

Figure 4.1 Homeopathy 1800–1900: the main approaches, their attributions and decade of appearance

In practice, many have regarded function and lesion as complementary, neither less 'real' than the other. And although some neo-Kentian homoeopaths use a single-remedy version of the acute 'general' model heavily weighted towards mental symptoms and 'constitution', even in chronic disease (Vithoulkas 1980; Seghal 1994; Candegabe 1996), reanalysis of Kent's own published cases has shown that, because of limitations in nineteenth-century pathological knowledge, he often thought he was prescribing for the individual when we now know he was actually prescribing – successfully – for the lesion (Eizayaga 1989).

The generally pragmatic approach found in British homeopathy is typified by Burnett and Clarke, who both managed to use high-potency simillima, nosodes, and isopathy, with low potency combination and organ remedies. Clarke (1900) compiled an important materia medica based on classical semiology, which also did justice to clinical nosology. More recent methods, such as those of Eizayaga and Elmiger, systematically traverse the whole field in any one chronic case. Present-day clinical trials of individualized homeopathy have hardly begun to reflect this widespread synthetic approach, as shown in Part III.

A.N. Whitehead famously said that Western philosophy was a series of footnotes to Plato, and Campbell (1984: 22) has pointed out that present-day homeopathy bears the same relationship to Hahnemann. With the exception of occultist homeopathy (e.g. Evans 2000), most of the different trends within the therapy are traceable to Hahnemann's own guidelines, but brought into sharper focus by his immediate followers and their descendants. It is easy to overstate the differences between homeopaths, as if each belongs to a separate warring sect, when in fact they share much common ground. However, it is reasonable to conclude that the possibility of many different approaches within the field of homeopathy is less problematic than is sometimes thought; even the most pessimistic reading must perceive an underlying unity: a shared belief in the efficacy of Hahnemannian potentized medicines in many different contexts, and chosen by many different heuristics.

Meanwhile, the preoccupation of orthodox internal medicine has been to establish treatments of causation in the species–lesion and extra-species areas (antibiosis), while disputing the need to bother with functional semiology once the solution has been found in the laboratory. Early homeopaths claimed the appropriate arena for testing their system versus its dominant rival was not the debating hall or the press but the field of experience, i.e. in clinical trials, at a time when allopathy was generally uninterested in or opposed to trials. Evaluation of the results of those early trials forms the subject of Part II.

Part II: Homeopathy and the development of clinical evaluation. A systematic review of clinical trials of homeopathy, 1821–1953

5. Why look at historical trials of homeopathy?

Background: The history of the evolution of the clinical trial has been surprisingly neglected considering the centrality of the trial in biomedicine. The early trials of homeopathy have been particularly neglected.

Questions: Are the historical trials of homeopathy relevant to present-day concerns? Is a review warranted?

Argument: An account of the historical trials of homeopathy is essential because:
- they were an important component in the evolution of the clinical trial;
- the judgements made by influential nineteenth-century opponents of homeopathy, ostensibly based on evidence from clinical trials, still colour debate today;
- valid trials of homeopathy in clinical contexts dramatically different from those found in the present day may increase our understanding of the therapy's potential, and indicate areas for future research.

5.1. The neglect of the pre-modern clinical trial

Clinical trials are a neglected area in the historiography of pre-twentieth-century medicine. This is particularly surprising considering that evidence from controlled trials is regarded today as a fundamental precondition for the practice of effective medicine and healthcare. The lacuna is explained most obviously by the fact that not many trials were carried out until randomized clinical experiments became accepted as a central dogma of scientific medicine in the second half of the twentieth century. There are two principal reasons for the late acceptance of trials compared with the institutionalization of the scientific experiment. First, they constitute an empirical procedure which tends to undermine the traditional Galenic authority of the physician and his institutions. Only a profession transformed or willing to be transformed by the penetration of empirical thinking could accept impartial trials which might overturn received wisdom, and would be expected to inform subsequent clinical decisions. The prospect of constant revision of working practices was unwelcome for most of history, and was resisted strongly in medicine, long after experimentation became the guiding principle of the scientific worldview during the seventeenth century (Bacon 1620). Second, even though the idea of therapeutic comparisons and controlled trials became tentatively established in the early nineteenth century, aggregated results of treatments imply probabilistic rather than certain knowledge of efficacy in individual patients. However unlikely the latter objective may seem now, it was the basis for the widespread rejection of empirical trials in the mid to late nineteenth century, and was endorsed by Claude Bernard's (1813–78) project to place clinicophysiological science on an equal footing with nineteenth-century positivist physics (Canghuilhem 1991).

Although there undoubtedly were some trials before the twentieth century, medical historians have continued to reflect a general lack of interest in the topic. There appear to be three main reasons. First, the groundwork of medical historiography had been put in place before the randomized clinical trial emerged after the 1939–45 war as the 'gold standard' of contemporary clinical research (Garrison 1917; Singer 1928; Castiglioni 1941; Guthrie 1945; Shryock 1948; King 1958). Second, Bernardian doubts about the scientific and ethical validity of empirical evidence from controlled trials were common well after then, even among historians who were themselves trialists. For instance, Bull (1959) wrote a history of the clinical trial, but then cast doubt on the importance of his contribution by comparing trials to uninductive technological advances, because

> the full sequence of observation–theory–hypothesis–experiment– validation is not usually invoked. The 'hypothesis' is usually very simple – that the test treatment is better than some other treatment.

Lastly, although a 'new' history of medicine emerged in the final third of the century, often originating from outside the medical profession, it has been concerned – like Foucault (e.g. 1963) who was influential in establishing the orientation – principally with the sociology of medicine, rather than its internal methodological processes.

Even when early clinical trials have been considered, they have been sidelined. For instance, although several extensive treatments of the emergence of statistical thinking have appeared recently (MacKenzie 1981; Porter 1986; Stigler 1986; Gigerenzer, Swijtink, Porter et al. 1989), clinical trials have been presented, if at all, as a mid twentieth-century, post-Fisherian development. In contrast, the 'numerical method' of P.-C.-A. Louis (1835), in which survival rates under competing treatments were collected and compared, has been presented as a false start, and subordinated to the much more impressive applications of statistical inference developing outside medicine in the first half of the nineteenth century.

Recent authoritative and systematic coverage of the history and historiography of medicine has reflected and perpetuated this lack of interest in trials as a distinctive medical domain (e.g. Porter 1993; Slinn 1995). Only in textbooks of epidemiology is the early clinical trial treated briefly, if at all, as a corollorary of the evolution of epidemiological method (e.g. Lilienfeld & Lilienfeld 1980). Typically, reference is made to the 1747 trial of limes and oranges versus other sour-tasting substances in the prevention of scurvy by James Lind (1716–94), and the 1847 trial by Ignaz Semelweiss (1818–65) of elementary hygienic measures in medical attendants to prevent puerperal fever (ibid.: 30f, 39).

Thus, as regards the early history and evolution of the clinical trial, the coverage is disappointingly thin. Even Shryock's (1961) otherwise important paper on quantification in medicine again mentions only Semmelweis's trial. Leaving aside brief popular overviews which have occasionally appeared (e.g. Rawlins 1990), the most sustained treatments of early clinical trials are those contained in academic theses. Bull (1951) includes a narrative account of the main historical experiments, later published separately from the main thesis (Bull 1959). Tröhler (1978) shows that priority for quantification in medicine belongs properly to eighteenth-century Britain rather than nineteenth-century France, as popularly supposed, but he is concerned with the emergence of statistics more than the trial. Two theses that were later published are mainly concerned with twentieth-century developments: Rosser Matthews (1995) on quantification in medicine, which focuses on selected case studies without aiming to be comprehensive; and Marks' (1997) study of US trial policy which challenges the notion that the modern clinical trial was solely or mainly a product of the medical profession's self-critical scientific advance (see Ch. 7 for discussion of this theory in the light of mid nineteenth-century homeopathic trials). Another national historical thesis (Cox-Maksimov 1998) explores the development of the controlled trial in Britain. Important papers include A. and D. Lilienfeld's review of case-control studies (1979), and A. Lilienfeld (1982) which places the emergence of the clinical trial within an evolutionary framework.

5.2. The neglect of homeopathic trials in particular

Although there were many nineteenth-century therapeutic trials which involved homeopathy, none of the above sources mentions them.

This notable neglect of homeopathic trials seems to be based on the general reasons given above, compounded by the hostile reception that homeopathy received from the allopathic profession. Jütte (1999) has recently pointed out that early positivist accounts of homeopathic history made little or no attempt to evaluate the system, but assumed that a statement of its tenets was enough to demonstrate its self-evident absurdity. It is undoubtedly true that the historiography of medicine was until recently overwhelmingly an internalist discipline, written by doctors for each other (e.g. Faber 1921) or occasionally in simplified form for the general public (e.g. Robinson 1931; Lloyd 1936). It was given above all to a Whiggish celebration of the triumphal advance of medical knowledge. This in turn rested on a rationalist conception of medical science which sought single overarching answers to clinical problems, as if medicine could be modelled on Newtonian physics and its search for a unified theory of physical forces. However embarrassing individual patients might be for this approach, a pluralist medical philosophy which could allow the possibility of divergent answers to specific therapeutic problems was inadmissable – a blindspot in the biomedical worldview noted in the early twentieth century by the allopaths Crookshank (1923 [1946]) and Bier (1925). Moreover, because it was believed that homeopathy had been shown conclusively in clinical trials to be a popular delusion like phrenology (Holmes 1842), there was clearly no need for the discussion of trials of non-medicine. Only one 'trial' was regularly mentioned in the century-and-a-half after its publication. This was Andral's observational study of 1834 (Anon 1834; Académie de Médecine 1835a), which constituted Holmes's top level of evidence against homeopathy, and was still being cited more than a century later as an example of how homeopathy had failed the test of 'exact, critical appraisal' (Shryock 1948).

In fact there were a number of genuine prospective clinical trials of homeopathy in the mid nineteenth century, which involved the medical establishment, but they have been entirely left out of orthodox histories. And once again, the sociological orientation of the late twentieth-century 'new' historiography of medicine meant that homeopathy was dealt with in terms of its spread, its clientele, its personalities, its political and economic conflict with allopathy, its relationship to other forms of alternative medicine such as herbalism and hydropathy, and its decline (e.g. Haller 1984; Barrow 1986; Roberts 1986; Brown 1987; Barrow 1988; Cooter 1988; Rankin 1988; Fye 1990; Gevitz 1994; Gijswijt-Hofstra 1996; Weatherall 1996; Jütte 1998). In this almost random selection of representative studies, clinical trials are mentioned hardly at all.

5.3. Homeopathic demands for trials

The widespread nineteenth-century indifference towards, and even rejection of, evaluation of allopathic procedures in clinical trials contrasts sharply with the homeopathic community's interest in and demand for trials. Internal and external factors seem to have contributed to this.

The early homeopaths rejected the standard accusations of charlatanry levelled at them, and stressed the scientific nature of their pharmacological research. The homeopathic drug proving bears an obvious similarity to the phase I clinical (screening) trial as it is known today. The need for lack of bias in the collection of signs and symptoms had been appreciated by homeopaths from the beginning (see Ch. 2), and placebo-controlled provings and reprovings emerged relatively early on, possibly influenced by the therapeutic use of placebo stemming from Hahnemann (see Ch. 8). The dilution and dosage experiments performed by the early homeopaths were another source of internal therapeutic comparison, and seem to have been far ahead of their time (see Ch. 7).

Equally importantly, homeopathy had emerged from the most comprehensive critique that nosology and therapeutics had received until that time, and it would have been inconsistent if it could not itself be subject to external comparison and evaluation. As noted in Ch. 2, Hahnemann (1817; 1852b) declared that homeopathy could only be validated by clinical experiment, not by argument. Homeopaths responded to the orthodox a priori rejection of their 'infinitesimal' doses (Holmes 1842; Routh 1852) by pointing to their success in practice, and insisted that 'Does it work?' was the relevant question, not 'Should it work?' (e.g. Bayes 1856: 22). Their advocacy, from the 1830s cholera epidemics onwards, of statistical comparison of mortality rates, time to recovery and drug costs under allopathy and homeopathy places them in the vanguard of evidence-based healthcare, as it is now known (Irvine 1844; Anon 1852; Ozanne 1853; Gallavardin 1860). The record shows that homeopaths and their supporters were anxious to conduct trials of homeopathy versus allopathy, confident that they would demonstrate the superiority of their therapy.

5.4. Historiography of homeopathic trials

5.4.1. Internal accounts

There are of course many internal histories of homeopathy, and nearly all commemorate a few of the better-known trials, but, as with orthodox medicine, there has been no comprehensive coverage of historical data from prospective trials.

J.-P. Gallavardin (1824–98) mentions a few of the trials conducted in the 30 years before he wrote, particularly those of the Paris school, and provides useful background data missing from some primary reports (Gallavardin 1860). Somewhat later, Wilhelm Ameke (1847–86) wrote about what he called 'trials of homeopathy by its opponents', including those by the Paris school, and others that Gallavardin did not mention (Ameke 1885: 312ff).

The historian of Russian homeopathy, Boyanus (1882), describes the setting up of various homeopathic hospitals, and mentions two prospective trials.

The first comprehensive presentation of a body of statistical evidence relating to the efficacy of homeopathy appeared at the end of the nineteenth century, when T.L. Bradford (1900), an American homeopathic librarian and biographer of Hahnemann, published *The Logic of Figures: or Comparative Results of Homoeopathic and Other Treatments*. This was not a review, but a compilation of reports from Europe and the USA that had appeared in the half-century after 1850. Many of these consisted of large-scale comparisons between mortality rates in orthodox and homeopathic hospitals during the numerous epidemics that swept Europe and America in the nineteenth century. The tabulated results are as much a commentary on the ineffectiveness of pre-modern orthodox medicine and public health as they are on the apparent efficacy of homeopathy. Bradford also included cost comparisons where they could be found, derived from reports by the administrators of public institutions that had employed the two systems in parallel or alternately for several years. These invariably show that the costs of homeopathic medication at that time were a small percentage of the costs of orthodox treatment. Unfortunately, however useful his compilation is as a starting point for the researcher, Bradford seems only to have included examples which favoured homeopathy, and thus cannot be considered to be an unbiased source. His references are mainly secondary reports from the English-language journals, and in some cases it has not been possible to trace his citations of secondary references, let alone the primary reports they were based on. Another problem with the majority of statistics presented by Bradford was his extensive use of mortality rates from institutions which were geographically remote – the treatment of cholera or pneumonia by homeopathy in Vienna cannot be compared directly with the results of allopathic treatment of the same diseases in Edinburgh, since, however accurate the diagnosis of the disease, the severity of the epidemic and baseline comparability of patients may well have been different. This incommensurability had been recognized long before by homeopaths more scientifically grounded than Bradford (e.g. Bayes 1856).

Some early twentieth-century trials were mentioned by Donner (1948), and more recently Coulter (1977: 552ff) described two trials undertaken by the Paris school, including Andral's.

5.4.2. External accounts

External accounts of homeopathic trials, other than the alleged falsifications of homeopathy by members of the Paris school such as Andral and Trousseau, are predictably scarce.

A systematic review of mid twentieth-century placebo research until 1959 contained a brief overview of historical pharmacological experiments, including the work of the Vienna Provings Union in the 1840s (Haas, Fink, Härtfelder 1959). A scholarly history of Italian homeopathy recounts in some detail the controversy surrounding two trials that took place in Naples in 1828–9 (Lodispoto 1961: 39ff).

Cassedy (1984) examined the debate over mortality rates under homeopathic and allopathic treatment in epidemics in North America and found evidence that some of the comparisons between homeopathic and allopathic treatment in the same institution at different times may have been flawed. For instance, there were (unproven) accusations that homeopaths had removed hopeless cases from the institutions, in order to improve their averages of cure. Although Bradford (1900) relied heavily on retrospective time-series data of this sort, it must be viewed with scepticism. Formal prospective trials do not seem to have been undertaken in the US until 20 years after Cassedy's study concludes, so a noteworthy trial of allopathy versus homeopathy which took place in Chicago in the 1880s is described only by Kaufmann (1971).

Some details of historical trials are given by Aulas (1991: 87ff), although the author's overtly anti-homeopathic stance undermines the objectivity of the account at many points, particularly where conflicting reports of the same trial exist (see Ch. 6). Appearing while the present review was in progress were two articles relating to the history of blind assessment and placebo controls which include some early experiments (Kaptchuk 1997; 1998a).

An exception to the generally disappointing neglect of historical trials, both orthodox and heterodox, is a very recent project designed to give them the coverage they deserve. The website set up by the Royal College of Physicians of Edinburgh jointly with the Cochrane Collaboration appears to be committed to an inclusive approach to the history of clinical trials, regardless of the therapy tested (Cochrane Collaboration & Royal College of Physicians of Edinburgh 1998). It already contains details of a few early ostensible or rhetorical tests of homeopathy (see Ch. 8) and will be updated as new material comes to light.

5.5. Justification for reviewing early homeopathic trials

From a present-day perspective therefore, it is important to review early homeopathic trials systematically. Historically speaking, this contributes to our knowledge of:

- the internal history of homeopathy;
- evaluation of the external judgements made on homeopathy;
- the historiography of the clinical trial;
- the reciprocal relationship between homeopathy and the growth of scientific clinical evaluation.

Clinically, because of the changing patterns of disease, it allows a search for evidence of:
- homeopathy's efficacy in diseases which are not prevalent now, or those where homeopathy would not be considered now;
- similarities and differences in homeopathic prescribing styles between then and now.

An overview of the early evaluations of homeopathy indicates a 'hierarchy of evidence', comparable to that recognized today (Last 1995: 76). In ascending order of probable bias this comprises:

1. Prospective clinical trials with concurrent controls, such as the quasi-randomized trial at the Ste Marguerite hospital, Paris (Tessier 1852).
2. Quasi-experiments (a) – Prospective clinical trials with closely comparable historical controls, as above (Tessier 1850).
3. Quasi-experiments (b) – formal large-scale prospective comparisons of mortality rates under concurrent homeopathic and allopathic treatment in epidemics in the same location, such as the 1854 London cholera epidemic (House of Commons 1854–55).
4. Quasi-experiments (c) – prospective interrupted time-series comparisons of therapies in the same institution at different times, e.g. trials of different potency regimes (Eidherr 1862).
5. Prospective observational studies with protocols for admission, dispensing and reporting (Schmit 1831).
6. Retrospective consecutive case series and statistics from epidemics, e.g. during the influenza pandemic 1918–20 17 000 cases were treated by homeopathy in the USA, with a mortality rate of 0.3% compared with the expected 20% (Foubister 1989: 11).
7. Individual case reports, widely distributed throughout the literature for illustrative and teaching purposes.

A systematic review of all this material would be impossible within the constraints of this thesis, especially since the bulk of reports exist in unindexed nineteenth- and early twentieth-century journals, monographs and textbooks. For this reason, it is proposed to look only at prospective evaluations.

5.6. Method

A systematic literature search, without language restrictions, was undertaken for published reports of trials that took place before 1965 (the date Medline starts). The designs had to correspond with levels 1–5 in 5.5 above, which comprise:

- prospective comparative therapeutic trials of homeopathy versus another treatment or
- prospective observational studies with or without historical controls.

In the light of the historical importance of placebo controls in clinical evaluation, the search was extended to include nineteenth-century placebo-controlled provings (see Ch. 8).

Modern and historical homeopathic texts and their bibliographies, and early homeopathic journals were handsearched for reports of nineteenth- and early twentieth-century clinical therapeutic trials. Embase, Hominform, Medline and Psychinfo computerized databases were queried for articles on the history of homeopathic and placebo research. *ReferenceWorks* computerized database (Warkentin 1994) of nineteenth-century homeopathic materia medica and provings was searched, using the terms 'control', 'placebo', 'saccharum lactis', 'sac. lac.', 'test' and 'trial'. Historians, researchers and librarians in the field were contacted.

Details from identified trial and study reports were entered into a standard computer database. The extracted data included location, principal trialists, size, design, condition, type of homeopathic and other treatment, evaluation, problems – and reception where traceable.

5.7. Results

The search for prospective clinical evaluations of homeopathy uncovered 45 relevant studies and trials from 1821–1953. Four groups are identified and covered in Chs 6–9, an analysis which respects their chronological evolution. Brief details of the 44 hospital-based trials found in the literature search are shown in Table 5.1.

With few exceptions, the trial designs fall into three clearly distinguishable phases:

1. Observational studies of classical homeopathy in mixed conditions (1821–35);
2. Pragmatic open-label comparisons of classical homeopathy with allopathy or no treatment, for mixed or specific conditions (1844–86);
3. Controlled trials of clinical homeopathy (nosological specifics) (1914–53).

This demonstrates a clear chronological evolution in the design of prospective therapeutic trials of homeopathy towards what became the accepted 'gold standard' in clinicopharmacological research after 1950. In view of these natural divisions, the most appropriate method of evaluation would seem to be to respect the evolutionary categories and divide the sample into three. This contextualizes the trials, allowing them to be evaluated in historically appropriate terms, and most importantly allows avowedly evidence-based judgements on homeopathy made at the time of, and in response to, the trials to be evaluated as well. Accordingly, the three phases are dealt with separately in Chs 6, 7 and 9.

Placebo was only used as a control in one hospital-based therapeutic trial (Lichtenstädt 1832). Because of the importance that the issue of placebo controls had in nineteenth-century clinical evaluation of homeopathy, this trial is discussed separately in Ch. 8 along with an abortive placebo-controlled trial in general practice (Potter 1880), 5 placebo-controlled provings and 3 trials of placebo alone (as a presumed or rhetorical equivalent of homeopathy), which were also uncovered in the literature search.

Table 5.1 Prospective hospital-based evaluations of homeopathy 1821–1953

Trialist, Date	Source	Condition	Design	Model	Control
Stapf, 1821	Ameke, 1885: 312	Mixed	Case series	Classical	None
Wislicenius, 1821	Ameke, 1885: 312	Mixed	Case series	Classical	None
Marenzeller, 1828	Schmit, 1831	Mixed	Case series	Classical	None
de Horatiis, 1828	de Horatiis, 1829	Mixed	Case series	Classical	None
de Horatiis, 1829	Panvini, 1829; Esquirol, 1835; Peschier, 1835; Rapou, 1847	Mixed	Case series	Classical	None
Herrmann, 1829	Herrmann, 1831	Mixed	Case series	Classical	None
Herrmann, 1829–30	Lichtenstädt, 1832; Seidlitz, 1833	Mixed	Open label	Classical	Allopathy Expectant + placebo
Attomyr, Ringseis, 1830–31	Attomyr, 1832	Mixed	Case series	Classical	None
Guéyrard, 1832	Guéyrard, 1833a; Guéyrard, 1833b; Pointe, 1833; Gallavardin, 1860	Mixed	Case series	Classical	None
Simon, Curie, 1834	Académie de Médecine, 1835; Simon & Curie, 1835; Gallavardin, 1860	Mixed	Case series	Classical	None
Andral, 1834	Anon, 1834; Irvine, 1844	Mixed	Case series	Naive	None
Andral, 1835	Académie de Médecine, 1835	Mixed	Case series	Naive	None
Stern, 1844	Stern, 1845	Mixed	Case series	Classical	None
Stender, 1847–54	Johannsen, 1848; Boyanus, 1882: 123–124	Mixed	Open label	Classical	Allopathy

Table 5.1 Prospective hospital-based evaluations of homeopathy 1821–1953 (cont.)

Trialist, Date	Source	Condition	Design	Model	Control
Tessier, 1847–49	Tessier, 1850	Pneumonia	Historical	Classical	Allopathy
idem	Jousset, 1862 [Re-analysis of Tessier (1850) + 10 unpublished cases]	Pneumonia	Historical	Classical	Expectant
Tessier, 1849	Tessier, 1850	Cholera	Cohort control	Classical	Allopathy
Tessier, 1849–51	Editorial, 1849; Ozanne, 1850; Tessier, 1852; Ozanne, 1853; Ozanne, 1857; Gallavardin, 1860	Mixed	Open label	Classical	Allopathy
Casper, Wurmb, 1850–59	Eidherr, 1862	Pneumonia	Time series	Classical	3 potencies
Balfour, 1854	West, 1854: 600	Scarlet fever	Open label	Clinical	No treatment
Chargé, 1854	Chargé, 1855; Sirus-Pirondi, 1859; Gallavardin, 1860	Cholera	Open label	Classical	Allopathy (see Ch. 7)
London Hom. Hospital, 1854	General Board of Health (1854–55); House of Commons, 1854–55; Medical Council, 1854–55a, b, c, d	Cholera	Open label	Classical	Allopathy
Burnett, 1870s	Burnett, 1888: 1–10	Fevers	Open-label	Clinical	Allopathy
Cook County Hospital, 1880–86	Chicago Herald, 1881; Cook County Hospital, 1885; 1888; Chicago Medical Society, 1922; Cook County Board of Commissioners, n.d.	Mixed	Open label	Unknown	Allopathy
Chadwell, 1914	Wesselhoeft, 1917	Scarlet fever	Quasi-random	Clinical	Placebo

Table 5.1 Prospective hospital-based evaluations of homeopathy 1821–1953 (cont.)

Trialist, Date	Source	Condition	Design	Model	Control
Wesselhoeft, 1914–16	Wesselhoeft, 1917	Scarlet fever	Open label time series	Clinical	No treatment
Wesselhoeft, 1915	Wesselhoeft, 1925	Diphtheria	Open label	Clinical	Antitoxin
Wesselhoeft, 1917	Wesselhoeft, 1917	Scarlet fever	Open label	Clinical	No treatment
Wesselhoeft, 1921–23	Wesselhoeft, 1924	Orchitis from mumps	Historical	Clinical	Classical / allopathy
Bier, 1925	Bier, 1925	Furunculosis	Case series	Clinical	Allopathy
Joachimoglu, 1925	Donner, 1948 34	Skin conditions	D-b p-c	Clinical	Placebo
Simonson, 1938	Donner, 1948 54–57	URTI, (5 trials)	S-b p-c + Open label allopathic	Unknown	Placebo; allopathy
Schilsky, 1938–39	Schilsky, 1941	Whooping cough	Open label	Classical	Allopathy
Paterson, Boyd, 1941	Paterson, 1941	Diphtheria immunity	Historical	Isopathy	Untreated population
Hess, 1942	Hess, 1942	Diphtheria	Open label	Clinical	Serum
Paterson, Templeton, 1941–42	British Homoeopathic Society, 1943	Mustard gas burns, (4 trials)	Random, d-b p-c	Clinical; Isopathy	Placebo
Ledermann, 1951–53	Ledermann, 1954	Surgical tuberculosis	Random, d-b p-c	Classical	Placebo

Key: d-b, s-b, double- or single-blind; p-c, placebo-controlled

6. The earliest observational studies, 1821–35

Background: The rejection of homeopathy by the medical establishment has been portrayed as a watershed in medical history because it is deemed to have been based on evidence rather than prejudice: homeopathy was given a fair trial, especially by the pre-eminent Paris School, and was found wanting. This belief forms the basis of an influential thesis that the development of modern scientific medicine, as a unified discipline, can be dated to that rejection in the 1830s and 1840s.

Questions: How valid was the trial evidence used by sceptics such as the French Académie de Médecine (1835) and Holmes (1842) in their rejection of the claims of homeopathy? Was their use of evidence biased in any way?

Argument: A systematic review of prospective trials of homeopathy that took place before 1842 shows not only that the individual trial evidence used by the most notable critics was wholly invalid, but also that virtually no fair trials of homeopathy had taken place by that time.

6.1. Introduction

In March 1835 the Académie de Médecine in Paris debated homeopathy (Académie de Médecine 1835a; 1835b). It was decided that homeopathy should on no account be accepted into the newly self-constituting body of scientific medicine, and a recommendation was made to the government that permission for a free homeopathic hospital be denied. Among the heated opinions informing this seminal judgement, some mention of evidence from clinical trials could be heard. The celebrated Gabriel Andral (1797–1876) gave an account of trials he had conducted in the Pitié in Paris, and Bailly, medical director of the Hôtel-Dieu, spoke of another trial at his own institution. A review of an account of an earlier trial in Naples was also prepared for the debate by Edouard Esquirol. All the evidence brought forward appeared to support the contention that homeopathy did not cure patients. A few years later, in a tract whose extraordinary influence since that time has been noted above (see Ch. 3), Holmes (1842) wrote that homeopathy was a delusion. Not only was the system completely implausible; most crucially in his hierarchy of evidence, it had also been falsified by clinical experiment. The examples used by Holmes were Andral's trials, and Esquirol's review.

These seemingly evidence-based judgements have been echoed ever since. A century later, discussing the emergence of the scientific biomedical world-view, Shryock (1948: 138f) could write:

> The manner in which critical methods undermined the old order is well illustrated by the history of homeopathy. This system was established in Germany during the last days of the *Naturphilosophie*, and was characterized … by a monistic pathology and therapeutics … Hahnemann was as 'regular' a medical philosopher as Brown, Rush or Rasori, but unfortunately was born just too late. The views of Brown could neither be proved nor disproved by the rationalistic controversies of 1800 … but Hahnemann's works appeared just in time to be subject to exact and critical analyses.

Holmes's top level of evidence against homeopathy is then cited:

> The French clinicians seemed willing to give homeopathy a trial. Andral, in particular, checked the system with care, trying it out in his wards in Paris with negligible results, and reporting to the Academy of Medicine that he had systematically experimented with the *materia medica* without finding any of the results Hahnemann reported.

Shryock, a founder of modern scientific historiography of medicine, then makes his largest claim:

> It was as a result of such apparently inductive checks on the new school that that it was eventually forced out of regular medicine … this expulsion, this transfer from the status of a system to that of a sect, affords one of the best criteria for dating the final advent of modern medicine. When a monistic pathology and a related therapeutics were no longer tolerated in regular medicine, that medicine had come of scientific age.

Leaving aside Shryock's mischaracterization – as monistic – of homeopathy's fundamental requirement of a constantly recalibrated therapeutics to match constantly varying pathologies, there can be little doubt of the importance of this judgement – if true. The question underlying a review of the first phase of homeopathic trials is therefore: did these clinical trials show conclusively that homeopathy was, as the Académie and Holmes thought, a delusion? Was it as we would say nowadays (less rhetorically, no doubt) no more than a placebo?

6.2. Results

Table 6.1 shows 12 studies conducted between 1821 and 1835. All the trials used homeopathic medicines for mixed conditions, acute or chronic, with little attempt at selection of patients. Half were terminated abruptly, either because of external opposition, or because of internal problems with allopathic staff compliance.

Table 6.1 Prospective observational studies of homeopathy in mixed conditions 1821–35

Trialist Date	Sources	Hospital	Model Control	N Length
Stapf 1821	Ameke, 1885: 312	Berlin, Charité	Classical None	? ? !
Wislicenius 1821	Ameke, 1885: 312	Berlin, Garrison Hospital	Classical None	? ?
Marenzeller 1828	Schmit, 1831	Vienna, Garrison Hospital	Classical None	43 40 d !
de Horatiis 1828	de Horatiis, 1829	Naples, Trinità	Classical None	200 5 mon
de Horatiis 1829	Panvini, 1829; Esquirol, 1835; Peschier, 1835; Rapou, 1847	Naples, Trinità	Classical None	60 40 d
Herrmann 1829	Herrmann, 1831	Tulzyn, Military Hospital	Classical None	164 3 mon !
Herrmann 1829–30	Lichtenstädt, 1832; Seidlitz, 1833	St Petersburg, Military Hospital	Classical Allopathy Expectant + placebo	395 341 521 5 mon
Attomyr, Ringseis 1830–31	Attomyr, 1832	Munich, General Hospital	Classical None	>100 5 mon
Guéyrard 1832	Guéyrard, 1833a; Guéyrard, 1833b; Pointe, 1833; Gallavardin, 1860	Lyons, Hôtel-Dieu	Classical None	15 (10) 4 d !
Andral 1834	Anon, 1834; Irvine, 1844	Paris, Pitié	Naive None	54 5 mon
Andral 1835	Académie de Médecine, 1835	Paris, Pitié	Naive None	140 3 mon?
Simon, Curie 1834	Académie de Médecine, 1835; Simon & Curie, 1835; Gallavardin, 1860	Paris, Hôtel-Dieu	Classical None	? ?

Key: ! = terminated prematurely.

The trials fall chronologically into two subgroups: firstly those taking place in Germany and German-dominated areas (Austria, Italy, Russia), and secondly the French studies. Most of the first group employed some form of protocol for conduct and evaluation, but the second group did not. None of the French trials was the subject of an authorized, published report.

6.3. Germanic trials

6.3.1. Berlin 1821: Stapf, Wislicenius

The earliest prospective public trials of the new system seem to have taken place in 1821. J.E. Stapf, one of Hahnemann's personal students and closest allies, was invited to demonstrate the clinical benefits of homeopathy at the Charité hospital, Berlin. According to Ameke (1885), the trial was abruptly halted by the hospital authorities as soon as it became apparent that Stapf was successfully treating patients with chronic diseases.

Wislicenius, another close colleague of Hahnemann, undertook another public series in 1821 also in Berlin, at the Garrison Hospital. Again according to Ameke (ibid.), Wislicenius achieved success, but the trial was not halted this time. Instead, the journal kept by Wislicenius detailing his treatments and observations was taken away by the allopathic doctors in charge of the trial and never returned. The military surgeon responsible said that it was not the business of the highest functionaries to give an account of the experiments, but that some day the results would be made known. The results were still unpublished 60 years later, when Ameke pointed out that if the trial had contained the slightest evidence against homeopathy it is doubtful whether the same functionaries would have lost any time in publicizing the fact.

6.3.2. Vienna 1828: Marenzeller

The trial at the Garrison Hospital, Vienna, was conducted by imperial decree, and a real effort was made to establish acceptable conditions for a valid study (Schmit 1831). The objective was to conduct a preliminary trial to see if homeopathic medicines were efficacious in any respect, not to evaluate its effectiveness in life-threatening conditions. A formal protocol for supervision, admission, consultation, prescription, dispensing and reporting was created. Marenzeller, the homeopath, was a surgeon-major recalled from active duty in Prague. 43 patients were admitted, and of these 32 were cured, 1 died, 5 passed to other departments, and 5 were recuperating on day 40 when the trial was mysteriously terminated. Seven of the eight allopathic commissioners called for further trials, saying that the study had shown nothing that could be held against homeopathy, but that the short duration and small number of patients meant it could not be conclusive. The eighth commissioner was implacably opposed. The main problem seems to have been that allopaths in the same hospital tried to subvert the trial by threatening patients with dire consequences from homeopathy, and they had to be excluded as happened later in Naples. The report and tables were written by J. Schmit, who attended every visit of Marenzeller but does not seem to have been a homeopath. The validity of the report can also be gauged from the fact that it was communicated by Hahnemann himself to a journal for publication, with an endorsement of Schmit's trustworthiness.

6.3.3. Naples 1828: de Horatiis

Homeopathy was introduced into Italy in the 1820s following the Austrian invasion of Naples, when Necker, the Austrian commander's personal physician, taught the system to four Italian doctors. During a trial from 14 March to 10 August 1828 at the Trinità hospital, Naples, the Royal physician Cosmo de Horatiis treated 180 patients with diverse illnesses, acute and chronic. There was only one death, from smallpox. According to the primary report, nearly all experienced relief, and a large number were cured (de Horatiis 1829).

6.3.4. Naples 1829: de Horatiis

Following the encouraging results of the first Naples study, de Horatiis got permission from Ferdinand, King of Naples to conduct a second trial in front of a commission of allopaths headed by Pasquale Panvini. The Neapolitan allopaths made repeated attempts to subvert the study, apparently trying to influence patients against homeopathy by spreading untrue rumours of many deaths, and they had to be excluded from the open wards. This was partly due to nationalist opposition to the Germanic medical system, and partly from the economic threat posed by homeopathy (Rapou 1847, 1: 136ff). Because of the conflict, the King attended the hospital in person, and is alleged to have remarked drily: 'These patients must all have risen from the dead' (ibid.). A hostile report by Panvini (1829) appears to have been deliberately and systematically biased, even claiming that the trial was terminated after 40 days because of the large number of deaths. In fact, the homeopaths withdrew because of the impossible working conditions, even though of 60 patients, 52 were declared cured, 6 significantly improved, and only 2 had died.

6.3.5. Tulzyn 1829: Herrmann

Herrmann (d. 1836) received a 1-year contract in February 1829 to test homeopathy with the Russian military (Lichtenstädt 1832). His first study took place at the Military Hospital in the market town of Tulzyn, in the province of Podolya, Ukraine. At the end of three months, 164 patients had been admitted, 123 cured, 18 were convalescing, 18 still sick and 6 had died (Herrmann 1831). The homeopathic ward received many gravely ill patients, and the small number of deaths were shown at autopsy to be due to advanced gross pathologies.

6.3.6. St Petersburg 1829–30: Herrmann

Following the Tulzyn trial, Herrmann was ordered to remove to the Regional Military Hospital in St Petersburg, where he again participated in a trial from September 1829 until February 1830, supervised by a Dr Gigler. At the same time that the homeopathic ward was set up, Gigler allocated another ward to expectant treatment – the then medical euphemism for no treatment over and above normal nursing care (Lichtenstädt 1832). During the 5 months of the trial, Herrmann treated 395 patients, of whom 341 were cured, 23 died, and 31 were transferred to other wards. The expectant arm received 341 patients, of whom 260 were cured, 53 transferred (9 of whom subsequently died), and 28 unaccounted for. During the same period, the general mortality in the allopathic wards was the same as under homeopathy – of 521 patients, 60 died. Seidlitz (1833) later selected 47 unfavourable homeopathic cases as the basis of a hostile and at times abusive report. As a result of the report by Gigler, homeopathy was banned in Russia for some years. (See also Ch. 8 for further discussion of the role of placebos in this trial.)

6.3.7. Munich 1830–31: Attomyr & Ringseis

The difficulties faced in the trial at the General Hospital, Munich, seem extraordinary (Attomyr 1832). There was a smallpox epidemic during the study period, and all the patients were vaccinated. There was serious allocation bias – simpler cases were invariably sent to the allopathic wards, while homeopathic wards received no-hopers and malingerers who wanted to overwinter in hospital. Two doctors were overtly hostile to homeopathy, and the dispensing physician was supposed to administer the medicines, but instead gave them to nurses who mixed them up. There was further lack of compliance from nurses, who provided the patients with tobacco, wine etc. The patients' food was tampered with to make it inedible, or served cold, and the hospital water supply was so tainted that patients often got diarrhea after drinking it. Attomyr notes that the conditions were so bad that a 99% mortality rate could not have been held against homeopathy. However, he claims Dr Ringseis and he did effect cures which allopathy couldn't approach. Details and prescriptions for 33 individual successful cases are given, many of which had not responded to previous allopathic treatment, including syphilitic lesions, gonorrhea, epilepsies, pneumonias and migraines. A series of 40 cases of scabies was also mentioned. (See also Ch. 8 for further discussion of the role of placebos in this trial.)

6.4. French trials

6.4.1. Lyons 1832: Guéyrard

The professor of clinical medicine at the Hôtel-Dieu in Lyons, Dr Pointe, wrote an article published on 12 October 1833 in the *Gazette Médicale de Paris*, which declared that recent calls in the French medical press to test homeopathy were superfluous – such a trial had already taken place:

> During April 1832, I made a ward of 30 beds available to Dr Guérard [sic], one of the most renowned doctors in our city. He was free to choose the number of patients he placed, and to prescribe anything he needed for the success of the Hahnemannian doctrine. I made one condition, that the visits would be made at a prespecified time every day, so that any assistants he required would be free. 15 acute and chronic cases – fevers, pneumonia, erysipelas, pulmonary catarrh, measles, jaundice, diabetes and so on – were chosen by Guérard, and each day, in front of 60 students and several of the town physicians, he examined the patients with care, gave them homeopathic medicines himself, and prescribed the regime. The trial lasted 17 days, and only stopped when Guérard voluntarily withdrew. During this period no benefit or noteworthy change was observed that could be attributed to homeopathy alone … What then is the use of a method which fails in precisely the most necessary places, where it is most frequently needed, and where the brilliant success of the old school is seen every day? (Pointe, 1833)

Naturally Guéyrard was compelled to reply to this, in spite of the difficulty of giving details of a trial that had taken place 20 months earlier. In the *Gazette* of 9 November he pointed out that, after being invited by Pointe to conduct the trial with promises of support for homeopathy, he found the conditions at the Hôtel-Dieu were appalling (Guéyrard, 1833). As in Munich, it had been impossible to get the staff to co-operate, and nurses would give the medicine prescribed for one patient to another, since they believed it was just sugared water. He prescribed for about 10 patients only during the first 3 days, and withdrew from the trial on day 4, when he found that a patient had been bled in his absence. Pointe's account was therefore substantially incorrect. As regards Pointe's assertion concerning the brilliant success of orthodox medicine in these circumstances, Guéyrard points out that the hospital statistics tell quite another story.

The editor of the *Gazette* gave Pointe the space to reply to Guéyrard in the same issue – a courtesy he had not extended to Guéyrard when Pointe's original account was published. However, Pointe avoided all mention of Guéyrard's specific allegations about the unacceptable conditions and conduct of the trial, or its true duration and abrupt cessation. Instead he concentrated on the question of the usual cure and mortality rate at the Hôtel-Dieu.

6.4.2. Paris 1834: Andral

Andral's first observational study took place in the Pitié, Paris, in 1834. Published anonymously, the report congratulated Andral's assistant Maxime Vernois for his meticulous observation, but Vernois later admitted he had written the report himself (Anon 1834; Vernois 1835). It briefly describes 35 mixed cases, from 54 admitted to the trial, and the prescription for each case. It is clear from the report that treatment was given in complete ignorance of homeopathic methodology: Andral believed that out of the many signs and symptoms presented by any patient, he was required to select a single important one to prescribe for. The chosen symptoms themselves often appear arbitrary – an incipient smallpox described as gastritis, for example – and most bear no recognized homeopathic relationship to the prescription. The reasons for this are discussed below.

6.4.3. Paris 1835: Andral

Andral's report of further trials in the Pitié, made orally to the Académie de Médecine (1835), is worth quoting extensively, in view of the enormous weight given to it in the rejection of homeopathy:

> I have submitted this doctrine to experiment; today I can count 130 to 140 cases collected in good faith, in a large hospital, with many witnesses.

Andral was sensitive to the criticisms made of his earlier study:

> To avoid any objection, I have obtained the medicines from M. Guibert, a stringently exact homeopathic pharmacist. The regime was scrupulously observed as required by Hahnemann. It has been said that for several months I did not faithfully observe all the precepts of this doctrine. I therefore took the trouble to begin again; I studied the practice of the Parisian homeopaths just as I studied their books, and I am convinced that they would act in no other way than I did, and that I was as rigorous as any.

After mentioning an unsuccessful attempt to conduct provings, he indicates his highly selective mode of evaluation:

> I took for this [second] series the most clear-cut cases; and firstly intermittent fevers. Some of these were treated with globules of quinine;[19] some recovered, but they would have recovered anyway; these partial successes don't prove anything. Others resisted stubbornly, and finally I was forced to resort to the usual method [blood-letting] which quickly brought them out of it. A case like this is still in my wards.

He had still not grasped the fundamental principle of individualization. In the following series he refers to an equally vague fever awarded a discrete nosological category by Pinel, but unrecognized by Hahnemann:

> A crowd of patients presented with the symptoms of Pinel's angiotenic fever. According to Hahnemann, this always requires aconite regardless of the nature and seat of the affection which accompanies it. I gave aconite in more than 40 cases, without the least effect; pulse and temperature stayed the same. It was unnecessary in these cases to wait a week for the effects of the medicine, and then say: The fever has gone. One knows that it would have gone anyway in that time.

---

[19] Andral used quinine sulphate, not the *Cinchona* of the homeopathic materia medica.

After wrongly attributing a doctrine of specifics to Hahnemann, Andral confounds syphilis with gonorrhoea, even though Hahnemann (1828–30) had clearly distinguished them:

> I fought syphilis in all its forms, ulcers, excrescences, and so on, with Mercurius solubilis Hahnemannii, and above all with Thuja, in which the German reformer has such great confidence. The disease did not stop progressing. I dressed the ulcers with Neapolitan ointment, and healing was rapid.

Just as in the earlier trial, each patient was given one dose of one medicine, for one symptom only. The patient was then left without treatment for a few days, and if recovery was not apparent, the case was transferred to orthodox treatment and counted as a failure for homeopathy:

> I treated rheumatisms, with or without fever, with Bryonia, Colchicum and so on. The pain was never reduced by these means. Three days later I bled and returned completely to the usual method, which promptly cured.
> Hahnemann does not recognize pneumonia, properly speaking. He sees only a collection of symptoms from which he chooses the predominant to fight. I did likewise ... sometimes with Aconite, sometimes Belladonna. Mild pneumonias progressed as usual; grave cases went from bad to worse, and soon forced me to finish with this illusory therapy.

In fact, Andral's renewed study of homeopathy had not advanced his understanding at all (see below).

6.4.4. Paris 1834: Simon, Curie

During the 17 March session of the Académie, at which Andral's account was heard, another appeal to clinical evidence against homeopathy was made. Dr Bailly, director of the Hôtel-Dieu, rose and said that although he had not made tests personally, he had requested that experiments be performed. Trials had been conducted by the homeopaths Léon Simon and Curie, and were unsuccessful according to Bailly. He claimed that the record of these failures was available on demand. After the debate, Simon and Curie disputed his verdict and publicly demanded that the full record of the trial be produced, publishing at the same time the objections they had made in writing in 1834 to Bailly about the conditions of the study (Simon 1835). Incredibly, Bailly claimed in response to have lost the hospital journal while rearranging his library (Gallavardin 1860).

6.5. Discussion

The early attempts to evaluate homeopathy by observational studies in public hospitals are interesting, mainly for what they reveal about the difficulties of introducing rational clinical evaluation into medical practice in the period 1820–35. It is hard to avoid the conclusion that early and later critics of homeopathy who cited these trials as conclusive evidence of the inefficacy of the system vastly overrated the validity of uncontrolled studies that were carried out by unskilled allopaths, or, when performed by experienced homeopaths, were frequently subverted. Revealingly, the one trial from before 1835 that seems to have avoided the worst excesses of the others and managed to reach a valid conclusion, Marenzeller's in Vienna, was not mentioned anywhere.

The chauvinistic attitude of the Neapolitan allopaths was seen again in the Paris School's reaction to homeopathy, and is another factor which must be included in discussions of the emergence of the clinical sciences. For instance, an article bearing the initials of Edouard Esquirol appeared in 1833 in the *Gazette Médicale de Paris* (E. E. 1833). The author objected to homeopathy because it originated from across the Rhine, and he expressed his revulsion at the contamination of Gallic medicine: 'This mystical system has already invaded our *belle France.*'

The Académie relied on the trials mentioned by Andral, Bailly and Esquirol to justify their recommendation that the French government should expel homeopathy from the body medical. In fact, the transparent inadequacy of Andral's grasp of homeopathic method make his experiments some of the least reliable clinical studies to have been performed. Bailly never produced the case records that Simon and Curie insisted showed his account was biased. And Esquirol's review of the trial in Naples was a double travesty: Panvini's polemic was systematically biased, and Esquirol's 'review' consisted of nothing more than a single case history extracted from Panvini's hostile report, by way of illustrating how homeopathy was killing patients. It was left to the homeopaths to introduce some genuine statistics: they pointed out that the 'opinion that homeopathy was lethal had been given the most formal refutation possible by the [Neapolitan] registrar of deaths' (Peschier 1835a).

The French debate was also coloured by Pointe's subsequently refuted (and undefended) account of Guéyrard's aborted Lyons trial, and Trousseau's (1834) trial of placebo alone, without control (see Ch. 8). Making his case against homeopathy in 1842, Holmes's highest level of evidence consisted once again of Esquirol's review and Andral's trials. Many critical accounts of the latter had appeared in the homeopathic press in Europe and America before 1842, but shortly after Holmes's intervention and partially in response to it, Irvine (1844) wrote by far the most devastating critique of Andral's Pitié trials. He showed that Andral was unable to apply the homeopathic materia medica, not only from a complete misunderstanding of the method as demonstrated by the published cases and comments, but because he had no knowledge of German: Hahnemann's *Reine Arzneimittellehre* had not been translated into French in 1834, and although *Die chronischen Krankheiten* had been translated (Hahnemann 1832), Andral failed to use any of the 22 new medicines listed there. Thus he

> *abstained from using the only medicines of which he had the means of making a right application.* (original emphasis)

Andral's incompetence had even been admitted by his own assistant, Vernois (1835). Irvine continues that Vernois,

> while admitting … the incapacity of his professor to perform homeopathic experiments from not knowing the action of the medicines, excuses his ignorance by saying it was unavoidable … surely the consciousness that he did not possess the means of testing the system, should have prevented him from stating before the Academy that he had given it a fair trial in his wards. (Irvine 1844)

As noted in Ch. 2, homeopathy was not the only subject to suffer from the low level of ostensibly evaluative debate at this time. The discrediting of Broussais came about from the death of a single celebrity, rather than from his general mortality rates in cholera (Hacking 1990: 84)

Be that as it may, Andral's trials have retained their status as foundational exemplars of the vaunted rigour of the biomedical worldview. It would appear, in fact, that if homeopathy is the target any evidence is adequate, however biased or unreliable. But what did Andral think of homeopathy, after Vernois's later admissions? Carroll Dunham, the eminent American homeopath, used to attend Andral's clinic at the Charité in 1850–51, and one morning asked if he hadn't once published a report on homeopathy (Dunham 1852). Andral replied that nothing had ever been published with his authority, but Vernois's anonymous 1834 report was substantially correct. He had come to believe homeopathy deserved the closest examination by every physician, and volunteered that he no longer thought his trials had been at all conclusive. Perhaps the early homeopaths' protests to the government that they wanted, above all,

> *judges*, but ones that are true not counterfeit; – trials, that are real, logical, and replicable in front of rigorous but knowledgeable witnesses; – in a word, truthful information with the power to allow a judgement to be deduced (Simon 1836),

had not been entirely in vain.

7. Comparisons with allopathy, 1844–86

Background: The middle years of the nineteenth century saw significant advances in the application of statistics to the evaluation of medical treatments. It has been forgotten that homeopathy also played a part in this stage of the development of the modern clinical trial, and was evaluated pragmatically by comparison with orthodox treatments.

Problems: How did trials of homeopathy come to be performed in the latter half of the nineteenth century, given the exclusion of the therapy from medicine? How valid is the evidence from these trials? How did these trials disappear from the historical record?

Argument: Authentic trials of homeopathy took place – against allopathic opposition – because of interest shown by governments and hospital administrations. Homeopathy was compared with allopathy in treatment of serious conditions such as cholera and pneumonia, and some good quality fair trials provide confirmation of evidence that had been dismissed when obtained retrospectively. Contemporaneous attempts to suppress or discount the homeopathic results show that they constituted a serious embarrassment to orthodoxy, which reacted by attempting to outlaw homeopathy.

7.1. Introduction

The verdicts of the Académie and Holmes discussed in Ch. 6 are generally believed to have closed the door on the nineteenth-century investigation of homeopathy in clinical trials (a view endorsed by, among others, Coulter 1977; Poitevin 1987; Aulas, Bordelay, Royer 1991). Their summary judgements, which had such a devastating and long-lasting effect on the acceptance of homeopathy, led to rifts in the medical professions that were emerging in most advanced countries. Nevertheless, prospective clinical trials of homeopathy continued to appear in surprisingly high-profile environments, making it possible to identify two periods of nineteenth-century evaluation. The first, reviewed in Ch. 6, lasted from 1821–35 and comprised trials by early adopters and opponents of homeopathy; the second wave, from 1844–86, involved trials of the system by more experienced practitioners, from a variety of backgrounds. The earlier phase looked at uncontrolled applications of the system as a whole in the treatment of many conditions within a single study; phase two saw the acceptance of the need for controls, historical or active, and the emergence of trials for specific conditions, and even of specific medicines for named conditions – clinical homeopathy, as described in Ch. 4. This development seems inevitable enough when seen against its historical background. After Louis's (1835) simple enumeration of survival rates in tuberculosis under bleeding and without, more advanced statistical activity spread through medicine from the late 1830s onwards:

> Humboldt reported statistical observations on yellow fever to the Prussian Academy, and Dupuytren performed a like service for the French Academy. Numerical studies of the causes and remedies for various diseases – for cholera and scurvy, as well as for typhoid and tuberculosis – began to appear. During the forties there followed dramatic demonstrations of the role played by doctors in spreading puerperal fever … based on statistical evidence first suggested by Holmes in Boston, and later independently collected in a systematic manner by Semmelweis in Vienna. (Shryock 1948: 141)

Homeopaths were quick to seize the opportunity that the emergent acceptance of empirical statistical evaluation offered, and demanded comparative trials. The results of the second phase of trials are examined in this chapter, and reasons for their neglect advanced.

7.2. Results

Details and results of the 11 trials (and 1 re-analysis with a different historical control) are shown in Table 7.1. It will be seen that nearly all involved some form of comparison: historical at first, followed by simultaneous controls. Four trials can be classed as large, involving comparisons of several thousand patients. Notes about the individual trials follow.

Table 7.1 Prospective hospital-based clinical trials of homeopathy 1844–86

Trialist **Date**	**Sources**	**Hospital**	**Condition**	**Design** **Duration**	**Model** **Control**	**n (†)**
Stern 1844	Stern, 1845	Miskolz, Temporary	Mixed	Case series (patient prefer- ence) 15 mon	Classical None	121 (0 †)
Stender 1847–54	Johannsen, 1848; Boy- anus, 1882: 123–124	St Petersburg, Women's	Mixed	Open label cf cf 7 y	Classical Allopathy	5999 (756 †) 2789 (413 †)
Tessier 1847–49	Tessier, 1850	Paris, Ste Marguerite	Pneumonia	Historical 2 y	Classical Allopathy	41 (3 †) 106 (32 †)
idem	Jousset, 1862*			Historical	Classical Expectant	50 (3 †) 100 (31 †)
Tessier 1849	Tessier, 1850	Paris, Ste Marguerite	Cholera	Cohort control 1 mon	Classical Allopathy	20 + 80 (48 †) 100 (59 †)
Tessier 1849–51	Editorial, 1849; Ozanne, 1850; Tessier, 1852; Ozanne, 1853; Ozanne, 1857; Gallavardin, 1860	Paris, Ste Marguerite	Mixed	Quasi-random Open label cf 3 y	Classical Allopathy	4663 (399 †) 3724 (411 †)
Casper, Wurmb 1850–59	Eidherr, 1862	Vienna, Leopoldstadt	Pneumonia	Time series 9 y	Classical D6 D15 D30	140 (8 †) 31 (19.5 d) 54 (14.6 d) 55 (11.3 d)
Balfour 1854	West, 1854: 600	London, Royal Military Asylum	Scarlet fever prevention	Quasi-random Open label cf <1 mon	Clinical (bel- ladonna) No treatment	76 (2 cases) 75 (2 cases)

Table 7.1 Prospective hospital-based clinical trials of homeopathy 1844–86 (cont.)

Trialist **Date**	**Sources**	**Hospital**	**Condition**	**Design** **Duration**	**Model** **Control**	**n (†)**
Chargé 1854	Chargé, 1855; Sirus-Pirondi, 1859; Gallavardin, 1860	Marseilles, Hôtel-Dieu	Cholera	Open label cf 3 d	Classical Allopaths using homoeopathics	26 (21 †) 31 (18 †)
London Hom. Hospital 1854	General Board of Health, 1854–55; House of Commons, 1854-55; Medical Council, 1854–55a, b, c, d	London, Golden Square	Cholera**	Open label cf 2 mon + 1 y retrospective	Classical Allopathy	87 (16 †) 3188 (1467 †)
Burnett After 1872	Burnett, 1888: 1–10	Barnhill Parochial, Glasgow	Unspecified fevers	Open label cf ?	Clinical (aconite) Allopathy	?
Cook County Hospital 1880–86	Chicago Herald, 1881; Cook County Hospital, 1885; 1888; Chicago Medical Society, 1922; Cook County Board of Commissioners, n.d.	Chicago	Mixed	Quasi–random Open label cf 6 y	Unknown Allopathy	1242 (8.2% †) 4692 (8.6% †)

* Re-analysis of Tessier (1850) with a further 10 unpublished cases from Tessier's series, compared with expectant treatment instead of allopathy as the historical control.

** Form B cases only: see Table 7.

7.2.1. Miskolz, Austro-Hungary 1844: general

Although this observational study in a specially set-up prison hospital at Miskolz, Hungary, appears to belong methodologically to the previous group of trials reviewed in Ch. 6, it also marked a conceptual advance: patients entered the study only after having been allowed to choose whether to undergo allopathic or homeopathic treatment. The report by F. Stern (1845), an orthodox doctor who had become convinced of the value of homeopathy, mentions vehement prior allopathic opposition, in the press and elsewhere, but the trial appears to have run smoothly for 15 months. Of 121 patients treated for many conditions, including gastric fevers and a considerable number of pneumonias and other inflammatory lung diseases, 96 were cured and 22 were significantly better when discharged because their sentence was completed. There were no deaths. Stern believed the success of the trial warranted making homeopathy available as a regular part of the hospital service, but allopathic agitation succeeded in obtaining a government decree forbidding it. Reasons given include the unsuitability of homeopathy to treat the conditions which Stern was curing, and the cost of building a new clinic and funding homeopathic treatment. Stern points out that the building already existed, and the salary of a homeopath was less than a quarter of the amount saved by using homeopathic medicines.

7.2.2. St Petersburg 1847–54: general

In an article on the state of homeopathy in Russia, Johannsen (1848) wrote that the new system suffered no discrimination there, and doctors were free to practise it, unlike in several other European countries. Although there were few medical services of either school, homeopathy appeared to be particularly popular with the large estate owners, who purchased medicines in bulk from the two licensed suppliers. As an example of the lack of discrimination in Russia, Johannsen mentions that an official in the Ministry of the Interior had wished to devote the Women's Hospital in St Petersburg to homeopathy. However, the Minister believed that it would be more useful if the 100 beds were divided equally between homeopathy and allopathy, so that a valid comparison could be made. Johannsen gives brief details of the experiment which had been going on for 2 years at the time of writing. It is clear that a great deal of effort had been expended to ensure a fair trial, in contrast to nearly all the previous studies in Europe.

Boyanus (1882) allows the proponent to be identified as Dr. Vladimir Dahl (whose conversion to homeopathy in the 1830s is mentioned below in Ch. 8), employed in the Ministry of Interior from 1841–49. The pro-homeopathic Minister was Count Lev Perovsky, and the homeopathic trialist was Dr Stender, assisted by Drs Lindgren, Johansen, Rosa, Gastfreund and Villers. The large-scale trial took place over 8 years, and as well as crude mortality rates, average length of stay and drug costs were computed. Table 7.2 (under 7.2.5 below) gives a tabulated comparison with a similar large-scale trial in Paris. Unlike that trial, no details of the homeopathic prescriptions are available, and Boyanus claimed that Stender's homeopathy was compromised by his desire to avoid conflict with officialdom.

7.2.3. Paris 1847–49: pneumonia

Jean-Paul Tessier (1811–62), a former student of the physiologist François Magendie (1783–1855) and the surgeon Guillaume Dupuytren (1777–1835) – and apparently the favourite of the latter, who left him a medical legacy in his will (Milcent 1862) – was one of the most highly regarded younger members of the orthodox Paris school when he began his exploration of homeopathy in 1846 or 1847. This was more than a decade after interest in testing homeopathy had died down in Parisian allopathic circles, although the therapy itself continued to win converts all over France (Garden 1992). In fact, Tessier had been advised to investigate homeopathy by Magendie, just as William Henderson (1810–72) had by his teacher John Abercrombie (1780–1844), in Edinburgh.[20]

Tessier published the report of his consecutive case series in the treatment of pneumonia and cholera after 3 years of research (Tessier 1850). There he recounts with great thoroughness and precision the steps he took in his evaluation of homeopathy and its eventual incorporation into his hospital practice. Beginning with a preliminary study of the general principles from the works of Hahnemann and his disciples, he moved on to accounts of treatments for specific illnesses. After he had 'grasped the spirit' of the new doctrine he began a 6-month test of the medicines to ascertain their safety and biological activity, on patients who he was sure would not be harmed by their use. Although he

[20] Henderson was the second Professor of Pathology at Edinburgh, and a pioneer microscopist. His researches included the first minute examination of the lung in pneumonia (1841), and he is credited with distinguishing typhus from relapsing fever in 1843 (Comrie 1932, 2, p. 623). He published details of 500 cases that he had treated homeopathically (Henderson 1845), causing one of the biggest storms in British medical life before or since, and was nearly forced from his chair. Nicholls (1988) describes the affair in detail. Only the fact that his case series was retrospective prevents its inclusion in this review.

became convinced of the activity and harmlessness of the ultramolecular homeopathic medicines after a few days, he continued the experiments for the full 6 months he had originally planned, in both acute and chronic cases. Only after this period did he feel able to begin his evaluation of the '*therapeutic* value' [original stress] of homeopathy.

He says that he chose pneumonia for the first prospective series because it was a well-known, unambiguous disease with clear diagnosis and prognosis. Although there are now many identifiable etiological factors, Tessier's description fits 'classical' community pneumonia from *Streptococcus pneumoniae* infection, which still accounts for 50% of cases in the UK (Davies 1990). In the 1840s the standard therapy consisted of up to 4 bleedings, blistering with vesicants, and dosing with antimony tartrate. His cautious approach was to substitute homeopathic *Phosphorus* for antimony, while leaving the other elements of the treatment unchanged. When he found that this was successful in every case, he began to reduce the number of bleedings, one at a time, until it was evident that they could be stopped altogether without detriment to the patient. After this he moved to purely homeopathic treatment.

The main medicines used by Tessier in individualized treatment were *Aconitum napellus*, *Bryonia alba*, *Phosphorus*, *Sulphur*, *Atropa belladonna*, *Arsenicum album* and *Iodum*, given in centesimal potencies – 6, 12, 15, 18, 24 and 30. Medication was usually administered as 4–6 globules dissolved in 4 oz filtered water, one teaspoonful hourly for 2 or 3 hours, following Hahnemann's latest instructions (see Ch. 8). *Aconitum* was given as one drop of C6 medicating tincture.

The case histories and assessment of the 41 patients treated purely homeopathically are given in detail. To counter bias in reporting the effects of treatment, Tessier arranged for the observations and reports to be made by two allopathic interns, Timbart and Guyton.

Tessier anticipated the argument that the same results would have been obtained from expectant treatment (no treatment except ordinary nursing care). He admits that there were no available statistics of mortality under expectant treatment to compare with those he had produced for homeopathy, but he rejects the argument on the basis of five observations:

1. In every case, the illness progressively worsened until the moment treatment began.
2. Soon after treatment began, a predictable homeopathic aggravation was experienced, of generally less than 24 hours duration, followed by rapid remission. Sometimes remission began within a few hours without aggravation.

3. *Bryonia* had an extraordinary effect on pulse rate, which could drop 20 or 30 beats from one day to the next.
4. Not a single old person died, even though they might have had pneumonia for a week before seeking help, or have reached the stage when consolidation was inevitable. In fact, old people recovered scarcely more slowly than the others.
5. Suppuration did not occur in any patient who had not presented with it, and it was arrested in most of those who did, with one exception (excluding the two terminal cases).

Tessier concluded that homeopathy appeared to be equally beneficial as regards the symptoms, progression and duration of pneumonia, and reasonably called for the method to be tested further in the crucible of observation and experiment. He also provided a case control: the statistics collected by Louis (1835) on the mortality of pneumonia in institutional care in Paris at that time had shown that a death rate of one in three could be expected with orthodox treatment. Tessier included in his series two cases that were terminal on admission and which he felt should have fallen outside the conditions of the experiment. Without them, there would have been only one death to report, but nevertheless, three deaths from 41 cases under homeopathic treatment was still less than 7.5%.

7.2.4. Paris 1849: cholera

Tessier (1850) next presented a consecutive series of the first 20 cholera cases he had treated. In all he saw nearly 100 cases in the 1849 epidemic, and compared his mortality rate with that in the allopathic wards in the same hospital. Although the homeopathic mortality rate was 10% lower, his results do not approach those found elsewhere. Reasons for this may include Tessier's unfamiliarity with the disease, and his use of potencies (C3 and C6) that, although lower than those that had worked so well in pneumonia, were higher than used elsewhere in cholera (see 7.3.2 Generalizability). His account is mainly important for the accurate clinical picture of cholera he gave.

7.2.5. Paris 1849–51: general

Tessier's experiments in pneumonia and cholera led to a large-scale prospective comparison of homeopathy and allopathy (Tessier 1852). The trial also took place at the Sainte-Marguerite Hospital, and pragmatically attempted to compare and evaluate homeopathy and allopathy as complete systems of internal medicine, rather than limiting the field of action to specific conditions.

The trial is historically remarkable because of the means used to avoid allocation bias. As seen in Ch. 6, allopathic doctors had generally assigned whom they liked to homeopathic treatment, but the potential for manipulation was minimized during this trial. One in 5 patients could be selected by either the allopathic and homeopathic doctor, but only in the presence of the other and, crucially, for treatment in their own ward, not that of their opposite number. More importantly, the great majority of patients were independently assigned to treatment. Each morning the central hospital administration of Paris received a list of available beds at the suburban hospital. New patients were allocated to a ward of 100 homeopathic or 99 allopathic beds strictly on the basis of the first empty bed; and the hospital administrators made clear at the time that 'the test of the two methods takes place as far as possible under the same conditions' (Gallavardin 1860). Reference was made to this arrangement in the medical press. A leading article on the front page of the *Union Médicale* for 8 December 1849 expressed outrage that patients were being sent by the central bureau to Sainte-Marguerite, where a doctor employed by the administration was 'openly practising homeopathy' (Editorial 1849).

As well as the quasi-randomization, several other features are noteworthy for the time. The trial was conducted over 3 years (1849–51), accepted more than 8000 patients, and used objective outcomes including costings for drugs and medical supplies as well as rates of bed occupancy and mortality. The administration reported a higher throughput and lower mortality rate in the homeopathic ward, for a hundredth of the cost in medical supplies, paralleling and improving on the results of the St Petersburg trial, as shown in Table 7.2.

Table 7.2 St. Petersburg 1847–54, Paris 1849–51. Large-scale pragmatic economic evaluations of classical homeopathy vs allopathy

Trialist **Dates**	**Hospital**	**N († or case-mortality)** **Mean days of bed occupancy** **Total trial drug cost (mean cost per patient)**	
		Homeopathic	Allopathic
Stender 1847–54	Women's Hospital, St Petersburg	• 5999 (756 † or 12.6%) • 24.75 d • 930 roubles (0.15 r)	• 2789 (413 † or 14.8%) • 27.5 d • 5600 roubles (2.01 r)
Tessier 1849–51	Sainte-Marguerite, Paris	• 4663 (399 † or 8.6%) • 23 d • <300 francs (<0.06 fr)	• 3724 (411 † or 11.0%) • 29 d • 23,552 francs (6.32 fr)

7.2.6. Vienna 1850–59: pneumonia

As well as external comparisons, there were questions of homeopathic method that required answers. For instance, the homeopathic community itself was aware that internal arguments about the activity of high potencies could not be resolved on the basis of conflicting and subjective accounts of success and failure from proponents or opponents. It even seemed that the higher potencies were more effective in pneumonia, but less so in cholera. A protracted interrupted time-series study comparing the relative efficacy of molecular and ultramolecular potencies, particularly in pneumonia, was carried out at Leopoldstadt Hospital, Vienna, from 1850 to 1859 by the doctors Casper and Wurmb (Eidherr 1862). During three consecutive 3-year periods, a single potency only was used in the trial: D30 from 1850–52; D6 from 1853–55; and D15 from 1856–59. The outcomes measured were the classical diagnostic stages of infiltration, resolution and exudation, as well as total length of stay. The individual patient data was tabulated, and mean times for each group calculated, as shown in Table 7.3. These appear to be inversely related to the potency used: the higher the potency, the speedier the recovery. The argument that the results may be biased because the trialists would have become better at prescribing over time seems invalid: the best results were obtained in the first period, the least good in the second, with the third intermediate. Interestingly, the experimenters were low potency prescribers by persuasion, and the superiority of higher potencies in pneumonia went against their assumptions, although it confirmed Tessier's findings. The trial was impressive enough for it to be cited by the low potency advocate Hughes (1893: 89) as evidence of the biological activity of ultramolecular potencies. (See also Ch. 4.)

Table 7.3 Vienna, pneumonia 1850–59. Results of prospective comparison of 3 potencies of indicated medicines: mean time in days to clinical stages of pneumonia

Years	Potency	N	Infiltration	Resolution start	Resolution complete	Infiltration signs gone	Exudation signs gone	Length of stay
1850–2	D30	55	3.0	3.0	4.9	7.1	12.3	11.3
1853–5	D6	31	4.1	3.5	6.9	9.3	20.5	19.5
1856–9	D15	54	3.0	3.2	6.3	10.3	18.1	14.6

7.2.7. London 1854: scarlet fever prevention

The homeopathic recommendation that belladonna could be used to treat the 'mild smooth scarlet fever of Sydenham' (Hahnemann 1801b) was taken up in medicine generally – Hufeland even wrote a literature review of case series that appeared to support the hypothesis. It was also believed to have a preventive effect, although Hahnemann's strictures about the uselessness of specifics that had not been worked out on the basis of the symptomatology of each fresh epidemic were forgotten. The allopath T.G. Balfour tested the prophylactic virtues of belladonna during an outbreak of scarlatina at the Chelsea Royal Military Asylum (West 1854). He assembled a group of boys who had probably not had the disease and dosed every alternate one, although nothing is known about the preparation or form of the medicine. Only two cases occurred in each group, and Balfour used the trial to make the methodological point that if he had not alternated but given belladonna to all he would probably have erroneously attributed the small number of cases to successful treatment. Clinically, he drew the lesson that the trial could show little about the efficacy of belladonna because it was clear that the epidemic was on the wane by the time the experiment was conducted. This reasonable interpretation stands in marked contrast to the conclusion of the epidemiologist and statistician W.A. Guy (1860). In the fifth of his Croonian Lectures on medical statistics, Guy gratuitously called Hahnemann's sanity or honesty into question, and cited Balfour's trial as all the refutation that was needed to demolish anything as fanciful as a homeopathic hypothesis.

7.2.8. Marseilles 1854: cholera

In 1853, Chargé had reported the success of homeopathy in treating cholera in Lyons. The following year, it was decided to compare the two schools during an outbreak in Marseilles. Unfortunately, the 1854 outbreak seems to have been more virulent than the previous year, and as in previous trials (see Ch. 6), the homeopaths withdrew after only 3 days complaining of exceptional allocation bias at the Hôtel-Dieu: 21 dead from 26 treated would have been a bad result whatever method used, and Chargé (1855) seems to have been expected to treat only patients in a state of collapse. The validity of the comparison is further undermined by the revelation a few years later that the allopaths in this trial had in fact used well-known homeopathic medicines (Sirus-Pirondi 1859): indeed they claimed the most effective of their treatments were ipecacuanha, nux vomica, chamomilla and veratrum album – unused in the allopathic treatment of cholera at that time, as the London returns make clear (see 7.2.9) – as well as camphor, although nothing is known of how the medicines were prepared or the mode of administration. This appears to be the first wholesale appropriation of homeopathic materia medica by allopathy, a phenomenon generally associated with the 1870s and later, as discussed in Ch. 3.

7.2.9. London 1854: cholera

The General Board of Health under Sir Edwin Chadwick (1801–90) had been a non-governmental organization. Chadwick's crusade for administrative reform as the necessary springboard to bring about improved public health, allied with a zealous lack of tact, had been enormously unpopular with the laissez-faire elements in mid nineteenth-century British society, and led to his removal in August 1854 (Lewis 1952). The Board was reconstituted, with greatly reduced powers, as a government ministry on August 12, on the lines of the Poor Law Board. In charge was Sir Benjamin Hall (1802–67) – a Member of Parliament and bureaucrat of the class that had provoked Chadwick's scorn, and previously known mainly as a supporter of mild ecclesiastical reform. Incongruously, given this inauspicious background, Hall's first act on August 12 was to set in motion a coordinated public health and medical response to the 1853–54 cholera epidemic then in full spate. By September, Hall had gone on to commission a major epidemiological survey of the epidemic. He was also anxious to know which treatments were most efficacious. His letter circulated at the beginning of September to all practitioners appearing in the Medical Register for 1854 states that he had established a Medical Council 'representing all branches of the medical profession' because of

> the great want that is now felt of some systematic record of cases of choleraic disease, their treatment, and results, with a view to determine, in so far as may be possible, the best mode of meeting this formidable epidemic. (Medical Council 1855b suppl. I: 67)

The Council consisted of 12 members nominated by Hall, the Royal Colleges and the Society of Apothecaries, under the chairmanship of John Ayrton Paris, President of the Royal College of Physicians. Three committees would facilitate the survey: Scientific Inquiries, to look into the nature, extent and probable causes of cholera; Treatment, to assess the relative advantages of rival methods; and Foreign Correspondence, to glean relevant information from scientists abroad.

But it was Hall, not the profession, who produced the first draft of the form used to collect the data required for a comparative clinical evaluation, as his letter of September 6 shows (General Board of Health, 1854–55). All probable cases seen in London hospitals were diagnosed and entered into newly printed record sheets. These used a 5-level clinical staging: Form A was reserved for levels 1 and 2 ('mild' and 'choleraic' diarrhea), while cases classed as cholera proper were entered into Form B – levels 3 and 4 were for those admitted without or with 'collapse' respectively, and level 5 for cholera terminating in 'consecutive fever' (Medical Council 1855b suppl. I: 80ff). As well as biographical data and dates of admission, details of previous treatments were noted. Cases could move from one form to the other, an arrangement which allowed an analysis of the progression of the disease and assessment of response to prescriptions made in hospital. The Medical Inspectorate set up in August was also required to visit each hospital regularly during the epidemic to ensure that accurate and truthful records were maintained, and to verify the diagnoses.

The Medical Council's report devoted much of its analysis to the possible causes of cholera: meteorological factors were most prominent, in keeping with the prevalent (pre-Hahnemannian) miasmatic theory of noxious vapours (Medical Council 1855a). The state of the water supply was also examined, and recommendations made for improving its quality.[21] As the report made clear, the historic importance of the treatment evaluation was not lost on the Medical Council:

[21] Remarkably, considering the priority usually given to Robert Koch's 1883 discovery, the report presented evidence from the microbiologist and food safety expert Arthur Hill Hassall of 'myriads of vibriones ... in every drop of every sample of rice-water discharge', on the soiled clothing and bed linen of cholera victims, and in the water supply (Medical Council 1854–55: 289ff). One of Hassall's illustrations, Plate 26, Rice water evacuation of cholera, (ibid. following p. 90) is an engraving of a composite slide showing shreds of muscle fibre, mucus and other fragments (x 220) surrounded by many vibrios singly and clumped together (x 350); other plates clearly distinguish the much smaller vibrio from countless other unicellular organisms found in the water supply. There were two reasons why Hassall and the Medical Council considered and rejected the vibrio as a causal factor: it was believed to be a *product* of enteric decomposition; and it was also found in samples from those who had died from other diseases (ibid.: 56). The understanding that the cholera vibrio was (a) the pathogen, and (b) must be present in the gut in sufficient numbers to poison its host lay in the future.

> The duties of the Treatment Committee consisted … in the invention of a mode by which the individual experience of practitioners might be brought under one comprehensive view, and thus has the science of statistics, for the first time, been applied on a large scale to medical treatment. (Medical Council 1855c: 7)

The tables presented in the report showed that 46% of those treated as in-patients or out-patients in London hospitals had died in the epidemic, and that treatment of whatever kind had been largely useless: the expectation of mortality in untreated cholera was approximately 50%, then as now (Medical Council 1855b suppl. II, table I).

The epidemic is best remembered for the activity of John Snow (1813–58), epidemiologist and pioneer of anaesthesia, whose theory that cholera was waterborne had been published after the 1848 epidemic (Snow 1849). In 1854 he visited the epicentre of the new outbreak, the Golden Square area of Soho where 500 deaths occurred in 2 weeks. As well as his celebrated removal of the Broad Street pump handle, he began correlating the pattern of mortality with the water supply to each house. It could not be denied that the Southwark and Vauxhall Company supplied water full of untreated sewage, or that the mortality rate in the homes it supplied was eight or nine times that of the homes in the same area supplied by the Lambeth Company – which had begun to draw its water from higher up the Thames. Nevertheless, Snow's empirically plausible explanation of a waterborne 'cholera poison' was still rejected in 1855 by the Committee for Scientific Inquiries. This was in spite of William Farr (1807–83) – one of Hall's appointees to the Medical Council – having written not long before in his official report on the 1848–49 epidemic that Snow's was 'in many respects the most important theory that has been propounded' (Farr 1852: lxxiv).

By coincidence the London Homoeopathic Hospital in Golden Square had been set up as a charitable foundation in 1849 by the many well-connected and aristocratic patrons of homeopathy, and had opened its doors in 1850. During the 1854 epidemic it was decided to waive the usual requirement of letters of recommendation, and to turn the tiny 30-bed hospital over to the treatment of the 'indigent poor' of the district. The hospital had to make several requests to be sent the forms to make the official returns, and even after it succeeded found its returns were omitted from the report of the Medical Council. The report listed the names of those who had contributed returns, and pointed out that:

> Among the names occur some of homoeopathic practitioners, from whom returns were received; but the Committee for Scientific Inquiries desire it to be

> understood that none of these communications have been used in the construction of the report. (Medical Council 1855b suppl. I: 68)

This omission was raised in a parliamentary question from Lord Robert Grosvenor and the matter was laid bare in the extensive correspondence that ensued (House of Commons 1854–55). Asked by Hall to explain its suppression of the homeopathic results, the Council's chairman[1] reported the unanimous resolution of the gentlemen of the Medical Council:

> That by introducing the returns of homoeopathic practitioners, they would not only compromise the value and utility of their averages of cure, as deduced from the operation of known remedies, but they would give an unjustifiable sanction to an empirical practice alike opposed to the maintenance of truth and to the progress of science. (ibid.: 194)

As noted in Ch. 2, in the mid nineteenth century the term 'empirical' still had a pejorative connotation. At the same time, useless or dangerous allopathic treatments were sanctioned by virtue of the categories they were held to belong to: calomel, chalk, ether and castor oil acquired therapeutic dignity, if not efficacy, when classed respectively as 'alterative', 'astringent', 'stimulant' or 'eliminant' (Medical Council 1854–55d) – the very same rationalist terms satirized half a century earlier by Hahnemann (1801d).

The returns from the homeopathic hospital in Golden Square showed a mortality rate in both Forms A and B decidedly below that obtained elsewhere in London, and in line with the homeopathic results reported in Europe since the 1832 pandemic. The Medical Council's suppression of the superior results of the heterodox treatment ironically undermined its intended outcome: the homeopathic returns were then formally published in far greater detail than the allopathic statistics, in a Parliamentary Return of May 1855, ensuring their survival long into the future (House of Commons 1854–55). A comparison of the results is shown in Table 7.4, broken down by clinical stage, and it can be seen that fewer died in each stage under homeopathy. The Medical Council report includes a few extra-metropolitan results for stages 4–5 only (underlined in the table) making it impossible to separate the London returns, but since the provincial mortality rate of 45.6% was virtually the same as the metropolitan rate of 46.02%, the comparison is informative.

[22] Paris was already well-known as a vitriolic opponent of homeopathy. Previously, when Frederic Hervey Foster Quin (1799–1878), who introduced homeopathy to Britain, tried to join the Athenaeum Club, Paris had organized a notorious blackball.

Table 7.4 London, cholera 1854 Diarrhea (Form A) and cholera (Form B) cases and mortality 1 July 1853 to 31 December 1854 from completed hospital returns

	Homeopathic hospital			Allopathic hospitals		
	N	†	%	N	†	%
Form A Stages 1–2	481	1	0.2	17460	109	0.6
Form B Stages 3–5	87	16	18.4	3188	1467	46.0
Stages 4–5 only	48	16	33.3	2672	1653	61.9

Sources:
Medical Council (1854–55b suppl. II, table III); House of Commons (1854–55)

Complete data are given for 568 individuals – identified by age, gender and occupation – treated by homeopathy during the general evaluation period, including prescriptions, with appended comments. From these it is possible to see that the doctors of the homeopathic hospital used a full range of individualized medicines such as *Veratrum album*, *Arsenicum album*, *Cuprum* and *Secale*, given singly. They were prepared according to the first British homeopathic pharmacopeia (Quin 1834), and were administered as drops of the first three decimal potencies repeated every 10, 15 or 30 minutes, or every 1, 2 or 4 hours. In addition, tincture of camphor (1 part to 6 of pure spirit) was prescribed in many cases at the beginning of treatment, a few drops every few minutes.

How valid are the homeopathic returns? Although the Inspector appointed for the district refused to visit, another commissioned Inspector, David Macloughlin, agreed – reluctantly, according to his unsolicited letter of 22 February 1855 to the Homoeopathic Hospital, included in the Parliamentary Return:

> You are aware that I went to your hospital prepossessed against the homoeopathic system; that you had in me, in your camp, an enemy rather than a friend, and that I must therefore have seen some cogent reason there, the first day I went, to come away so favourably disposed as to advise a friend to send a subscription to your charitable fund, …

As important as his prior hostility towards homeopathy was the fact that he had spent 20 years in India:

> I need not tell you that I have taken some pains to make myself acquainted with the rise, progress, and medical treatment of cholera, and … claim for myself some rights to be able to recognise the disease, and to know something of what the medical treatment ought to be; …

This experience makes his comments on the homeopathic results particularly valuable. He went on:

> That there may be no misapprehension about the cases I saw in your hospital. I will add, that all I saw were true cases of cholera, in the various stages of the disease; and that I saw several cases which did well under your treatment, which I have no hesitation in saying would have sunk under any other.

He concludes with what he had already told the homeopaths,

> and what I have told everyone with whom I have conversed, that although an allopath by principle, education and practice, yet was it the will of Providence to afflict me with cholera, and to deprive me of the power of prescribing for myself, I would rather be in the hands of a homoeopathic than an allopathic adviser.

In a postscript Macloughlin also mentions his research into the premonitory diarrhea of cholera. He had claimed for some years, against the opposition of the rest of the profession, that if treated early enough it could prevent development of full-blown cholera. Now there was renewed interest in his theory, and he had been asked to submit his work as a prize essay to the French Imperial Institute. Observing that all the homeopathic cases of cholera had suffered diarrhea first, he ensured in his essay that the homeopathic results were placed 'for accurate observation of the disease by the side of St Thomas's, St Bartholomew's, St Mary's, the Westminster and the University College hospitals' (House of Commons 1854–55: 93).

A possible objection to the comparison was that the allopaths only recorded the more serious cases; the homeopath Joseph Kidd made this point at a meeting of the British Homoeopathic Society at the time (cited in Leary 1987). Table 7.4 makes it clear that the proportion of Form B cases was similar under both systems: 18.1% in the homeopathic hospital, 18.3% in the others. Apart from the Inspector's testimony, and the comparable proportions of the clinical stages treated, another clue to the reliability of the homeopathic returns is their use of intention-to-treat as a fundamental principle: even patients who died in the street before admission were included as if they were homeopathic failures. This was not the policy of all London hospitals, some of which discharged hopeless cases to improve their own mortality rates, as Florence Nightingale objected a decade later in *Notes on Hospitals* (cited in Iezzoni 1996).

7.2.10. Glasgow 1870s: mixed fevers

James Compton Burnett (1840–1901) was a brilliant student with medical degrees from Vienna and Glasgow. During his internship at Barnhill Parochial Hospital and Asylum, Glasgow, he was in charge of a fever ward where children were admitted for assessment before being passed to other wards for treatment. Dissatisfied with allopathy, he read about homeopathy but was unable to believe the reports of its successes, and decided to expose it as a sham. *Aconitum napellus* appeared to be suitable for many of the fevers, and accordingly Burnett instructed the nursing sister to give Fleming's aconite tincture (a proprietary non-homeopathic dilution) to the boys on one side of the ward only, while the others received treatment as usual. The homeopathic group appeared to benefit, and Burnett continued the experiment for some time, always finding the same result. However, he arrived one morning to find that the boys on both sides of the ward appeared decidedly better than the previous evening. The sister explained that she had decided to bring the 'cruel experiment' to an end, and dosed both groups from 'Dr Burnett's Fever Bottle'. Burnett (1888) later recounted this anecdotally as the first of his *Fifty Reasons for Being a Homoeopath* – the name of the book in which he recorded his conversion from allopathy.

7.2.11. Chicago 1880–86: general

A randomized pragmatic trial was planned in the Cook County Hospital, Chicago, but the allopaths objected on the grounds that the patients might be assigned to an unwanted treatment. However, it was soon found that the patients did not know the difference between allopathy and homeopathy, so a compromise was reached involving alternate allocation. Two sets of results from two separate years show an approximate equivalence between the two methods. Unfortunately, nothing is known about the sort of homeopathy on offer, or the extent to which homeopathic medicines were used in the allopathic wards at this date.

7.3. Discussion

7.3.1. Planning and design

The traditional interpretation of the evolution of the clinical trial sees it as a product of the internal transformation of medicine from craft to science. Marks (1997) has challenged this notion – that the modern randomized clinical trial was solely a product of the medical profession's self-critical scientific advance – and put forward the idea that controlled trials assumed their pre-eminent position in the latter half of the twentieth century as much because of governmental and bureaucratic requirements designed to keep the medical profession in check. Whether ultimately accepted or not, Marks's thesis appears to find a remarkable pre-confirmation in the pragmatic homeopathic trials of the mid nineteenth century. Although homeopaths were vocal in their demands for statistical comparison of their results with allopathy, it is unlikely that the more important trials would have taken place without the active involvement and encouragement of hospital administrations or governments. Bureaucrats, commissioners and boards of guardians were often uninterested in the doctrinal component of the battle between the two principal medical systems of the day, and saw it as their duty to serve the best interests of their patients, and the communities which funded their hospitals.

In fact hospital statistics had been collected in Britain since the sixteenth century, often as a way of showing benefactors the value of their contributions (Iezzoni 1996). The comparisons of homeopathy and allopathy in the mid nineteenth century can now be seen as an interesting development in a long tradition of ad hoc cost-benefit analysis. This is true not only of trials in this review, but can be found in many other contemporary sources where comparisons were made retrospectively. For instance, an allopath alleged in a French political journal that the administrators of the hospital at Thoissey near Lyons were about to forbid a Dr Gastier from practising homeopathy there, as he had been doing since 1832. The hospital board, which included the mayor and priest of Thoissey, replied in a letter of 2 January 1846:

> We cannot remain silent about a purely gratuitous allegation, which supposes we do not know the limits of our competence … Hospital administrations exist to regulate the goods and revenues of these establishments, to see they are well kept, to ensure that each member of staff meets his obligations exactly, but not to order doctors how to practise … Our records attest that since Dr Gastier has practised here, the number of deaths relative to the number of admissions is less than before; that pharmacy expenses are almost zero; and the hospital ser-

> vice, simpler and more efficient, has been demonstrably improved. (cited in Gallavardin 1860: 28f)

It was clear to many such impartial administrations that homeopathic medicines cost a small fraction of allopathic drugs, yet seemed no less effective. The large trials in St Petersburg and Paris explicitly incorporated economic evaluation in their design, as shown in Table 7.2, and the later large trial in Chicago occurred after the hospital commissioners had already allowed homeopathy into the service in the belief that it would

> be beneficial in increasing the efficiency of the hospital work, and reducing very materially the expenditure for drugs and liquors. (Chicago Herald 1881)

Hospital boards also seem to have been aware of the need for impartial assignment of patients to treatments. The quasi-randomized allocation to the first empty bed in either ward at Sainte-Marguerite seems to have been an elegant pragmatic solution to something which might have posed problems for strict alternation or randomization, because of the reduced length of stay in the homeopathic ward. Opposition to pragmatic trials per se and to randomization came mainly from the allopaths: as noted, calls to halt Tessier's trial were prominently featured in the allopathic medical press; the Medical Council's Treatment Committee obstructed the London Homeopathic Hospital's request for the forms needed to return their results, and suppressed the returns once they were made; and a proposed randomized design in Chicago was abandoned because of allopathic protests. It would seem that allopaths were only in favour of trials of homeopathy when placebo was used as the comparator, rather than orthodox medicine (see Ch. 8). Nevertheless, the results in Paris so impressed the administrators that they allowed Tessier to continue – in the face of non-stop allopathic hostility – what became in effect a 15-year open trial of homeopathy, first in Sainte-Marguerite, then Beaujon and finally the Enfants Malades (Milcent 1862). As in Thoissey, the Paris hospital administration refused to participate in a professional dispute and answered the allopathic attacks solely by citing the mortality rates, bed occupancy and drug costs under the rival systems (as shown in Table 7.2). Moreover, they added,

> far from hindering medical freedom by forbidding M. Tessier to use homeopathy in his ward, we urge him to pursue his studies for the benefit of humanity. (Gallavardin 1860: 26)

7.3.2. Generalizability

Not all reports specify the type of homeopathy used, so it is impossible to comment on the validity of many results. Nevertheless, several of the studies are exemplary in this respect, including full details of the prescriptions made for each patient. Were the results found in these trials comparable with those found elsewhere? It would seem that in most cases they were. The pneumonia mortality rates reported in Paris and Vienna seem entirely representative: for instance, the London Homoeopathic Hospital returns for 1850–55 show the results of treatment and mortality in scores of conditions, from tuberculosis to heart disease, and only 3 of 60 pneumonia patients died (Editorial 1857). In other words, the most reliable evidence found in this review endorses a phenomenon reported throughout Europe and America, from many independent sources. Even opponents were forced to admit the startling efficacy of homeopathy in pneumonia (e.g. Routh 1852).

The cholera statistics appear equally plausible. Although Tessier had found that high potencies worked well in pneumonia – a phenomenon later confirmed by Casper and Wurmb in Vienna – their use in cholera was less successful. In fact, a consensus emerged among homeopaths to use low potencies and tinctures in cholera, as shown in the London returns. Why there should be such empirical differences in the efficacy of the potencies best adapted to different diseases has never been explained. Nevertheless, the London results happen to be the best controlled ones available, and occurred in the area of London where the epidemic hit hardest; there, treatment exclusively with low potencies achieved results that are in line with those reported by experienced practitioners elsewhere. The clinical staging of Forms A and B, and the testimony of an independent Inspector with expert knowledge of the disease, make it possible to conclude that these are among the most reliably diagnosed cholera cases of the time. More successful results reported elsewhere under homeopathy no doubt conflated full-blown cholera with less serious and earlier manifestations.

To what extent can the apparent superiority of the homeopathic results be attributed to the mere absence of harmful allopathic procedures, such as blood-letting, blistering and dosing with calomel? Cholera and pneumonia were homeopathic *causes célebres* of the day, and it is reasonable to use them here as test cases. The natural case fatality rate in untreated cholera remains close to 50%, the same as in the earliest untreated epidemics in nineteenth century (Gale 1959: 67f), and very close to the aggregated returns from British hospitals in 1854 under various forms of allopathic treatment (7.2.9). Louis (1835) found a case fatality rate in conventionally-treated pneumonia of >30%, and in the next 3 decades observational studies of no treatment other than nursing care showed similar losses (7.3.3).

Political will and public health measures consigned cholera to the history books well before the end of the century – in northern Europe at least – but accounts such as the *Report of the 13th Annual Meeting of the Children's Homoeopathic Dispensary (1927)* indicate that the apparent superiority of homeopathy in pneumonia was being demonstrated well into the twentieth century: deaths of children treated at the London Homoeopathic Hospital were still half of those elsewhere (Leary, Lorentzon, Bosanquet 1998). Not until 1938 and the introduction of sulphapyredine did orthodox treatment of pneumonia approach homeopathic rates of cure: 46% of those aged over 45 with the disease were still expected to die before then (Cruikshank 1942).

7.3.3. Reception

Allopathic attempts to prevent trials taking place, or to suppress results when these emerged, are the strongest evidence of the reluctance to allow the results of homeopathic treatment to influence the development of medical science.

Tessier's results were doubly embarrassing for allopathy: he was a highly respected allopath, and homeopathy had been declared to be a placebo. The earliest reactions to all homeopathic results in pneumonia, not just Tessier's, were to dispute the diagnosis. When this became impossible, and the positive results could be denied no longer, the only possible conclusion for sceptics – homeopathic efficacy being an impossible conclusion, of course – was that orthodox treatment actually killed patients who would survive without treatment. Tessier's former student Pierre Jousset (1862) tells us that in 1860 the Académie de Médecine even offered a prize for a study of expectant treatment in pneumonia. In response, Jousset republished Tessier's 1849 results plus 10 cases from the same series that had remained unpublished, along with a detailed account of several case series of expectant treatment drawn from the international literature. As Jousset showed, the trials of no treatment had failed completely to support the sceptical hypothesis: they had returned mortality rates of 31%, strictly comparable with the expected rate under allopathy.

As seen in the quotation from Shryock in the Introduction (7.1), this came against a background in which all sorts of statistical comparisons were emerging. What Shryock's Whiggish account of the canonical examples of statistics in the service of biomedical progress completely neglects to mention is the professional reaction that these comparisons attracted when changes in medical practice were indicated – ranging from tight-lipped denial to hysterical opposition. Louis's demonstration of the inefficacy of bloodletting was ignored – it was still recommended in pneumonia in the most authoritative textbooks in the twentieth century (e.g. Osler 1912: 99); and Semmelweis was sacked from his job in Vienna for showing that the unsterilized hands of surgeons fresh from dissecting cadavers were infecting the women they handled in the delivery room (Semmelweis 1861). Homeopathy was not alone in enraging the old guard.

Given the way medical historiography has evolved and the unreliability of nearly all external accounts of homeopathic treatment until very recently, it should be no surprise that of all mid nineteenth-century statistics, those from large successful homeopathic trials have been forgotten or are left out of accounts of the development of the clinical trial, or medicine in general. While Semmelweis is rightly honoured for reducing the mortality from puerperal fever from 18.27% to 1.27% in his clinic (ibid.: 170), the comparable homeopathic achievement in reducing the mortality in pneumonia from over 30% to around 5% or better is ignored. This is in marked contrast to the earlier invalid trials of homeopathy which are still held to have demonstrated the illusory nature of the therapy. Tellingly, the 1854 cholera treatment evaluation in London has even been recognized as a defining moment in the evolution of the clinical trial by Lilienfeld (1982), but the existence and suppression of the superior homeopathic results is not mentioned – presumably because they were unknown to him. It is doubly unfortunate that internal homeopathic accounts of the affair have tended to confuse the issue by attributing the suppression to the Board of Health, rather than the Medical Council which was in fact responsible (e.g. Mitchell 1975; Coulter 1977; Leary 1987).

The administrators of the Thoissey hospital made a further point about the regulation of professional medical practice in their eloquent dismissal of the claims of their allopathic detractor:

> Medicine is a liberal art, and at the same time perfectly liberal in its application. Never, and it is this which proves our point, never, at any time, in any country, under any regime, has the most absolute public power tried to forbid or dictate to doctors, this or that treatment … . (Gallavardin 1860: 29)

Predictably, homeopathy *had* been outlawed by imperial decree in Austria from 1819 onwards, a ban that was lifted only after Fleischmann's mortality rate at the Gumpendorf Hospital, Vienna, in the cholera epidemic of 1836 was half that of the allopaths. And even mid nineteenth-century liberal democracies could not prevent the rapidly professionalizing allopaths from conducting their own witchhunts. Serious embarrassment coupled with an inability to put patient care ahead of professional politics seem ultimately to have hardened allopathic opposition. In France, Tessier was ostracized and passed over for promotion in spite of his extraordinary single-handed achievements, and died a disappointed man (Milcent 1862). In Britain, the allopaths failed to get homeopathy outlawed in the Medical Act of 1858 despite some vitriolic lobbying – the memory of the cholera episode would still have been fresh in both Houses. Instead the British Medical Association imposed its own internal rules forbidding any member to practise homeopathy, or even to consult professionally with homeopaths. The American Medical Association was constituted in 1847 specifically to control and regulate medical practice in opposition to the recently formed homeopathic association, and imposed even more draconian restrictions on its members than the BMA's. Notorious incidents followed on both sides of the Atlantic. In 1865, the American Surgeon General narrowly escaped prosecution for saving the life of the Secretary of State (seriously wounded at the same time as the Lincoln assassination), having collaborated with a homeopath (Coulter 1973). And in 1881, during Disraeli's final illness, when Queen Victoria asked the leading allopathic chest physician Richard Quain to consult with the only doctor Disraeli had ever respected – the homeopath Joseph Kidd – Quain at first refused. The Queen's advisers forced him to reconsider by letting him believe he was guilty of disloyalty to the Crown, but he only gave way with the permission of his trade union leader, who allowed him to take the case on condition that Kidd signed a paper ceding responsibility to the allopath, and – implausibly – swearing that he had not used homeopathy to treat Disraeli (Buckle 1920: 609–611).

Homeopaths and their supporters continued to press the case for comparative trials, but were rebuffed. An offer of £5000 (equivalent to approximately £1 million today) was made by Major Vaughan Morgan in the 1860s to establish a homeopathic ward in a London hospital for 5 years, to allow a genuine prospective evaluation of the system. It was refused by St George's and every other hospital that it was subsequently offered to (Ameke 1885: 321). The public had little say in matters of professional conduct, and homeopathic practice came to mean professional suicide for all but the most dedicated or foolhardy doctors. Empirical statistics counted for as little as they had 50 years earlier when the *Bulletin Général de Thérapeutique* announced that the clinical results of homeopathy were irrelevant, however successful, because the end could not justify the means (Editorial 1834). The script could have been written by Molière: 'Better to die according to the rules, than to pull through against them.'[23]

---

[23] 'Il vaut mieux mourir selon les règles, que de réchapper contre les règles. ' *L'Amour Médecin* (II, v: 58–59).

8. Placebo controls – in trials and in practice, 1810–1920

Appeared as: Dean M.E. (2000). A homeopathic origin for placebo controls: 'An invaluable gift of God'. *Alternative Therapies in Health and Medicine.* 6(2): 58–66; Dean M.E. (2000). Debate over the history of placebos in medicine. *Alternative Therapies in Health and Medicine.* 6(4): 18–20.

Background: Placebo controls were used in drug trials by homeopaths well before they were considered necessary in orthodox medicine. This practice is acknowledged by medical historians, but is currently thought to have been prompted by prior external use of placebo controls to discredit the system.

Question: Is it possible to locate the origins of, and assign priority in, the use of placebos in homeopathic research?

Argument: The normative claim of external prompting is reexamined in the light of a comprehensive literature search for nineteenth-century homeopathic therapeutic trials and provings using placebo. Single-blind placebo controls, used in a similar manner today, are shown to have originated independently within homeopathy's own disciplinary matrix before the first external evaluations. They are the most likely source for the first allopathic placebo-controlled evaluations of homeopathy as well as later placebo-controlled crossover and parallel group experiments by homeopaths.

8.1. Introduction

'Placebo: A medicine having no pharmacological effect, but given for the purpose of pleasing or humoring the patient' (Jones, Hoerr, Osol 1949). The medical dictionary entry dates from 1949 when well-meaning fraud was still the conventional use for placebo, as it had been for centuries – for example in the treatment of troublesome patients, or to mask the lack of valid remedies in palliative care. The dictionary omits any mention of sham comparison treatments in clinical research, an evaluative use of placebo generally believed to have arisen only in the 1930s. It is true placebo controls were not common until the 1950s when randomization, blind assessment and statistical analysis finally came together to determine the form of the present-day clinical trial (Lilienfeld 1982), but in fact blind assessment has been traced back to the emergence of scientific pharmacology in the nineteenth century, as Haas and colleagues (1959) showed in a comprehensive early review of placebo research. A more recent general history of placebo controls and blind assessment by Kaptchuk (1998a) cites even earlier placebo tests of new therapies in the late eighteenth and early nineteenth centuries, and advances the theory that they were first introduced to expose allegedly quack systems, such as mesmerism and homeopathy. This helped to define and legitimate the territorial claim made by orthodox medicine, at a time when it often did more harm than good, and was losing face (and patients) to novel and more attractive therapies (Daniels 1971: 171ff).

Although the early adoption of placebo controls in trials by homoeopaths has been cited in support of a progressive outlook (Kaptchuk 1997), the same author has also suggested that they probably incorporated placebo in response to external rather than internal pressure (Kaptchuk 1998a). The evidence for this normative hypothesis consists of studies using placebo in parallel with homeopathy, or alone (as a presumed equivalent), conducted by sceptics and critics of homeopathy, dating from as early as 1834.

As an assessment of the validity of this argument, an account is given here of all published nineteenth-century placebo-controlled therapeutic trials of homeopathic medicines, or 'homeopathic' placebos without active controls found in the comprehensive literature search. As described in Ch. 5, the general literature search was widened in this instance to include any nineteenth-century placebo-controlled therapeutic trials or drug-tests. The review presented here is followed by earlier evidence which showed that the comparative and evaluative use of placebo had arisen and was well-accepted within homeopathy's own disciplinary matrix before the first external evaluations took place – and is still used in an identical manner today.

8.2. Placebo-controlled provings

As already noted (see Ch. 3), Hahnemann came to use higher potencies in treatment during the 1820s, and standardized this at C30 in 1829. Crucially, he also standardized the proving potency at the same level, and the symptoms from these ultramolecular tests were included in the materia medica without supporting evidence from material doses. Since healthy provers were presumably still as insensitive compared to the sick as Hahnemann had found originally, the rationale for this leap of faith was elusive to some homoeopaths and most sceptics.

Their doubts were compounded by Hahnemann's later bad habit of deriving indications from medicines tested on sick patients rather than healthy volunteers, which led to the inclusion in the materia medica of some symptoms obviously due to prior illness and not the test substance (Hughes 1893). As a result, placebos were introduced into homeopathic trials. The five placebo-controlled provings found in the literature search are summarized in Table 8.1, and discussed below.

Table 8.1 Placebo-controlled provings, 1834–1901

Report	Provers	Design	Proving drug	Placebo	Result
Seidlitz, 1834	Hospital staff	Crossover s-b	Carbo-veg C30	Similar tablets	0
Löhner, 1835	General public	Quasi-random parallel d-b	Natrum-mur liquid potency	Snow water	n/a
Wesselhoeft, 1877	Medical students	Time series and crossover s-b	Carbo-veg potencies	Identical powders	0
Potter & Storke, 1880	Homeopaths	Parallel d-b	Aconite C30	Identical tablets	null
Bellows, 1906	Homeopaths and medical students	Parallel d-b	Belladonna ø and potencies	Identical tincture and powders	+ (ø) 0 (potencies)

Key: d-b, s-b, double- or single-blind.; +, 0, – placebo-controlled results

The earliest account of any placebo-controlled proving that historians have so far found must be counted as evidence for the normative hypothesis. It took place at the Naval Hospital, St Petersburg in January 1834. Seidlitz, the allopathic physician in charge, had been contacted by Dr Dahl (see 7.2.1) about the new therapy taking root in Russia. Seidlitz (1834) countered Dahl's enthusiasm by offering to demonstrate the illusory nature of homeopathy, and asked a Dr Gödechen to give potentized *Carbo vegetabilis* (vegetable charcoal) or dummy tablets to healthy medical staff. Each prover received a verum tablet once daily for a few days followed by placebo. The tablets were all dispensed single-blind by Gödechen, and according to Seidlitz's account the appearance or non-appearance of symptoms was unrelated to whether placebo or verum was taken, but correlated with the psychological characteristics of the prover. Seidlitz later repeated the experiment but dispensed the tablets himself, and got substantially the same results. His report is sarcastic throughout, so the objectivity of his data collection and reporting cannot be taken for granted, any more than in his abusive account of the 1829–30 clinical trial by Herrmann, also in St Petersburg (Seidlitz 1833) (see Ch. 6, as well as 8.4.3 below).

Further external pressure on homeopathy to adopt placebo controls came in a double-blind test of potentized *Natrum muriaticum* (common salt) in liquid form with distilled water as control from 1835. It was not organized by allopaths but by G. Löhner (1835), a journalist in Nuremberg, and Kaptchuk (1998a) notes that the atmosphere seems to have resembled a séance more than a sober scientific experiment. This inconclusive study even attempted random assignment, by haphazardly shuffling the verum and placebo vials.

In contrast to these external evaluations, the scientific importance and quality of the work of the Vienna Provings Union, in the 1840s, was favourably appraised more than a century later in Haas and colleagues' (1959) review of historical and contemporary placebo research referred to above. The Vienna experiments included single- and double-blind tests of many potencies of the same medicines in the same subjects with washout periods of no treatment. Their reprovings (of *Aconite*, *Bryonia*, *Colocynth*, *Natrum muriaticum*, *Sulphur* and *Thuja*) and primary provings (of *Argentum nitricum*, *Coccus cacti* and *Kali bichromicum*) are preserved in Hughes and Dakes's *Cyclopaedia of Drug Pathogenesy* (1886–91), an important late nineteenth-century recension of the homeopathic materia medica which aimed to include only reliable proving and toxicological symptoms: high potency data was admitted on condition that it was supported by information derived from more material doses.

Following this type of internally-generated comparison of different potencies and no treatment, homeopaths elsewhere began the regular employment of placebo controls in provings, well before they were considered necessary in medicine generally. This seems to have started at Boston University Medical School in 1877. At that time it was a homeopathic institution, and Conrad Wesselhoeft Sr, a professor of materia medica, performed a single-blind crossover trial specifically 'for the purpose of demonstrating the necessity of countertests in drug-proving' (Wesselhoeft 1877). His students knew they were reproving *Carbo-veg*, but not that some of them received unmedicated lactose to begin with. There is little quantitative or qualitative difference between the symptoms produced in the two phases of the crossover, and 50 provers failed to show any symptoms at all.

This experiment was probably the inspiration for the Milwaukee Academy of Medicine's double-blind placebo-controlled reproving of *Aconitum napellus* C30 (monkshood) in 1879–80 (Potter and Storke 1880). The 25 homeopathic physicians who volunteered as provers were invited to distinguish between vials of verum and identical placebo; only nine replied, none correctly. However, a contemporary comment by the homeopath Samuel Swan (1888) about idiosyncrasy and provings is still relevant: 'In this varying sensitiveness of individuals to different potencies and different drugs lay the entire failure of the Milwaukee Test.' The Milwaukee Academy also conducted a similar therapeutic trial mentioned below.

During the 1880s, placebo controls were used increasingly, as the following references to saccharum lactis (milk sugar) in zinc provings indicate. They are quoted here as they appeared in the *Cyclopaedia of Drug Pathogenesy* (Hughes & Dake 1886–91):

> JOSEPH RHODES, aet. 24, health good. Proved 3x [D3] trit. [iodide] in 2 gr. powders. 1st, 2nd and 4th d.—Took powder in m., which caused temporary nausea (as sac. lac. does), soon relieved by food. On latter d. repeated dose at 3 p.m., when nausea was followed by burning in stomach and cramp-like pains in bowels. These soon passed off while walking. Doses were repeated on 6th and again on 19th d., with no further effect. (Trans. of Amer. Inst., 1888: 167.)
>
> CHAS. H. WELLS, aet. 29, health good. Sac. lac. test negative. Took several 3 gr. doses of 6x [D6] trit. of phosphate without effect. Then, after an interval of two weeks, began the 2x [D2] trit. On 1st d., at 9.30 a.m., he took 3 gr., and soon began belching a gas resembling sulphuretted hydrogen. At 1 p.m. repeated dose, which made belching more marked, and soon slight disturbance of stomach bordering on nausea was experienced. Later, felt weakness in bowels, as if diarrhoea would come on. Some confusion of ideas. 2nd d.—Passed comfortable n. At 5 p.m. took 3 gr., and soon experienced the belching; then nausea and a diarrhoeic stool ensued, with confusion of mind. (Trans. of Hom. Med. Soc. of Pennsylvania, 1889: 202.)

These low-potency reprovings support Hahnemann's much earlier findings published in *Chronic Diseases* (1828–30, iii), and it is worth noting that gastric irritation, vomiting and diarrhoea are acknowledged side-effects of present-day oral zinc salts (Fastner 1980). Paradoxical benefit from zinc sulphate in the treatment of benign gastric ulcer has also been found in a double-blind placebo-controlled trial (Morgan 1978).

The culmination of the late nineteenth-century American efforts to eliminate suggestion was undoubtedly a multicentre double-blind placebo-controlled crossover reproving of *Atropa belladonna* (deadly nightshade) in molecular and ultramolecular potencies, which took place between 1901 and 1903 (Bellows 1906). It provided some confirmation for the accepted *Belladonna* drug picture, mainly from provers taking large doses of mother tincture.

8.3. Therapeutic trials involving placebo

8.3.1. Placebo-controlled trials

The second trial by Herrmann in St Petersburg in 1829–30 has been discussed in Ch. 6 (Lichtenstädt 1832). As well as comparison with the usual allopathic treatment, another control group was established by the trial supervisor, Gigler: patients received expectant treatment – nursing care, tisanes, baths and so on. This group was also prescribed placebos consisting of such things as bread pills or lactose powders. The significance of this is discussed below (8.3.2).

Following Herrmann's second trial, no further deliberate parallel or cross-over placebo controls in therapeutic trials of homeopathy were found before 1879, when the Milwaukee Academy of Medicine (at the same time as its proving referred to above) asked homeopaths in private practice to distinguish identical vials of verum and placebo by assessment of their patients' response to treatment (Potter & Storke 1880). Out of 47 physicians who agreed to participate, only one returned a result – correct as it happened.

8.3.2. Trials of placebo without homeopathic treatment

There were at least two early prospective placebo trials considered by opponents and sceptics of the day to provide evidence against homeopathy, included here even though they did not in fact involve treatment with homeopathic medicines. Three such trials were found altogether, and are listed in Table 8.2.

Table 8.2 Trials of placebo alone as presumed or rhetorical equivalent of homeopathy

Report	Condition	Design	Equivalence	Control	Result
Pigeaux, 1834; Trousseau & Gouraud, 1834	Mixed	Case series	Presumed	None	n/a
Forbes, 1846	Diarrhea	Parallel s-b p-c	Rhetorical	Allopathy	no difference
Lisle, 1861	Mixed	Case report	Rhetorical	None	n/a

Key: s-b, single-blind; p-c, placebo-controlled

At the Hôtel-Dieu, Paris, in 1834, Armand Trousseau (1801–67) and colleagues gave an uncontrolled single-blind placebo treatment to patients with various illnesses (Pigeaux 1834; Trousseau and Gouraud 1834). It consisted of bread pills, labelled as if they contained one or two decillionths of a grain of valerian, a herb popular in the folk and orthodox treatment of anxiety and depression. As Hughes (1893) notes, it was hardly ever used in homeopathy, although *Valeriana* had been one of Hahnemann's earliest provings to be published (Hahnemann 1805b). Some patients responded to the bread pills and others did not, although there is no indication whether any reported symptomatic improvements – in tuberculosis for instance – were more than transient. Trousseau seems genuinely to have believed this was a valid test of homeopathy – a system whose absurdity he was in no doubt of. It has been pointed out that he was equally capable of errors of design and inference in his own sphere of orthodox pharmacology, even dismissing one of the most effective specifics known to history – colchicum for gout – as a placebo, in the same way that he did homeopathy (Goodwin & Goodwin 1984; Reubi 1986).

Another account of a trial involving alleged homeopathic treatment appeared from the pen of Sir John Forbes (1783–1861). Unable to decide which allopathic treatment was best (or worst) in a diarrhea epidemic, Forbes (1846) claimed to have prescribed bread pills to half his patients, with no difference in outcome from treatment as usual. He gives an elaborate description of the manufacture of the bread pills as if they were homeopathic medicines – and for all his readers knew, they were – but it is Dickensian tongue-in-cheek, and the therapeutic comparison was intended to be as unflattering to allopathy as to homeopathy. His readership seems to have realized this: in spite of his position as Fellow of the Royal Society and Household Physician to the Royal family, cancellation of subscriptions forced the closure of the journal Forbes edited in the months following the publication of his – by then notorious – review article.

Forbes also mentions the existence of placebo-controlled experiments in German hospitals, prior to 1846, which were apparently 'unfavourable to the claims of homeopathy'. Unfortunately his article lacks any details of these trials, and it was not possible to identify them conclusively in the literature search. However, a possible solution to the mystery of Forbes's missing German trials is offered below (p. 151, footnote 25).

The rhetorical use of the term 'homeopathic' to denote 'illusory' or 'placebo' can also be seen in a report by Lisle (1861), who recounts some experiences giving bread pills to patients with neurotic symptoms. Lisle called this 'orthodox homeopathy', because, as he said, 'Bread pills or globules of Aconitum C30 or C40 amount to the same thing.'

8.4. Placebo in homeopathic practice

There is no doubt that placebo had begun to be used in the evaluation of homeopathy by sceptics and opponents as early as 1829, first in therapeutic trials then provings. It is hard to find another example of drug placebo controls in any field at this date, adding weight to the proposition that homeopathy only adopted them as early as it did because of external pressure. Left out of any account of interactions between homeopathy and orthodoxy, though, is a standard homeopathic practice dating from before then. This involves the deliberate use of placebo in case-taking and prescribing for chronic and non-urgent medical conditions. The practice was undoubtedly made possible because lactose (discovered in 1615) was used in both the preparation of homeopathic medicines (insoluble substances were triturated with lactose), and as a carrier for dispensing liquid potencies when the process was complete, in the belief that it was pharmacologically inert. This meant it was easy for homeopaths to employ a surrogate treatment indistinguishable from verum, at a time when allopathy would have found it difficult. Hahnemann's developing use of placebo reveals an alternative route to placebo controls, originating in homeopathic practice rather than allopathic exposé.

8.4.1. Hahnemannian usage

Hahnemann's publications mention placebo in discussions of case-taking, -assessment and -management. As early as the first edition of the *Organon* (§ 75), Hahnemann (1810) discusses psychosomatic reactions, such as exaggerated responses to placebo or no treatment. It is clear that he is referring here to the traditional use of placebo, but the sophistication and holism of his concept of illness is apparent when he urges that the tendency to exaggerate sufferings should not be disregarded or palliated with placebo, as was usual, but should be included as an important psychological factor in the patient's overall symptom picture.

Hahnemann also stresses that a patient's presenting symptoms may well be confounded by previously-prescribed allopathic medication. In an essay of 1805, *The Medicine of Experience*, he had advised discontinuing any medication for a few days to allow an accurate symptom picture to emerge (Hahnemann 1805c), and he repeats this in §70 of the 1810 *Organon*, which grew out of the earlier essay. In the equivalent section (§ 97) of the second edition he additionally suggests providing a placebo during the washout (Hahnemann 1819a).

There is even evidence from this period that Hahnemann began to use placebo during homeopathic treatment itself. In 1813 he was personally responsible for treating many patients in a typhus epidemic which broke out in Leipzig during the Napoleonic wars. After the first stage of the illness, for which he gave a single dose of *Bryonia*, he waited for the second stage to manifest, which was then treated with a single dose of *Rhus toxicodendron*: 'In this interval, before the second medicine is needed, we may, in order to meet the demands of the patient for medicine and to put his mind at rest, give a placebo every day, such as a few teaspoonfuls of raspberry juice, or some powders of milk-sugar' (Hahnemann 1814). In the article on *Rhus-tox* in *Materia Medica Pura* (1811–21) he notes the huge allopathic mortality rate in this epidemic and comments: 'Of 183 cases treated by me in Leipzig, not one died: this created a great sensation among the Russians (then ruling in Dresden), but was ignored by the medical establishment.'

Ten years later, in the theoretical part of *Chronic Diseases*, Hahnemann (1828–30: 215ff) expands the role of placebo. He had maintained for three decades that a single dose of the indicated medicine, however attenuated, should not be repeated until it had 'worked itself out' over days or weeks if necessary, and he reiterates that here. Recommending that numbered medicated doses should be followed with numbered placebo powders, Hahnemann makes it clear that this was not only to harmonize with current dosage expectations, but also to address his concern about the tendency of patients to produce psychosomatic reactions to the single homeopathic doses. He states that intercalated lactose powders help to reduce non-specific responses, allowing a more accurate assessment of the patient's progress. Hahnemann enthuses that lactose used in this manner is 'an invaluable gift of God'.

8.4.2. Early adoption by followers

This phrase appeared unchanged in the second edition of *Chronic Diseases* (Hahnemann 1835: 161ff), but a new footnote refers to an internal debate between the 'purists', who worried that lactose used as a substrate might be pharmacologically active or become so during trituration and potentization, and those like Hahnemann who were convinced that it remained inert. As far as I have been able to discover, the debate originated with the Swiss homeopath C.G. Peschier, who informed the Congress of the Universal Homeopathic Association, held at Leipzig on 10 August 1832, that his patients often produced new or worsening symptoms after unmedicated lactose (Peschier 1835b). After the congress, Peschier put this to Hahnemann, who said it needed experimental replication. Indeed Hahnemann himself went on to conduct a proving of lactose in potencies up to C18 which, according to his footnote, failed to produce symptoms in reliable subjects. Peschier's account of the debate also refers to the ensuing discussion in the German homeopathic press. Although some practitioners attributed the appearance of new symptoms to the natural course of the disease, or to carryover effects from previous medicines, G.W. Gross (1794–1847), one of Hahnemann's closest associates, seems to have summed up majority opinion when he wrote: 'Patients look for something in the powders that is not there.' Unconvinced, Peschier substituted sucrose and his Genevan patients apparently had no further problems from placebo.

8.4.3. Hahnemannian placebos in trials

Reports of three prospective trials by the homeopaths Attomyr and Herrmann (discussed in Ch. 6) make it clear that Hahnemann's indications for the use of placebos in homeopathic treatment were swiftly adopted by his followers, and medicated and unmedicated powders were routinely used before the lactose debate.

The first study by the German homeopath D. Herrmann (1831), contains the earliest evidence of the use of placebo in addition to verum. It took place in 1829 at the Military Hospital in Tulzyn, province of Podolya, Ukraine, on the instructions of the Russian Tsar, Nicholas I. Herrmann faced a number of difficulties in this trial, and not just from the allopathic evaluators as was expected. His patients were hard-living Russian soldiers unwilling to give up their tobacco and absinthe to follow the minimalist homeopathic regimen. Their distrust of the distinctly unheroic white powders was not tempered by the intercalated doses of unmedicated lactose that Herrmann provided.

The second trial by Herrmann in St Petersburg in 1829–30 included a parallel group receiving expectant treatment at the instigation of Gigler. According to the report by Professor Lichtenstädt (1833) these patients not only received baths, tisanes, good nutrition and rest: they also received placebos modelled on those used as part of normal homeopathic practice:

> During this period, the patients were additionally subjects of an innocent deception. In order to deflect the suspicion that they were not being given any

medicine, they were prescribed pills made of white breadcrumbs or cocoa, lactose powder or salep infusions,[24] as happened in the homeopathic ward.

Interestingly, a second report on this trial was published by Seidlitz (1833) who then went on to conduct the first known placebo-controlled proving four years later (Seidlitz 1834; see above 8.2.).

Attomyr's trial at the General Hospital, Munich, in 1830–31 provides evidence not only of the use of Hahnemannian placebos, but also an unintentional interrupted time-series comparison of homeopathy and placebo (Attomyr 1832). Noting that the first 10 of a series of 40 patients with scabies had recovered within 10 to 14 days after treatment with *Sulphur*, Attomyr was at a loss to understand why the next 30 patients took much longer to recover – typically, three to four weeks. It turned out that the second group had been given unmedicated lactose or nothing at all. Whether the comparison favouring homeopathy was due to negligence or malice is unknown, since it was not part of the trial protocol. Attomyr's report mentions many serious threats to validity: the worst seem to have been allocation bias (the sickest patients were always assigned to the homeopaths), and non-compliance of regular staff. The allopathic dispensing physician was openly hostile, and instead of administering the prescribed medication himself as per protocol, gave it to nurses – who then either failed to deliver it or gave it to the wrong patients. Problems like these were commonly faced by homeopaths invited to conduct trials in allopathic hospitals, as discussed in Ch. 6.

8.4.4. Divided doses and placebo

As discussed in Ch. 2, Hahnemann's scrupulous concern not to inflict avoidable iatrogenic harm on patients had led him to abandon allopathy before 1790, and subsequently to reduce homeopathic medicines to infinitesimal dilutions given in single doses. It seems that he could be equally fastidious concerning harmless surrogate medication. A letter of 5 August 1830 from Hahnemann to his trusted associate Stapf observes: 'The homeopathic physician must come to

---

[24] Salep and saloop are English corruptions of *sahlep*, Arabic for the starchy extract of the ground tubers of various species of orchid. It was popular in the nineteenth century and earlier when prepared and served as an infusion in boiled water, and was often given to invalids (Grieve 1931). I am indebted to Roger Britt of the Institute of Translators and Interpreters for the translation and definition of *Salepabkochung*.

the point when he refuses to give placebos and will only give the helpful remedy when and where it is required' (Haehl 1927, 1: 327).

He eventually reached a possible resolution of his dilemma in his revised instructions for administration of potencies (Hahnemann 1837: iiiff): a single medicated powder or globule was to be dissolved in a glass of water and succussed before each administration of a teaspoonful. Hahnemann believed the extra succussion, referred to nowadays as the 'plus' method, meant patients did not receive a harmful identical stimulus, allowing safe repetition of medicines. The procedure was adopted by many homeopaths throughout Europe. For example, an appreciative mention of the 'new and wise rule' for repetition of doses is included in a balanced critique of Hahnemann by J.-P. Tessier (1856). In spite of this opportunity to abandon the use of placebo during treatment, Hahnemann's case-notes from 1842 show that he continued to prescribe intercalated lactose – but dissolved and succussed in the new manner – until the end of his career (Hahnemann 1852b: 773ff).

Hahnemann also retained placebo for washout. §281 of the 1842 revision of the *Organon* (unpublished until 1921) even extends this to homeopathy: placebo should follow a course of treatment, to establish whether any remaining symptoms are an expression of the natural disease or reactions to the homeopathic medicines (Hahnemann 1921).

8.4.5. Later evidence

Notwithstanding Hahnemann's later divided doses, single dry doses intercalated with lactose continued to be used. The plus method appears not to have been well-known in North America, and did not usually find favour with the ultrahigh-potency school which came to prominence there at the end of the nineteenth century. For instance, J.T. Kent (1888), the best known exponent of 'metaphysical' homeopathy, acknowledged that divided doses given in water were 'in harmony with correct practice', but appears not to have used them. 'Sac. lac.' is frequently referred to in his case reports, itself often given in single doses at long intervals (e.g. Kent 1912c) and he believed it was impossible to practise homeopathy without knowing how to make use of placebo.

Later evidence of placebo used as washout and run-in can be found within the European repeated-dose tradition. In the 1920s, for example, the German homeopath and teacher Erwin Scheidegger regularly prescribed numbered powders of unmedicated lactose for one or two weeks in chronic and non-urgent cases before changing to numbered powders of verum; his student Fritz

Donner (1948: 61) cited this approvingly as an instance of the ease with which homeopathy can incorporate scientific controls against bias. Donner subsequently became bitterly critical of homeopaths because of what he believed were their anti-scientific tendencies, unaware that Scheidegger had adopted a historic practice which predated emergent biomedical evaluative procedures by a century (Donner 1969).

Placebo is still prescribed by many homeopaths today, to judge by its frequent (and unremarked) occurrence in the single case reports readily found in most classical homeopathic journals. It is discussed in standard modern textbooks with varying emphases. One author in the classical tradition regards it as indispensable, given still-current expectations of medication repeated daily (Dhawale 1985: 418ff). Another recent author, associated with the critical tendency in homeopathy, advocates repeated doses of verum, following the later Hahnemann, and concludes that the practice of giving placebo may alienate patients who discover they have received it (Eizayaga 1991: 251).

8.5. Discussion

As discussed in Chapter 6, a received idea in medical historiography indicates that the development of modern scientific medicine, as a unified discipline, can be dated to the rejection of homeopathy in the 1830s and 1840s. The notion advanced by Kaptchuk (1998a) that placebo controls in trials of homeopathy were first adopted in 1834 to expose the system seems to be a corollorary of that argument.

Nevertheless, the evidence of placebo in early therapeutic trials reviewed here shows a clear priority of internal homeopathic usage. The chronology of trials mentioning placebos before 1835 – given either as part of Hahnemannian practice, unintentionally, or as deliberate external controls – is shown in Table 8.3.

Table 8.3: Occurrence of Hahnemannian (internal) and external placebo controls in homeopathic trials 1829–35

Location Date	Report Language	Design	Placebos		Comments
			Internal	External	
Tulzyn 1829	Herrmann, 1831 German	Observational therapeutic	Yes	No	Hahnemannian usage
St Petersburg 1829–30	Lichtenstädt, 1832; Seidlitz, 1833 German	Parallel therapeutic	Yes	Yes	Hahnemannian usage; placebos identical to those used in the homeopathic arm were also given to an expectant group.
Munich 1830–31	Attomyr, 1832 German	Observational therapeutic	Yes	No	Hahnemannian usage, but unmedicated lactose also given to some patients negligently or maliciously instead of verum.
St Petersburg 1834	Seidlitz, 1834 German	Time series proving	No	Yes	Seidlitz had reported the 1829–30 St Petersburg study.
Paris 1834	Pigeaux, 1834; Trousseau & Gouraud, 1834 French	Observational therapeutic	No	Yes	Placebo only, no verum.
Nuremburg 1835	Löhner, 1835 German	Parallel proving	No	Yes	No clear relationship to above.

The normative thesis of external pressure prompting the adoption of placebo controls in trials by homeopaths seems difficult to sustain given the diffusion of within-patient placebo controls in homeopathy before 1830, their explicit imitation in the first known trial with a separate placebo arm in 1829–30, and the poor design and conduct of later allopathic challenges.[25] The early homeopaths' own disciplinary matrix was fertile enough to generate research into the system's internal validity, such as time series provings and trials in the 1850s, and there can be little doubt that placebo-controlled provings by homeopaths in the 1870s, as well as single-blind n-of-1 trials in the 1920s, sprang from the same source. Outside everyday practice, homeopaths only used placebo in provings, and then specifically to test problem areas in their discipline, such as high potencies or substances with low toxicity. The results seemed to bear out the doubts of the critical homeopaths about Hahnemann's nomination of C30 as the exclusive proving potency after 1828, since lower potencies were a more reliable source of clinical indicators when applied to healthy provers. Unfortunately, the debate that should have followed, on whether the pure pathogenetic symptoms of the earlier materia medica had been contaminated or enriched by uncontrolled high potency provings, never really took place. The definitive statement of the critical position was given by Hughes (1884: Ch. XII) in his lecture on 'The future of pharmacodynamics' to the Boston University Medical School. But, as Hughes points out, the other side had been unwilling to counter the critique, or were too easily refuted when they did. All too typically, high potency enthusiasts such as Samuel Swan (1888) retorted that provers who showed as many symptoms from placebo as verum were actually proving *Sac-lac.*

However, by contrast with proving data, higher potencies continued to be found as or even more effective in treatment of some clinical conditions such as pneumonia (see Ch. 7). Convinced of the fundamental soundness of their therapy, homeopaths seem to have been uninterested in placebo-controlled

---

[25] Table 8.3 also shows, incidentally, the likely candidates for Forbes's unspecified and allegedly placebo-controlled German trials (see 8.2.2.2, above). Nearly all the reports were published first in German, and were conducted by German doctors. Russia has been spoken of as an intellectual dependency of German thought in the second quarter of the nineteenth century (Berlin 1978: 122). A French 'exposé of German trials' (Martins 1835), which actually contains a translation of the 1834 *Carbo-veg* proving in St Petersburg by Seidlitz, demonstrates geographical and medical dependency also. This group of trials and provings could well have been remembered as 'trials in the German hospitals' by Forbes (1846), writing more than a decade later.

therapeutic trials at this date, but instead demanded pragmatic trials of homeopathy versus allopathy.

In reply to this argument (Dean 2000), Kaptchuk (2000) has emphasized the relevance of the – undisputed – priority of parallel group placebo controls in tests of mesmerism which occurred in the 1780s, and the fact that homeopaths were aware of this. There is no doubt that influential homeopaths were not just passive observers of the mesmeric debate, but conducted their own investigations. Hahnemann's ally G.W. Gross – who wrote about nocebo effects in medicine as early as the 1830s, as mentioned above (8.4.2) – was well aware of the effects of suggestion. His earlier critical investigation of dowsing had demonstrated that the pendulum responded to unconscious muscular movements of the diviner's hand, and not to direct external influence from metals as the mesmerists thought (Gross 1822). But there is little hard evidence that the use of wooden rather than metal rods to test mesmerism as a system affected internal homeopathic practice or experimentation.

The designs of the earliest placebo-controlled experiments by homeopaths help to clarify the difference in outlook. The placebo-only trial by Trousseau in 1834, and the parallel group proving by Löhner in 1835 may have been the first of their kind, and may have been influenced by the design of mesmeric studies, but did they exert any direct influence on internal homeopathic trials? The first placebo trials by homeopaths were crossover and time series studies – as indeed was Seidlitz's proving in 1834 – using the single-blind washout and intercalated placebos that had been institutionalized in homeopathy since 1810 and witnessed by allopaths in hospital trials from 1829 onwards. Not until the late nineteenth century did homeopaths introduce parallel placebo arms. It can even be argued that the homeopaths adopted the more rational approach – using within-patient controls during treatment – at a time when it was scarcely possible to assemble equivalent parallel groups.

Kaptchuk (2000) also objects that all doctors had traditionally handed out placebos instead of medicine, and were aware that it could be used as a comparison. However, Kaptchuk's own earliest instance of 'occasional' orthodox within-patient placebo control dates from the 1950s (Shideman & Beckman 1958; Kaptchuk 1998b). In fact there is no evidence that anything like Hahnemannian usage was ever institutionalized in allopathy before the twentieth century: the first orthodox proposal for placebo-controlled n-of-1 trials is currently attributed to the German researcher Paul Martini in the 1930s (Martini 1932; Shelley & Baur 1999), who may even have been aware of Scheidegger and traditional homeopathic placebo usage. (Martini's subsequent placebo-controlled provings are mentioned in Ch. 9.) Equally noteworthy, homeopaths do not seem to have given placebo alone in the time-honoured manner, but always before, during or after treatment with verum. In the 1900s, when prominent orthodox doctors such as Richard Cabot (1909, 1, 23), were beginning to question the ethics of their 'innocent deception' of patients with placebo, others equally eminent could still argue that it was in the patient's best interest (Janet 1925, 1, 337f). Placebo as within-patient control was not even mentioned in that debate.

All the evidence points to the early homeopaths thinking they were more scientific than the regulars. They had pharmacological tests, fine discrimination of diagnoses at the symptom level and statistics on their side, and they used placebo as a control in everyday practice, not merely to palliate troublesome patients or to expose quackery.

9. Adoption of the biomedical research perspective, 1914–53

Background: The emergence of the clinical research orientation that came to define biomedicine in the twentieth century is believed to have sounded the death knell for homeopathy.

Questions: How did emergent models of scientific medicine affect the design of homoeopathic trials in the first half of the 20th century? Are the results contingent on the designs used in any way?

Argument: Early twentieth-century homeopaths quickly adopted the conventions of the controlled trial, ahead of orthodox medicine in some cases. Homeopaths were also able to adopt an explanatory research model, exposing the discipline to an internal critique.

9.1. Introduction

The marginalization of homeopathy was virtually complete by 1900. In the countries where clinical trials had been conducted during the nineteenth century – Germany, Italy, Russia, France, Britain and the USA – rigorous exclusion from clinical and academic debate ensured that Hahnemann's research programme was disregarded, even where quasi-legal sanctions designed to encourage allopathic guild monopoly had failed to suppress its practice (Ameke 1885; Lodispoto 1961; Coulter 1973; Nicholls 1988; Faure 1992a; Jütte 1998; Kotok 1999). Only the very greatest allopaths dared break ranks. Joseph Lister (1827–1912) said that if he had known earlier what the homeopaths knew about the vascular effects of aconite and belladonna he might have been able to save his father, who died after extensive blood-letting (cited in Haller 1984). Emil von Behring (1854–1917), the discoverer of antitoxin treatment and prophylaxis for diphtheria and tetanus, repeatedly cited Hahnemann's influence and importance in the development of immunology (Behring 1893; 1898; 1915). Behring even demonstrated the paradoxically enhanced immunogenic activity of continued serial dilutions to the Berlin Physiological Society in 1892, but was advised to suppress this experiment because it gave comfort to the homeopaths, and only recalled the event in public after becoming the first Nobel laureate for medicine (Behring 1905: xxvii).

Against a background of increasing biomedical hegemony the 30-year gap between the last homeopathic treatment trial of the nineteenth century and the first of the twentieth century found in the literature search becomes easier to understand.

9.2. Results

Twenty separate trials were reported in 10 publications in 2 languages, English and German (see Table 9.1).

The reports ranged from anecdotal to detailed, and the trial conditions ranged from boils to surgical tuberculosis, with acute infectious diseases constituting the majority. The trials were conducted in 3 countries only, USA, Germany and Great Britain, and are discussed here in relation to the homeopathic research climate in each country.

9.3. USA 1914–38

The unsatisfactory state of doctoring was obvious to many in late nineteenth-century America, and was satirized by Mark Twain (Ober 1997). The preservation of a free market in medicine – despite allopathic attempts to create a monopoly – had allowed a proliferation of medical systems, practitioners and the colleges that turned them out. However, with no externally imposed objectives, the standards of many institutions were deeply suspect (Hudson 1972). The report prepared for the Carnegie Foundation and the AMA by Abraham Flexner (1910) was designed to bring about root-and-branch reform of medical training and practice, in which the research perspective that had taken root in Germany would be institutionalized in the US (Berliner 1977). One of its immediate effects was the closure of many medical schools, and the casualties included lesser allopathic institutions, as well as some naturopathic, chiropractic and homeopathic colleges (e.g. Roberts 1986). This seems to have been less because of allopathic protectionism (which was already waning by this time, the battle against homeopathy won), than because of a fundamental ideological shift – henceforth, treatments required justification in practice, and practices could, in principle, be supplanted by others when supported by better evidence.

Table 9.1 Hospital based evaluations 1914–53

Reference (trial date)	Trialist Hospital	Condition Main outcome	Design	N	Model Control(s)	Result by group
Wesselhoeft, 1917 (1914)	Chadwell Massachussetts Homoeopathic	Scarlet fever; time to discharge	Parallel quasi-random	? ?	Clinical (Bell D3) Placebo? No treatment?	control slightly favoured
Wesselhoeft, 1917 (1914–16)	Wesselhoeft Massachussetts Homoeopathic	Scarlet fever prevention; incidence	Open label time series	26 26 28	Clinical (Bell D3) Atropine D3 No treatment	38.5% 38.5% 35.7%
Wesselhoeft, 1925 (1915)	Wesselhoeft Massachussetts Homoeopathic	Diphtheria; mortality	Parallel open label	56 252	Clinical (Merc-cy D3) Antitoxin	† 0% † 11%
Wesselhoeft, 1917	Wesselhoeft Massachussetts Homoeopathic	Scarlet fever; time to discharge	Parallel open label	114 113	Clinical (Bell D3) No treatment	46.4 d 50.2 d
Wesselhoeft, 1924 (1921–23)	Wesselhoeft Massachussetts Homoeopathic	Orchitis from mumps; incidence	Historical	67 428 8153	Clinical (Plumb-ac D3) Classical Allopathy	1.5% 28% 18%
Bier, 1925	Bier Berlin Polyklinik	Furunculosis; cure	Case series	34 0	Clinical (Sul-iod D6) Allopathy	100% 0%
Donner, 1948: 34 (1925)	Joachimoglu Berlin Polyklinik	Skin conditions; identify verum	Parallel d-b	? ?	Clinical (Sul-iod D3) Placebo	? ?
Donner, 1948: 54–57 (1938)	Simonson New York Flower (Children)	Acute and chronic URTI: 5 trials; cure by date	Parallel s-b + open label allopathic	314 95 448	Unknown Placebo Allopathy	72–87% 50–73% 19–80%

Table 9.1 Hospital based evaluations 1914–53

Reference (trial date)	Trialist Hospital	Condition Main outcome	Design	N	Model Control(s)	Result by group
Schilsky, 1941 (1938–39)	Schilsky Hamburg Rothenburgsort	Whooping cough; A. ≤ 1 y; B. ≥ 1 y duration;	Quasi-random open label	88 82	Classical Allopathy	A. 66.6; B. 54.8 d A. 67.4; B. 52.8 d
Paterson, 1941	Paterson, Boyd Glasgow Homoeopathic	Diphtheria; immunity after +ve Schick test	Historical control	33 3743	Isopathy (APT C30 or Diphtherinum C201) Untreated populations	20/33 (60.6%) 33%
Hess, 1942	Hess Missing	Diphtheria; mortality	Parallel open label	69 ?	Clinical (Merc-c, Merc-bi, Lach, Nit-ac) Serum	† 18.6% † 11.4%
British Homoeopathic Society, 1943 (1941–42)	Paterson Glasgow Homoeopathic	Mustard gas burns: 1trial; intact or me- dium/deep	Random d-b; partial crossover	14 14	Isopathy (Mustard gas C30) Placebo	Highly significant for homeopathy (see Apps 2.2, 2.4)
British Homoeopathic Society, 1943 (1941–42)	Templeton London Homoeopathic	Mustard gas burns: 3trials; superficial, medium or deep	Random d-b; chi 2 tests; meta-analysis	127 113	Clinical or isopathy Placebo	Highly significant for homeopathy (see Apps 2.2, 2.4)
Ledermann, 1954 (1951–53)	Ledermann Burton-on-Trent, Bretby Hall Orthopaedic	Surgical TB; progress: A. general; B. unexpected	Random, masked, chi 2 test	29 30	Classical Placebo	A: nsd B: 9/27 vs 3/24 (p=0.08)

Key: d-b, s-b, double- or single-blind

Although the example of homeopathy throughout the nineteenth century had been instrumental in bringing about this medical watershed, by the end of the century in many respects homeopathy itself had become far less forward looking and experimental than in Hahnemann's time. J.T. Kent was the best known homeopath of the day, and he expounded the texts of the previous hundred years as if they were evidence of divine revelation (see Ch. 4). From such a vantage point research facilities were irrelevant, and it is no surprise that Kent's Chicago college was closed following the Flexner report. However, from another point of view, the report can be seen as endorsing the attempts of the critical stream that emerged in homeopathy in the 1830s to evaluate the components of the discipline. The introduction of placebo-controlled provings in the USA in the 1870s was discussed in Ch. 8, and following Flexner an increasingly critical detachment can be noted in homeopathic debate of the day concerning therapeutics. Hospital statistics were no longer an automatic demonstration of allopathic brutality and inefficacy as mortality rates under the two systems began to converge in some illnesses (Askenstedt 1915). It is at this moment that therapeutic trials designed to test internal homeopathic hypotheses emerged in the USA. The principal exponent was Conrad Wesselhoeft Jr., a member of a prominent German-American homeopathic family stretching back to the introduction of homeopathy to the US in the 1830s. Wesselhoeft not only had a secure base in a Boston homeopathic medical school that survived Flexner, but was able to use his position as consultant physician at the Massachusetts Homoeopathic Hospital to compare clinical and classical homeopathy with allopathy and no treatment in prospective case series and parallel group trials.

At the same time, basic research into the effects of high potencies in animal systems was under way in the US. The geneticist Mary Stark collaborated with the homeopath G.B. Stearns in investigations into the genetic effects of clinical homeopathy and nosodes in hereditary tumours in fruit flies (Stearns & Stark 1925). Stearns (1932) went on to investigate objective physical reactions to potencies in humans, continuing a line of work begun by the San Francisco physiologist Prof. Albert Abrams (1863–1924), and developed and replicated in Britain (see 9.5). Abrams (1916) noticed that percussion of the abdomen of a patient with a cancerous lip emitted a distinctive note, only when the patient faced west. Patients with other pathologies showed similar reactions when facing in different directions. Abrams hypothesized this was an electromagnetic phenomenon, and constructed a circuit with variable resistance to investigate it. He found that specific diseases caused replicable changes in resistance: cancers reacted at 50 ohms, tuberculosis at 15, and so on. Drugs and other substances introduced into the circuit also caused changes in the reactions of healthy subjects. As a bitter opponent of homeopathy he thought this would be an ideal opportunity to demonstrate that its medicines were placebos, and was surprised to find that they appeared to be responsible for the strongest of all the reactions he was able to measure in his subjects.

9.3.1. Boston 1914: scarlet fever

According to the only source (Wesselhoeft 1917), Chadwell orally presented the results of a scarlet fever trial in Autumn 1914. There are no details of numbers treated, or indeed whether 'receiving no medicine' is intended to indicate 'no treatment' or 'treatment with placebo'. Chadwell gave every other case *Belladonna* D3 and found, if anything, a slight disadvantage from homeopathy. Wesselhoeft reports that these results were a shock to many in view of *Belladonna*'s reputation in scarlet fever, and Chadwell was censured in the ensuing discussion for his assumption that each case required the same medicine. However, Wesselhoeft says in defence that

> he was not examining the fundamental principle of homeopathy. On the contrary he was investigating the accuracy of one of the myriad of notions which have arisen in the past hundred and twenty years and which have become part of the practice and teachings of a large element of the homeopathic school. The notion he investigated concerned the much vaunted value of belladonna in scarlet fever. What he showed very conclusively was that this drug in the third decimal dilution was not as efficacious in the average case of scarlet fever as one is led to believe from homeopathic teachings. Further criticism as to the dosage employed was irrelevant to the proposition and to the conclusions drawn.

This trial may well have been the trigger for the series of literature reviews and trials in common contagious diseases that Wesselhoeft subsequently undertook.

9.3.2. Boston 1914–16: scarlet fever

Beginning in the winter of 1914, and in the two subsequent winters of 1915 and 1916, Wesselhoeft (1917) tested the prophylactic efficacy of homeopathy or no treatment in scarlet fever. The subjects were nurses in the fever wards of the Massachussetts Homoeopathic Hospital, and the first medicine to be tested was *Belladonna*. The same D3 potency tested by Chadwell was used in 1914 and again in 1915, when the test medicine was *Atropine*, the principal alkaloid of belladonna. In 1916 the nurses received no treatment. The incidence of the disease was virtually the same in each of the 3 years.

9.3.3. Boston 1915: diphtheria

In a paper read to the Bureau of Clinical Medicine, Cleveland in 1924, Wesselhoeft (1925) situates his review and trial of homeopathic treatment of diphtheria in the context of the available evidence in favour of Behring's antitoxin serum treatment, which was still fairly controversial. Wesselhoeft notes that *Mercurius cyanatus* had been recommended in the homeopathic literature, supported by published case series, and he therefore chose it for 56 cases out of 308 admitted with diphtheria to his hospital in 1915. There were no deaths or complications from treatment with *Merc-cy* D3; all made uneventful recoveries, while the mortality rate in those treated with serum at the same time was 11%. The report offers the opinion:

> It may be assumed that there were others that did not require antitoxin, but our judgement was certainly correct on this 17 per cent. In milder years it may have run to a much higher percentage.

Wesselhoeft still recommended antitoxin as the first line treatment in serious cases, and also hinted at the close family resemblance between antitoxin treatments and homeopathy, acknowledged by Behring (see 9.1):

> Like Schulz and Bingel, I am not an opponent of serum therapy. My interest in homeopathic therapeutics *in its widest sense* prompts me to seek the safest, the promptest, and at the same time the least disagreeable methods of dealing with cases of this dangerous disease. [added emphasis]

9.3.4. Boston 1917: scarlet fever

Chadwell's treatment trial of 1914 was repeated by Wesselhoeft (1917), and the numbers involved were large enough to discount random variation between groups. The main outcome was days to discharge, showing a slight trend in favour of homeopathy. As with Chadwell's trial, it is unclear from the report whether placebo was given; if patients were simply given no treatment any superiority of *Belladonna* could well be due to other factors. The report also tabulates the complications in each group: the most common were otitis, mastoiditis, nephritis and arthritis, and there was no difference between the two groups in incidence or type of complication. Wesselhoeft pointed out that this should surprise nobody, since *Belladonna* proving symptoms bore only a slight resemblance to the currently prevalent form of scarlet fever, or to its complications.

9.3.5. Boston 1921–23: mumps

In 428 adult cases of mumps treated by classical homeopathy in the Massachussetts Homoeopathic Hospital during 1917–18 no real benefits from the remedies were observed. In fact, the 28% incidence of orchitis, a common complication of mumps, was 10% higher than in 8153 male cases of mumps that Wesselhoeft (1924) was able to find in the orthodox literature. This disparity prompted him to investigate the materia medica along the lines proposed long before by Hughes and Burnett, to find if possible a pathological simillimum for the condition. Out of many medicines that affected the salivary glands and testes, only one produced the parotitis with orchitis and nervous symptoms that characterize mumps. That was lead, which interestingly was not mentioned in the homeopathic literature regarding mumps, but which deserved a trial. From 1921 until July 1923, when the paper was read to the Bureau of Pedology of the American Institute of Homeopathy, all cases of male mumps at or above puberty admitted to the Massachussetts Homoeopathic Hospital were given *Plumbum aceticum* D3 every 3 h for the first week. Of 67 cases so treated, there were no complications and the single case of orchitis developed 3 days after admission. Wesselhoeft continued:

> This is not individualizing our cases. It is crude homeopathy, but it is a closer approach to homeopathic prescribing in mumps than when untrustworthy symptoms in the materia medica are selected for indications. Routine treatment is a precarious thing, but in epidemics and in hospital work individualization is well-nigh impossible except in the severe cases. Unless subsequent results upset our results from plumbum in mumps, it would appear that the homeopathic school has found the first efficacious medicine in this disease, not so much for the acute symptoms as a prophylactic for the complications which render this disease dangerous.

9.3.6. New York 1938: URTI

The results of 5 trials of homeopathy vs placebo and allopathy in various acute and chronic upper respiratory conditions that took place in 1938 seem to be mentioned only in a series of lectures published in German 10 years later

(Donner 1948: 54–57). The trials were conducted by J.T. Simonson with children attending the Flower Hospital attached to the homeopathic New York Medical College. Details of the trial and homeopathic methodology are absent from Donner's report, although the number of children receiving each treatment was tabulated and percentages of cure given (see Table 9.2).

Table 9.2 Results from 5 trials in URTI conducted in 1938 at the New York Flower Hospital

Condition	**N**	**Homeopathy**		**Placebo**		**Allopathy**	
Outcome		n	(% cure)	n	(% cure)	n	(% cure)
Acute feverish headcold	37	12	(nd)	14	(nd)	11	(nd)
Acute rhinopharyngitis Cure at 2 w	207	34	(76)	22	(73)	151	(40)
Acute sinusitis Cure at 3 w	92	26	(85)	7	(72)	59	(66)
Chronic rhinopharyngitis Cure at 1 mon	327	118	(87)	52	(52)	157	(57)
Chronic sinusitis	194	124	(72)	←		194	(36)

Altogether, 857 patients were involved in the trials. There was no noticeable difference in efficacy between any treatment in acute feverish headcold, but homeopathy was superior to placebo or allopathy in the other 4 trials. The most notable homeopathic successes occurred in chronic conditions that resisted any of the several parallel orthodox treatments used such as ephidrine and silver nitrate. Trial 5, for chronic sinusitis, differed from the other parallel group trials: from the original intake of 194, 124 failed to progress under conventional treatment and were then given homeopathy. The German homeopath Fritz Donner, who late in life became one of homeopathy's bitterest critics (e.g. Donner 1969), wrote in 1948 that although numbers were small under some treatments, the statistics could not be gainsaid, and bore out the persistent claims of homeopaths that their daily practice showed homeopathy was sometimes superior to allopathy in sinusitis and upper respiratory infections.

9.4. Germany 1925–42

In Germany, high-potency individualized homeopathy had almost disappeared in the latter part of the nineteenth century, reemerging only after 1945, with the publication of Kent's works in German translations. Homeopathy had received some scientific endorsement around 1900, from independent researchers such as Hugo Schulz and Behring, but their results were violently repudiated by orthodoxy. Representative clinical homeopaths of the period are Alfons Stiegele (1941) and Otto Leeser (1936). A temporary renaissance of homeopathy in German *Schulmedizin* in the first half of the twentieth century can be dated from the publication of a substantial article by the leading Berlin surgeon, August Bier (1925), in the respected national journal, *Münchener medizinische Wochenschrift*. Bier's title asked 'What position should we take regarding homeopathy?', and, although by no means interested in Hahnemannian dogma, he answered by advocating general critical investigation of the similia principle. He based this on an historical review, and the successful experiments which he had himself undertaken in dermatology following Stiegele's advice (discussed below). Despite some fierce a priori opposition, homeopathy then began to enjoy a brief period with a comparatively high profile in Germany, and the review by Guttentag (1940) outlines the events following Bier's intervention which eventually led to the creation of two academic posts in homeopathy at Berlin in 1940. Fritz Donner also formed a link between clinical research in the US and Germany, translating several of Wesselhoeft's articles and commenting on their relevance to problems found in the treatment of infectious diseases (Wesselhoeft Jr 1928; 1929; Donner 1942).

Some indication of the level of orthodox interest in evaluating homeopathy at this time is shown in the pathogenetic drug tests (provings) performed by Paul Martini, a clinical pharmacologist whose claims as a pioneer of the modern clinical trial have been overlooked in English-language historiography, but are as strong as those of R.A. Fisher in Great Britain (Martini 1932; Shelley & Baur 1999). Whether the results of Martini's placebo-controlled provings provided any support for homeopathy is disputed – Haas et al (1959) claiming they did, and Donner (1969) the converse – but they are only relevant here as an indication of the seriousness with which the investigation of homeopathy was undertaken in the Third Reich as part of the *Neue deutsche Heilkunde* programme. Announced by Rudolf Hess at a homeopathic conference in 1938, this seems to have been inspired as much by a search for cost-effective (*rationell*) healthcare, as by nationalist pride in homeopathy's origins. Although it had previously been feared the results of the homeopathic investigations in the Nazi period were lost for ever (Ernst 1995a), the literature search for this review found reports of two clinical therapeutic trials, along with discussions of them in the contemporary homeopathic press.

9.4.1. Berlin 1925: furunculosis

Bier was not a homeopath, but a renowned skin specialist and surgeon. He notes (1925) that the well-known and uncontroversial toxic effects of high doses of sulphur taken internally – such as abscesses, eruptions and furunculosis – lent support to its use for those conditions in homeopathy. The choice of *Sulphur iodatum* D3 as the homeopathic medicine for chronic furunculosis was at the suggestion of the leading homeopath Alfons Stiegele, and Bier reports that this gave good results at his Polyklinik. He then went on to test *Sul-iod* D6, a much more dilute preparation, in a series of 34 cases, many of whom had constantly relapsed after orthodox treatments such as quartz lamp, yeast, arsenic, irritants and autohemic therapy. Bier reports that all were cured under homeopathy, including 3 cases who relapsed under D6 but then responded to D3. The success rate in 28 cases of acute furunculosis was equally good, but less convincing because of the unknown natural recovery time in the acute condition. Bier also reported good results in acne – vulgaris, indurata and rosacea – but notes that some cases did not respond, suggesting that sulphur was less generally homeopathic in those conditions than in furunculosis. He noted equally good results in dermal staphylomycoses such as pyodermia following scabies and impetigo. His conclusion was unambiguous and challenging: *Sulphur* was 'better, simpler and cheaper' than even the best of the other therapies, such as the Finsen quartz lamp, and

> An accurately chosen internal remedy, given in the proper dosage in a case of clearly infectious type, where other remedies are considered useless, will give a greater result than any other measure, including especially immunization, physical and surgical therapy. It is important to emphasize this in these days when internal drug therapy is looked down on with an air of condescension.

9.4.2. Berlin 1925: skin conditions

Joachimoglu, a researcher at the Berlin Pharmacological Institute, subsequently challenged Bier to distinguish coded vials of *Sul-iod* D3 and placebo, by assessing the clinical response of patients in his clinic. Bier apparently passed the test, but the anecdotal report gives no details of the numbers involved or Bier's success rate (Donner 1948: 34).

9.4.3. Hamburg 1938–39: pertussis

The trial of classical homeopathy for whooping cough at Hamburg's Rothenburgsort Hospital was interrupted by the outbreak of war (Schilsky & Bayer 1941). Patients were categorized into those below or above 1 year old, because of the difference in the normal course of the disease in those age groups, and were alternately assigned to homeopathy or treatment as usual. Nursing staff were trained to note the symptoms and record the number and severity of coughing fits. There was little difference in the length of stay between the two treatment groups. The report lists a series of problems in the trial which may have affected the result, most of which seem plausible: the hospital setting made prescribing difficult, mainly because the cases were taken by nurses who reported the symptoms to the doctor; a lot therefore depended on the temperament and memory of the data collectors; parents are normally more aware of the individualizing modalities; homeopathic treatment did not start on the day of admission; and all the patients were mixed together in the wards.

Contemporary homeopaths complained that the potencies used by Schilsky were not reported, evidently believing this held the key to the negative results (Schier 1942). Schilsky (1942b) had published details of the medicines and potencies he used in treatment of pertussis in the winter of 1940–41, and they are clearly the standard low potencies used in German homeopathy at that date (e.g. *Cuprum* D4, 6, 8; *Coccus cacti* D8; *Drosera* and *Ipecac* D15). Although these presumably bore some resemblance to those used in the trial, he replied that he would give details at a later date (Schilsky 1942a). However, when Donner (1942) came to write a review article on homeopathy for infectious diseases, later the same year, Schilsky had still not obliged his critics.

9.4.4. ? 1942: diphtheria

The trial of serum vs homeopathy plus serum in diphtheria by F.O. Hess (1942) was reported in an oral presentation to a meeting of the Medical Society of Oberlausitz, and the location of the trial was unspecified. The published details are scanty, giving no indication of assignment method, and omitting complete numbers of patients treated. Four homeopathic medicines are listed, without any indication of dosage or whether they were prescribed classically or clinically. Serum plus homeopathy was markedly less effective in reducing mortality than serum alone – suggesting either a danger from homeopathic medicines, or assignment bias. Hess also reported that homeopathy was totally ineffective in malignant diphtheria, a fact confirmed to him by Stiegele in a personal communication. Discussion of the trial in the homeopathic press raised the standard objections: the report gave no indication that Hess had any first-hand knowledge of homeopathic prescribing, nor why the medicines were chosen above others. One criticism seems highly pertinent: homeopaths had already observed that serum doses needed to be halved when given concurrently with homeopathic treatment (Schmitz 1942; Schwartzhaupt 1942).

9.5. Great Britain 1941–53

The decline of British homeopathy at the beginning of the twentieth century paralleled events in Germany and the USA. However, Kent's influence was introduced and perpetuated in the UK after it had begun to wane in the US as the result of a scholarship programme which enabled British homeopaths to study in Chicago. Inglis (1964: 85ff) described the effects of the Kentian 'take-over bid' for British homeopathy after 1912. An exclusive classical orthodoxy was promulgated by Sir John Weir, Margaret Tyler and a dwindling band of followers, and by the 1970s British medical homeopathy had become heavily involved with anthroposophy.

As noted, clinical research was not part of Kentian homeopathy, and the research figures to emerge in the inter-war years were somewhat unusual. John Paterson and William Boyd were both based at the homeopathic hospital in Glasgow. Both published regularly, and their presentations to the 11th Congress of the International Homeopathic League are representative of their individual work immediately before they collaborated on clinical trials. Paterson (1936) had continued the investigations of bowel flora and their relation to homeopathic treatment begun by Edward Bach and C.E. Wheeler. Boyd (1936) had conducted biochemical and biophysical tests into potency variation. The latter tests were done using equipment that Boyd had developed to refine the early investigations of Abrams into homeopathic action at a distance, and were thought to allow an objective test of the medicines and potencies suited to any individual. It is worth recounting some of the story since it contains details of an early British placebo-controlled test of human reactions to homeopathic potencies.

Boyd was interested in Abrams's techniques, but quickly realized that Abrams had wrongly identified resistance as the electrical factor and replaced the original resistors with variable conductances and a variable condenser. His more rigorous method, which involved placing the subjects in a Faraday cage, was tested by an independent committee, led by Sir (later Lord) Thomas Horder, in a fraudbusting exercise funded by the Royal Society of Medicine

(Horder 1924). In 5 blind test series Boyd's team was almost completely successful in distinguishing coded vials of substances such as sulphur or morbid matter from placebo or other substances. The only errors occurred twice in one series of 20 Bernoulli trials, and Whately Smith, the investigating scientist, believed this was probably due to operator error. In another series of 25 successful trials Smith calculated the odds against the results being due to chance as 33 554 432 to 1. Horder, who seems to have been unaware that some of the coded vials contained homeopathic *Sulphur* – which were also correctly identified – reported the results to a closed meeting of the RSM. According to a journalist from the *Morning Post* who managed to gatecrash, there was unanimous agreement not to discuss the matter further, and no further funds were made available to investigate the phenomenon, even though it pointed to a possible diagnostic test for cancer and other serious disease (Russell 1973: 44ff).

It is still not known whether the reactions were primarily electromagnetic, perhaps involving some form of quantum effect at levels excluded by mainstream biology, or whether they were primarily psychic (assuming such a distinction is valid). The whole area of dowsing effects, homeopathic action at a distance and related biophysical phenomena was thoroughly reviewed at the end of the period in question by a university physicist and geologist, and the title of his book, *Psychical Physics*, seems apt enough (Tromp 1949). In the 1940s Boyd also conducted a protracted series of more orthodox experimental tests of the effects of potentized substances, such as mercuric chloride on enzyme production by yeast. This work is still accepted as being among the most rigorous pre-clinical research conducted in homeopathy, and the cost of replicating it to the standards set by Boyd was estimated at £100,000 at 1982 prices by Kollerstrom (1982).

9.5.1. Glasgow 1941: diphtheria

At this time, the Schick test was widely used to ascertain acquired post-vaccination immunity to diphtheria. Paterson and Boyd (1941) designed an experiment using the test as a measure of whether high potencies were biologically active. They were explicit that it was not designed initially to test whether homeopathy might have a prophylactic effect in diphtheria, although claims of the prophylactic effects of isopathy have been common in homeopathy, and disputed equally frequently.

Four case series with a historical control were undertaken to explore whether homeopathic potencies of vaccine (alum-precipitated toxoid C30) or the diphtheria nosode (*Diphtherinum* C201) could bring about an increased proportion of negative tests in subjects previously testing positive. Out of 33 subjects originally testing positive, 20 (60%) tested negative after treatment. While acknowledging the problems inherent in the Schick test and in retrospective comparisons generally, the authors believed their preliminary result compared favourably with the (recent) historical control of 3743 untreated Glaswegian children, only 33% of whom were Schick negative when retested.

9.5.2. Glasgow & London 1941–42: mustard gas burns

Following its use during the First World War, mustard gas was known to cause not just the well-known signs of conjunctivitis and blistering, but to compromise immune functioning by attacking blood-cell production in the bone-marrow (Kurmbahaar 1919). The renewed threat of chemical attacks in the early years of the Second World War meant that research into methods of prevention and treatment of mustard gas lesions assumed a high priority. British homeopathic researchers and clinicians offered their services to the Ministry of Home Security, and this led a series of preventive and treatment trials at the homoeopathic hospitals in Glasgow and London (British Homoeopathic Society 1943). The 10% solution of mustard gas in benzene was supplied by the Ministry, and trials took place under carefully controlled conditions. Application of the solution to the forearm, area affected, room temperature, preparation of the skin and surgical dressing were all standardized, as was the age, sex and physique of the volunteers as far as possible. In Glasgow an ad hoc method of randomization to treatment was used. Coded vials were laid out on a table, alternately potentized *Mustard gas* C30 (prepared by London Homoeopathic Laboratories) and placebo, and volunteers were paired. The first of each pair took any vial, and the second any serial number above or below the one taken by his colleague. The London trials used what was to become the standard modern randomization method, in which vials were coded in advance by an independent source (in this case Nelson's pharmacy, London) that held the code until after the experiment was over. The two approaches are reflected in the equal numbers of verum and control in Glasgow, and unequal numbers in London.

The outcome measure used in all the trials was the appearance of the lesion 7 days after first application. Visual inspection and photographic records were used in Glasgow to categorize the lesions as either superficial (skin intact) or deep (breach of surface). The first 12 cases showed no deep lesions in the verum group and conversely no superficial lesions in the controls. Further volunteers were tested, with similar results, although the report is unclear whether the tabulated 'summary of 28 cases' (p. 5) represents new cases or includes the 12 original ones. 13 of the tested cases then took part in a randomized crossover, approximately 4 weeks later, also double-blind and placebo-controlled. This led to 4 groups: placebo–verum (7 cases) verum–placebo (3 cases), verum–verum (2 cases) and placebo–placebo (1 case). The results seem to confirm those found in the first series, even extending them: the verum–placebo group still produced superficial lesions a month after verum. The one placebo–placebo case produced marked and extensive dermatitis, suggesting sensitization to mustard gas. This was treated with *Rhus-tox* C30, matched to the presenting symptoms; intense itching was relieved quickly, and rash disappeared within 2 days.

Two medical officers in London used visual inspection only to grade each lesion on a 3-point scale of superficial, medium or deep. This difference, as well as the larger numbers involved in London, meant that the Glasgow figures were not included in the statistical analysis of results conducted by H.O. Hartley of the Statistical Computing Service. The first London series tested C30 potencies of *Mustard gas* (2 preparations), *Rhus toxicodendron*, *Kali bichromicum*, *Opium* and *Cantharides*, each against its own placebo group. Analysis was conducted for all groups combined, and each medicine separately, and the results are shown in more detail in Apps. 2.2 and 2.4. The combined analysis established a statistically significant positive result for verum (chi^2 = 8.44). *Mustard gas* (chi^2 = 3.58) and *Rhus-tox* (chi^2 = 5.24) approached significance on their own, despite the very small numbers involved (23 and 21 respectively). The second series retested *Rhus-tox* as a treatment and *Mustard gas* as prophylactic, adding *Variolinum* (smallpox nosode) and *Rhus-tox* as prophylactic. According to Hartley, further analysis confirmed the efficacy of *Mustard gas* as prophylactic (chi^2 = 10.39). Moreover, the efficacy of *Rhus-tox* as a treatment was 'definitely established' (chi^2 = 7.04), especially when the results from series 1 and 2 were combined (chi^2 = 11.78).

The Glasgow and London trials' homeopathic interest stems from their suggestion that isopathy (i.e. *Mustard gas*) can protect against but not treat mustard gas lesions, and that an unrelated natural substance which causes a clinical analogue of the lesions (i.e. *Rhus-tox*), can treat but not protect. This appears to support experimentally the traditional neglect of isopathy and nosodes in treatment of their source conditions, while allowing them a role as prophylactics (see Ch. 4). It was later shown that the original statistical analysis underestimated the efficacy of *Kali-bich* in series 1 because the placebo group in that experiment was atypical (Owen & Ives 1982). The conduct of the trials as a whole is remarkable for the era, and the London series included what are probably the first randomized double-blind placebo-controlled clinical experiments to incorporate not only individual statistical analysis but a simple meta-analysis as well.

9.5.3. Burton-on-Trent, 1951–53: surgical tuberculosis

A trial of classical homeopathy in tuberculosis of bones and joints was conducted by E.K. Ledermann in the early 1950s. Ledermann had previously published a case series of serious mixed chronic diseases including surgical TB, and later had argued that homeopathy was perfectly suitable for evaluation in clinical trials, but should be tested against placebo, not conventional therapies (1945; 1949). The randomized trial at Bretby Hall Orthopaedic Hospital, Burton-on-Trent, was a development of that research interest. Ledermann (1954) randomized patients single-handed by tossing a coin, and was aware which patient received verum or placebo, on top of treatment as usual – bedrest, immobilization, surgery, diet, antibiotics. However, the hospital staff, including R. Lunt, the orthopedic surgeon who made the clinical evaluation, were not aware which treatment had been given. The main outcome was 'general progress' measured on a 5-point scale, and showed no statistical difference between groups. A secondary binary measure of 'unexpected improvement' was applied to the first 51 patients only (27 verum, 24 placebo), and showed a trend in favour of homeopathy: 12 met the criterion, 9 of whom had received verum. There were many obstacles to the satisfactory conduct of the trial. Sutherland, the MRC statistician, noted that the homeopathy group appeared to contain more advanced cases at admission, and that concurrent antibiotics may well have masked longer term benefits from homeopathy. Ledermann himself had a 5-hour journey to the hospital from London, preventing consultations of the frequency and length normally expected. Lunt was anxious to try the new antibiotics, marsilid and isonicotinic acid hydrazide, and stopped evaluation of 'unexpected improvement' prematurely as noted.

9.6. Discussion

9.6.1. Conditions treated

Homeopaths had always claimed that chronic disease could be treated successfully, but after some early trials for mixed conditions (see Ch. 6), clinical trials had focussed almost entirely on acute illnesses. This represents the clinical concerns of the pre-antibiotic era, but also some of the administrative difficulties in conducting lengthy trials for chronic illness. The exceptions in this group were chronic furunculosis, chronic URTI and surgical tuberculosis.

9.6.2. National styles of homeopathy

National styles of prescribing are apparent in the trials found here, and reflect the research climate in each country. In Germany, the subject was approached from the clinical low-potency quadrant shown in Figure 4.1. In the USA, low- and high-potency advocates were both represented, but human clinical trials were only conducted using low potencies. The absence of French clinical trials in this period is notable, although in vitro and animal research into the physico-chemical basis of dynamization was more advanced there than elsewhere, as the result of the formation of three major research-orientated homeopathic pharmacies around 1930 [26]. In Britain, in the 1930s, basic research into potency variation paralleled the French and American efforts, and towards the end of the period British researchers managed to synthesize the different national trends of the previous 40 years, investigating the effects of ultramolecular potencies on healthy and sick humans, using clinical, isopathic and classical methods.

The content of the trials shows that some homeopaths at least were willing to expose homeopathy to an internal critique. The trial designs show a retreat from the pragmatism of the previous 50 years, and the development of a much narrower focus, testing hypotheses about specific treatments such as those seen in the American trials before 1923. Trials of increasingly clearly defined conditions became the norm, allowing the rejection of traditional clinical recommendations which had outlived their usefulness. However, the trialists were quick to point out that the average group effect of a specific was not a test of homeopathy per se, but only a test of the specific medicine and potency used.

It is worth noting the retreat from traditional ideas of individualizing treatments that created the need for these trials. Hahnemann repeatedly pointed out that each epidemic required a *genius epidemicus* to be worked out to match the current symptoms. Although he recommended *Belladonna* for the 'mild smooth scarlet fever of Sydenham' that was prevalent in about 1800 (Hahnemann 1801b), he warned later that the same treatment was not suitable

---

[26] Boiron (1990 Chs 3–5) reviews French basic research 1900–1950, as part of a broader historical treatment of the potency problem in homeopathy, culminating in the Beneveniste–*Nature* 'memory of water' controversy.

for a much more severe disease (probably hemorrhagic scarlet fever) that began to emerge in his lifetime, but which was still given the generic diagnosis and treatment for 'scarlet fever' by German physicians (Hahnemann 1808b). Records of the virulence of the disease in Great Britain from the mild, rarely fatal disease that Sydenham observed in 1675 until the 1950s, seem to confirm Hahnemann's observations:

> It seems clear that bad epidemics occurred in the eighteenth century, that there were quite long intervals between them, and that sometimes in the early years of the nineteenth century – probably about 1803 – the disease became milder, although it was still common. The mild phase ... lasted until about 1830, but from then on the disease began to increase in severity again ... In 1840 the number of deaths nearly doubled and, for a generation after, scarlet fever was the leading cause of death amongst the infectious diseases of childhood. (Gale 1959: 89ff)

Hahnemann called the more virulent disease purpura miliaris, and recommended *Aconitum* at one time. However, his continued emphasis on the need to recalibrate treatments was forgotten, and *Belladonna* was used, with little success, by homeopaths and allopaths for the rest of the nineteenth century (see Ch. 7). The three trials of *Belladonna* by Chadwell and Wesselhoeft Jr were clearly designed to test an outdated treatment they had reason to believe had become a millstone round homeopathy's neck. Wesselhoeft showed by reanalysis of the symptomatology that the *Belladonna* provings only corresponded to the mildest cases of the disease – as Hahnemann had pointed out. Wesselhoeft (1924) also went on to show that reanalysis of collective symptoms in mumps, according to the traditional method used in epidemics, could lead to an effective treatment that was unlisted in the homeopathic clinical guides. This was for a condition where classical individualization of symptoms had been found to be ineffective – and in fact with a higher complication rate than under allopathy – in the same hospital (see 9.3.5).

Nosological categories also determined the treatments in the earliest German trials of this group. A contemporary account by the homeopath Otto Leeser indicates the vehemence of some of the a priori allopathic opposition to Bier's trials, and also views the affair from a perspective of greater homeopathic experience than Bier's.

> In his polemic publication W. Heubner denies that the action of sulphur in furunculosis, even if it should be confirmed, is concerned with a homeopathic effect. He states: 'Because the introduction of a disease like furunculosis through the ingestion of large doses is not held possible even among the ho-

> meopathic profession and much less has not been demonstrated.' I must contradict him: In Hahnemann's *Chronic Diseases*, one finds under sulphur the symptom, boil. In the depiction of the action of sulphur by Hugo Schulz one finds: 'Increased sweating occurs, eruptions of the most diverse type develop, particularly furunculosis.' But we may permit a contemporary of Heubner who is unsuspected of any homeopathic conceptions to speak. L. Lewin states: 'After the ingestion of sulphur, occasionally an acne or miliaria-like eruption appears, very rarely swellings and carbuncle-like formations.' From more recent times the experiences of A. Bier as well as his pupil Abegg may be added.
>
> I have mentioned this controversy in order to show that the use of sulphur is well founded homeopathically and that A. Stiegele, who at one time recommended a retesting of sulphur iodatum to A. Bier, was entirely justified from the standpoint of the homeopathic method. But what Stiegele surely did not wish and what, as he himself has stressed repeatedly, would be entirely non-homeopathic, is the generalization to which Bier's reports gave occasion in the medical world, namely that sulphur is indicated for any furunculosis. With such an unselected procedure only a certain percentage of results will be obtained. It is not homeopathic when one proceeds to give sulphur on the basis of the diagnosis furunculosis. Only if the furunculosis stands on the soil of such skin and metabolic alterations which lie in the sulphur trend, will the homeopathic physician select sulphur. It might be that he would select arsenicum if there were a diabetic basis, or again arnica if there were a diabetic basis, or again arnica if there were a pyemic state in the degenerative condition of issue and skin, and a tendency to ecchymosis spoke particularly for it. To know the homeopathic use of sulphur means to know the homeopathic materia medica as completely as possible so that one may proceed differentially-therapeutically. (Leeser 1936: 368ff)

Later trials of clinical homeopathy in Britain screened a range of clinical medicines inductively in order to establish the most promising ones which were then retested with larger numbers. Isopathy was also used as a test of the biological activity of high potencies per se. The last trial in the review tested individualized high potency classical homeopathy demonstrably similar to that practised today.

9.6.3. Trial design

Received opinion states that the self-critical ideal of biomedicine was reflected in the gradual emergence of the modern clinical trial by about 1950, combining randomization, blinding and statistical analysis (Lilienfeld 1982). At the same time, the emergence of the clinical research orientation that came to define biomedicine in the twentieth century was also believed to have sounded the death knell for homeopathy.

Against this, early twentieth-century clinical trials show that homeopaths quickly adopted the conventions of the controlled trial, ahead of orthodox medicine in some cases. The use of placebos as a control was already institutionalized within homeopathy in a way that it had not been elsewhere (see Ch. 8), and homeopaths appear to have been eager to grasp the opportunity to apply more modern statistical analyses to their therapy than had been possible in the previous century. In particular the emergence of standard deviation was welcomed, since it helped to remove a notorious source of bias that had affected comparisons of unbalanced treatment groups (Guttentag 1940). Some British trials in the group reflect advanced experimental thinking for their day, and were designed with independent statistical analysis of the results in mind. Beginning in 1941, reports began to contain enough detail about experimental conditions and results for them to be assessed for internal validity using modern methodological quality scales. The era of modern clinical evaluation of homeopathy can be dated to circa 1940, and it is appropriate therefore to use that as the starting date for the review of contemporary trials in Part III.

Part III:
Is homeopathy clinically relevant? A systematic review of clinical trials, 1940–98

10. Rationale

Background: Public demand for alternative and complementary medicine has never been greater, and homeopathy is high on the list of sought-after therapies. Purchasers and providers looking for evidence to justify funding naturally turn to published reports of clinical trials or reviews of those trials.

Questions: What reviews have been conducted? Did their design and conduct affect the conclusions drawn? Is a further review justified? If so, what areas of interest should it explore?

Argument: Traditional narrative reviews are giving way to systematic literature reviews. With regard to homeopathy, these have mainly been limited to the placebo question. The most inclusive review was published in 1991, since which time many trials have been published. All of the reviews provide only scant detail of trial content. A new review of trials with placebo, orthodox and no treatment controls is justified. It should contain enough detail to provide the foundation for a searchable database of homeopathic trials, and should also look at areas neglected in previous reviews, such as intrahomeopathic differences, safety and clinical relevance.

10.1. Previous reviews of homeopathic clinical trials

Recent reviews of clinical trials of homeopathy fall into two main groups, narrative and systematic. Traditional narrative reviews, often found in textbooks and monographs, have tended to survey a variety of experimental evidence, including controlled therapeutic trials in humans (e.g. Sankaran 1978; Coulter 1981; Scofield 1984; Aulas, Bordelay, Royer 1991; Righetti 1991; Bellavite & Signorini 1995; Meyer 1996). The criteria for inclusion and assessment are not stated in any of these sources, and the most trials reviewed in any was 31 (Aulas, Bordelay, Royer 1991). Overall conclusions are generally declared to be positive or negative according to the number of trials that found statistically significant differences between homeopathy and placebo. Authors' allegiances regarding the plausibility of homeopathy sometimes interfere with the reporting and interpretation of evidence. Some sources attempt to explain away any positive results for homeopathy, in keeping with the authors' rejection of homeopathy's plausibility (e.g. Aulas, Bordelay, Royer 1991; Meyer 1996), while only interpretations favouring homeopathy are found in another source, coupled with overt anti-allopathic bias (Coulter 1981).

However useful discussions in sources not subject to peer review may be in other respects, narrative reviews are clearly open to many sorts of bias in the framing of study questions, literature search, data extraction from primary reports, interpretation of results and presentation of overall conclusions – a widespread problem by no means confined to reviews of homeopathy (Cook & Leviton 1980). The presence of any of these potential biases poses a threat to the purpose of literature review, which can be summarized concisely as the synthesis of results from individual studies with the intention of allowing generalizations to be made about, or from, an intervention or population of interest.

By contrast with narrative reviews, systematic reviews are expected to be conducted according to a transparent protocol from the outset, allowing method and results to be independently replicated, as in scientific experimentation generally (e.g. Oxman, Cook, Guyatt 1994; NHS CRD 1996; Mulrow & Oxman 1997). The literature is searched, and data extracted, in a predefined way, and quality scales are often used to allow comparison of individual trials and to give greater weight to results from trials with higher internal validity (Moher, Jadad, Nichol et al. 1995). Overall conclusions are either based on rigorous overviews, or increasingly on quantitative estimates of effect, coupled in both cases with sensitivity analyses of the robustness of evidence. It is generally regarded as unwise to dichotomize trial results into 'positive' and 'negative' on the basis of 95% significance tests, since p values of 0.04 and 0.06 indicate similar strength of evidence. The technique of meta-analysis tries to avoid this by converting a single (main) outcome from each study to an odds ratio, or similar. Ratios are then weighted for sample size and pooled. Combining results, especially of small studies which may have insufficient power to reject a null hypothesis, can allow a more definite answer to a question (Cook & Leviton 1980; Pogue & Yusuf 1998).

The science of conducting reliable systematic reviews is a recent one (Light & Pillemer 1984; Chalmers & Altman 1995; Russell, Di Blasi, Lambert et al. 1998), and developments typifying the evolution of the field as a whole can be traced even in the small sample of 5 found here after a literature search was undertaken for systematic reviews of homeopathy. The essential characteristics of those that were not restricted to specific conditions or medicines are shown in Table 10.1.

The earliest review (Hill & Doyon 1990) does not appear to have followed an explicit protocol, other than screening reports for adequate randomization. The authors extracted data concerning trial design, treatments and outcomes from 40 randomized trials of homeopathy vs placebo, orthodox or no treatment controls chosen from an unspecified number found in the literature search. No quality assessment instrument for grading internal or external validity was used. Results were displayed as positive or negative declarations of the original authors, presumably depending on whether statistical significance of $p \leq 0.05$ was found – 19 positive, 19 negative, 2 undecided. The reviewers declared that there was not enough evidence from large high-quality trials to support the idea that homeopathic medicines might be efficacious.

Table 10.1 Inclusive systematic reviews of clinical trials of homeopathy, 1990–98

Reference	Design	Homeo. type	N found	N incl.	Question	Quality tool	Result
Hill & Doyon 1990	Systematic review	All	?	40	General overview	no	–ve
Kleijnen, Knipschild and ter Riet 1991	Systematic review	All	107	105	General overview	yes	+ve (?)
Boissel, Cucherat, Haugh and Gauthier 1996	Meta-analysis	All	189	20	> than placebo?	no	p<.001
Linde, Clausius, Ramirez, et al. 1997	Meta-analysis	All	186	89	> than placebo?	yes	OR 2.45
Linde & Melchart 1998	Meta-analysis	Classical	35	32/19	> than placebo?	yes	RR 1.65

Kleijnen, Knipschild and ter Riet (1991) used an explicit protocol and a very extensive literature search for trials with placebo, orthodox or no treatment control (including historical controls, uniquely among these reviews). The quality assessment tool devised by the reviewers awards points for the usual internal validity factors such as randomization and masking, but imposes heavy discounting of positive evidence found in small trials, which immediately attracted adverse comment (Fisher, Huskisson, Scott et al. 1991). The scale (0–100) awards up to 30 points for trial size alone, and small trials are further penalized, as they can receive only 10 out of the 20 points possible for randomization – no matter how well they were randomized. Small trials with good internal validity are inevitably labelled as 'poor quality', inherently unable to surpass the 55 point cut point (as discussed in Dean 1998). The scale also deducts points if the manufacturing procedure for a test medicine was not described in full, which attracted further criticism from Fisher et al. (1991) who observed that most biomedical journals impose strict word limits that restrict the amount of detail that can be included in trial reports. The test medicine in the (small but well-conducted) trial by Fisher et al. (1989), for example, was made in accordance with the French national homeopathic pharmacopeia, but there was no opportunity to mention this in the space allowed. The vote count in the review was again based on individual significance tests, but showed evidence of homeopathic superiority in 81 of 105 of trials (77%), a trend which seemed independent of trial quality to the reviewers. They stated that they would be more likely to modify their prior incredulity about homeopathic efficacy – which led them to conduct the review – when independent replications of successful trials had been published.

Another very extensive literature search was conducted using a rigorous protocol for data extraction in order to answer the placebo question by meta-analysis, for the first time in reviews of homeopathy (Boissel, Cucherat, Haugh et al. 1996). No previously developed quality assessment tool was used, because trials were required to meet all the inclusion criteria – mostly standard internal validity points relating to masking and randomization. However, the decision to exclude any trial that was not explicitly analysed as intention-to-treat restricted the meta-analysis to only 20 trials of the 189 found. The criterion was adopted to exclude biases that can affect treatment-only analyses, but in this case left out many trials where the assigned and analysed numbers were the same because there had been no attrition. The authors acknowledged that their meta-analysis technique of pooled p values from separate trials was problematic, but a positive result survived sensitivity analyses such as exclusion of poor quality trials and the addition of hypothetical trials with null results ($p=0.5$) to the pool. An overall value of $p<0.001$ led the reviewers to conclude that at least one of the review trials must have shown superiority to placebo, although it was not possible to identify which one.

A parallel review with an explicit protocol designed to answer the placebo question also used an extensive search strategy and uncovered 186 trials, of which 133 were placebo-controlled and 119 were also randomized and/or double-blind (Linde, Clausius, Ramirez et al. 1997). The quality scale was again developed by the review team, and does not contain any of the contentious items or weightings noted in the scale devised by Kleijnen et al. (1991). Although only 89 trials results were reported in a manner allowing them to be expressed as odds ratios, the positive meta-analysis of those trials survived all the sensitivity analyses conducted: for each of classical, clinical, isopathic and complex homeopathy alone; for ultramolecular dilutions above Avogadro's constant (D24 and C12 or above in homeopathic potencies); for Medline-only trials; and for 26 high-quality studies only. However, the authors were clear that there were no implications for clinical practice, since they found no evidence that homeopathy was effective in any single clinical condition.

Two of these authors then reviewed trials of classical homeopathy, again to answer the placebo question (Linde & Melchart 1998). A refinement of their quality scale was used to assess 32 of 35 reports suitable for inclusion in the overview. A meta-analysis similar to that carried out in the sensitivity analysis for classical trials in the previous review was performed with 19 trials containing results that could be converted to rate ratios. Although an overall RR of 1.65 was found, little convincing evidence of superiority to placebo was found in trials with high quality scores – RR 1.12.

10.2. Is another systematic review of homeopathic trials justified?

In view of the evidence overviewed here, what is the justification for another systematic review? If it were to try to answer the placebo question once again, there would be little point. The painstakingly thorough meta-analysis by Linde et al. (1997) is generally regarded as the strongest evidence yet published of homeopathic superority over placebo. There is a case for updating it when a substantial number of new randomized placebo-controlled trials has emerged – ≥20% new trials are recommended to avoid the risk of Type 1 error (Pogue & Yusuf 1998) – but that is not the same as a new review.

However, all of the reviews discussed were explicitly or implicitly designed to answer the scientific question 'Are homeopathic medicines any better than placebo?'. Various eligibility criteria for study inclusion, such as placebo-controlled only, or randomized only, or intention-to-treat only, might have left out trials of interest from the point of view of planning further research and replications. Moreover, although the review with the least restrictive criteria assessed 105 trials altogether (Kleijnen, Knipschild, ter Riet 1991), many more trials with no treatment and orthodox treatment as control have been published or discovered since it was conducted. It must also be noted that all the reviews provide only brief details of the trials.

These observations taken together suggest the need for a comprehensive and systematic literature search to create a detailed database of prospective clinical trials of homeopathy with controls, including no treatment and orthodox treatment as well as placebo. From a number of recommendations concerning future research made by Scofield (1984), two in particular stand out as not having been addressed in any of the above reviews: (1) that the safety of homeopathy cannot be taken for granted, despite the assurances of many of its proponents; and (2) that homeopathy needs to provide evidence of clinical relevance, not mere statistical superiority to placebo. Questions about the following areas should therefore be posed in a new review:

Intrahomeopathic differences: Although some previous reviews have identified 4 basic homeopathic subgroups – classical, clinical, complex and isopathy – little attention has been paid to differences in content and treatment validity.

Safety: The safety of homeopathic medicines has often been assumed (Jonas 1998), and few empirical studies have been published (Hentschel, Kohnen, Hahn 1998). A new review should look for evidence of adverse treatment effects as reported in trials.

Holism: Classical homeopathy is claimed by its proponents to be a holistic therapy, dissimilar to biomedicine which tends to target the specific causes or symptoms of pathology. Global response to treatment as measured by effects on comorbidity and intercurrent illness should be included.

Efficiency: Homeopathy is often said to be economically efficient because of the low cost of medicines. Cost–benefit and cost–utility data should also be looked for in a new review.

Clinical relevance: Statistical superiority over placebo does not guarantee clinical relevance. Other points of comparison can be looked for in trials of homeopathy vs orthodox treatments, and in placebo-controlled trials for conditions where orthodox treatments are unavailable or of low efficacy.

In the light of these considerations, a new comprehensive database and review incorporating the points above as objectives seemed to be justified, and was therefore undertaken. The methods are discussed in Ch. 11.

11. Methods

11.1. Literature search and data sources

Medline, Embase and the Cochrane Library databases were searched for controlled clinical trials of homeopathy using the terms 'homeopat*' and 'homoeopat*' for the period to 31 December 1998, and the entire result of the searches was manually screened.

The great majority of alternative therapy reports are not indexed by the principal biomedical data extraction services such as Index Medicus and Embase, so a comprehensive search was conducted of the so-called grey literature, including:

- British Library AMED/CATS and RCCM CISCOM databases of references from alternative medicine journals not indexed elsewhere
- cumulative indexes of the principal international homeopathic journals not included in Medline or Embase
- the bibliographies of monographs (e.g. Sankaran 1978; Coulter 1981; Aulas, Bordelay, Royer 1991; Righetti 1991; Bellavite & Signorini 1995; Meyer 1996)
- international and national homeopathic congress proceedings (e.g. Liga Homeopatica Internationalis and GIRI – International Congress on Ultra Low Doses)
- the paper archive of 348 trial reports and review articles collected by Hominform (Glasgow Homeopathic Hospital Library) on behalf of the EU Homeopathic Medicine Research Group (Boissel, Cucherat, Haugh et al. 1996).

The bibliographies of original research reports and review articles cited in the sources above were also screened. Internationally, researchers and librarians in the field were contacted and asked to provide further references.

11.2. Language restrictions

Results of systematic reviews are highly susceptible to bias when based only on reports in English (Moher, Fortin, Jadad et al. 1996). Because of the international spread of homeopathy and the high proportion of non-English language reports, the literature search included reports irrespective of language.

11.3. Inclusion and exclusion criteria

The criteria established for selection and exclusion of trial reports are listed below.

11.3.1. Therapy definition

Homeopathy was defined as any of the methods described in Ch. 4, and their variants, and broadly classified as classical, clinical, complex or isopathy.

The definition did not include therapies or diagnostic systems related to homeopathy, such as anthroposophical medicine and radionics (Steiner 1948; Russell 1973), which sometimes employ homeopathic medicines but with fundamentally different reasons and methods for their selection.

11.3.2. Medicine definition

Homeopathic medicines were defined as substances prepared according to homeopathic pharmacopeia, and included in the homeopathic materia medica and repertory (e.g. Schroyens 1993). Although some reviews accept only potentized medicines (e.g. Linde, Clausius, Ramirez et al. 1997; Dantas & Fisher 1998), it was decided to include unpotentized mother tinctures (Ø) as well. The boundary between homeopathy and phytotherapy is fuzzy in certain areas, but the review relates to homeopathy as practised and its clinical relevance rather than the dilution–placebo question. A number of homeopathic medicines were adopted from folk medicine before being subject to provings, and are widely used in homeopathy as both mother tincture and potencies, with similar indications. An example would be marigold (*Calendula officinalis*) for wound healing.

The definition excludes electronically and radionically simulated potencies (e.g. Thomas 1994; Dittmann, Kanapin, Harisch 1999).

11.3.3. Trial design

Given the small number of trials found in previous systematic reviews (maximum = 189) for the field as a whole, the inclusion of pseudo- and nonrandomized trials meeting these criteria was felt to be justified, especially as a quality assessment instrument purposely designed for this was used (see 11.6).

Studies were eligible for inclusion if they were:

- prospective human clinical (curative, palliative or prophylactic) trials

with

- one or more concurrent or historical control groups that received either no treatment, placebo or an orthodox treatment
- a mean of ≥10 patients in each treatment arm.

Studies not eligible for inclusion were:

- retrospective
- single-group designs (including placebo-controlled time series or before-and-after designs)
- trials with surrogate outcomes only
- pathogenetic drug tests (provings) designed to elicit symptoms in healthy volunteers
- experiments to measure physiological effects of homeopathy on healthy subjects.

11.4. Data extraction

The primary data extraction form created for the review was successfully piloted in a review of trials of classical homeopathy, and was refined for the present review. It contains 43 fields which were filled in for all trials, and a further 7 relating to classical homeopathy only.

Studies were indexed under the following heads:

- *Bibliography* including publication type and language.
- *Clinical* including trial condition, clinical area, levels of disease (acute, chronic, subacute) and treatment (curative, palliative, symptomatic).
- *Population* including country, number assigned, number analysed, age, gender, inclusion and exclusion criteria.
- *Design* including number of centres, masking, randomization, overall follow-up period.
- *Pharmacy* including type of homeopathy, medicines, potencies, dosage and repetition, manufacture. Dilutions above N_A (equivalent in homeopathic potencies to ≥C12, D24) were also classed as 'ultramolecular', while those below were classed as 'molecular'.

- *Treatment* including the number of homeopaths required to decide a prescription, whether follow-ups were included, and the interval between them.
- *Outcomes* including primary and secondary outcome measures, in order of importance as far as could be ascertained; reporting of adverse reactions; effects on comorbidity and intercurrent illness.
- *Results* including authors' reports and estimates of effect; statistical tests (where given). Confidence intervals were not reported in most trials and were not collected here.

Trials of classical homeopathy were also assigned to 1 of 3 overall categories defined according to the accrual policy and initial availability of treatment options:

- *open* when therapists made a free choice from the homeopathic materia medica;
- *restricted* when individualization was limited to a choice from a pre-defined list of medicines intended to be used for all subjects whether appropriate or not;
- *selective* when subjects were admitted to a trial only provided they had previously been matched with a medicine from a pre-defined list.

The following fields were also completed for classical trials:

- degree of choice of initial potency: fixed, limited or free
- freedom or otherwise to change medicine, potency or repetition: fixed, limited or free
- the number of homeopaths required to decide a prescription
- the treatment rationale in the words of the original author or authors.

11.5. Representing strength of results

As noted, vote counts based on totalling dichotomized 'positive' and 'negative' results are not recommended (Cook & Leviton 1980). Yet in a review of widely different designs and treatments where pooled estimates of effect are not intended, an adequate means of summarizing results is required. A compromise was adopted based on the creation of a 5-point stratified vote which takes account of statistical trends and secondary outcomes as well as significant differences in a primary outcome. Trials controlled by placebo or no treatment were assigned to one of 5 levels:

+	significant result favouring homeopathy in primary outcome
(+)	statistical trend favouring homeopathy in primary outcome, or significant results in secondary outcome(s)
0	statistical equivalence
(-)	statistical trend favouring control in primary outcome, or significant results in secondary outcome(s)
-	significant result favouring control in primary outcome.

In view of the difficulties attached to the interpretation of equivalence in pragmatic trials of competing treatments (Jones, Jarvis, Lewis et al. 1996), trials of this sort were graphically distinguished from no treatment and placebo-controlled trials, and assigned to one of 3 levels:

>	significant result favouring homeopathy in primary outcome, or equivalence of primary outcome plus significant result favouring homeopathy in secondary outcome(s)
=	statistical equivalence, including insignificant trends in either direction
<	significant result favouring orthodox treatment, or equivalence of primary outcome plus significant result favouring orthodox treatment in secondary outcome(s).

For trials that compared homeopathy with more than one control treatment, the vote was based on a single comparison: orthodox treatment, placebo, no treatment, in that order of preference.

11.6. Methodological quality instrument

Instruments for evaluating the validity of clinical trial conduct, analysis and reporting have become popular since one of the first was published two decades ago (Chalmers, Smith Jr, Blackburn et al. 1981). However, methodological quality (MQ) scales can easily mislead, and their use is being increasingly questioned. Because many scales conflate reporting standards with internal validity in a single score, this can lead to separate reports of the same trial receiving widely different scores on the same scale (Dean 1998). Moreover, a comprehensive evaluated review of 25 MQ scales and 9 checklists – including Kleijnen et al. (1991) – showed that the same trial might score 20% or 70% depending on the scale used, and criticized all of the scales for not having been developed scientifically, with the exception of one developed by the reviewers (Moher, Jadad, Nichol et al. 1995; Jadad, Moore, Carroll et al. 1996). The conclusions were that many scales failed to define the constructs they sought to measure; and that checklists were probably of greater use to the authors of trials than to reviewers. Because of problems such as these, some sources now advise against quality scoring altogether, or suggest reviewers use them merely as a primary exclusion filter (NHS CRD 1996; Mulrow & Oxman 1997).

In a fresh attempt to develop a reliable and valid instrument, a preliminary wish list of 49 items thought to be indicative of internal validity was reduced to just 3 core items: randomization; double-masking; and analysis of dropouts and withdrawals (Jadad 1994). Although this scale is now used widely, a weakness is that trials that report randomization are scored as being properly randomized even when details of the randomization method are not given. This may be related to the scale's original development as part of an effort to review an archive of several thousand pain trial reports. It appears to have been designed at least initially as a simple primary filter to allow extraction of ostensibly high quality trials from a mountain of data.

The situation in homeopathy is completely different: with fewer than 300 trials found in all it seems wasteful to discard preliminary evidence of lesser quality which might nevertheless stimulate further more rigorous research. Bearing the above-mentioned problems in mind, it was decided that the use of a preexisting MQ scale would be justified if it allowed meaningful weighting of trials with widely different designs in a review not intended to include a post-filtration meta-analysis of results derived from one design alone. Moher et al.'s (1995) review of scales contained at least one instrument (Cho & Bero 1994) that appeared to have been developed and tested for interrater reliability in a similar manner to that by Jadad et al. Although this scale suffers from some of the shortcomings common to others – conflation of reporting with internal validity, scoring of precision of results – it was adopted here in preference to other scales reviewed for 3 compelling reasons:

1. It is designed to allow meaningful inclusion and weighted comparative evaluation of many different study designs, including prospective case series, case-controlled studies and longitudinal cohort studies, not just randomized, masked pharmacological trials. This would be important if a decision were

made at a later date to enlarge the database to include designs excluded from the present review.

2. It contains 23 questions (plus a further 7 on clinical relevance – see 11.7), corresponding in many respects to the revised checklist of 22 items prepared by The Consolidated Standards of Reporting Trials Group (CONSORT) (e.g. Moher, Schulz, Altman et al. 2001), in contrast to the streamlined 5-item tool developed by Jadad et al. The answers to these 23 (or 30) questions are worth retaining in any searchable database that might be created from this review, regardless of the plausibility of the combined scores.
3. All questions apart from no. 1 (study design) and no. 2 (study question) are scored on a 3-point scale of 0 ('no'), 1 ('partially') and 2 ('yes'), rather than the more usual binary 'yes', 'no'. This acknowledges the distance between trial conduct and reporting that sometimes exists, and is comparable with the checklist created by the original Standards of Reporting Trials Group (1994).

The MQ instrument used here is shown in Table 11.1.

Table 11.1 Methodological quality instrument, after Cho & Bero (1994)

AU (PY) TI

1 Study design (check 1 only) __

Experimental, randomized trial:	Experimental, unrandomized trial:	Nonexperimental:
___ Placebo-controlled	___ Placebo-controlled	___ Cohort, prospective
___ Comparative, no placebo	___ Comparative, no placebo	___ Cohort, retrospective
___ Time series	___ Time series	___ Cross-sectional
___ Crossover	___ Crossover	___ Case-control
	___ Natural experiment	___ Case reports or case series

2 What was the study question?

SCORES FOR Qs 3–23:
YES = 2 PARTIALLY = 1 NO = 0 Not applicable = strike through

3 Was the study question sufficiently described? __
4 Was the study design appropriate to answer the study question? __
5 Were both inclusion and exclusion criteria specified? __
6 Were subjects appropriate to the study question? __

7 Were control subjects appropriate? (If no controls were used, score 0) __
8 Were subjects randomly selected from the target population? __
9 If subjects were randomly selected, was randomization sufficiently well described? __
10 If subjects were randomly allocated to treatment groups, was allocation truly concealed? (If unrandom, strike out) __
11 If blinding of investigators to intervention was possible, was it reported? (If not possible, strike out) __
12 If blinding of subjects to intervention was possible, was it reported? (If not possible, strike out) __
13 Was measurement bias accounted for by methods other than blinding? __
14 Were known confounders accounted for by study design? (If no known confounders, strike out) __
15 Were known confounders accounted for by analysis? (If no known confounders, strike out.) __
16 Was there a sample size justification before the study? __
17 Were post hoc power calculations or confidence intervals reported for insignificant results? __
18 Were statistical analyses appropriate? __
19 Were the statistical tests stated? __
20 Were exact *P* values or confidence intervals reported for each test? __
21 Were attrition of subjects and reason for attrition recorded? (If no attrition, strike out.) __
22 For those subjects who completed the study, were results completely reported? __
23 Do the findings support the conclusion? __

Quality score [TOTAL /number of scored qs]: 0.______

In Question 1 each reviewed design receives a score of 1–5: 1 for case reports, 2 for time series or uncontrolled experiments, 3 for cohort or case-control studies, 4 for unrandomized controlled trials, 5 for randomized controlled trials. In this review, designs scoring lower than 3 were excluded. Questions 3–23 are scored as shown. Question 10 originally asked: 'If subjects were randomly allocated to treatment groups, was allocation sufficiently well described?'. It was felt the second clause could be modified to 'was randomization truly concealed?' with no loss of the authors' original intent, but a considerable gain in clarity and salience.

Final scores can be weighted in one of 3 ways, shown here with the inter-rater reliability of overall quality scores in tests conducted by the instrument's authors:

1. all questions equally weighted: $r = .81$ (95% CI, .58–.93)
2. Question 1 multiplied by 3: $r = .89$ (95% CI, .73–.96)
3. points for design, randomization, masking, statistical analysis, and support of conclusions by result given more weight: $r = .85$ (95% CI, .65–.94).

Scheme 2 was adopted for this review, giving possible design scores of 9, 12 or 15.

To ensure consistency, an extensive key to filling in the form was created for the review (efforts to elicit a response from the authors having failed). The key included rules for adjudicating difficult or borderline cases.

External comparisons between MQ scores obtained in this review and the scores of the same trials as rated by Kleijnen et al. (1991) or Linde et al. (1997) were made.

11.7. Clinical relevance instrument

A literature search revealed only one instrument for evaluating clinical relevance (Cho & Bero 1994). This was presented in the same source as the methodological quality instrument, and was developed in the same manner.

Table 11.2 Clinical relevance instrument (Cho & Bero 1994)

SCORES FOR Qs 1–7: YES = 2 Partially = 1 NO = 0

1 Were the therapeutic outcomes measured in the study important? __
2 Were subjects representative of those who would actually use the treatment? (Insufficient info = 0) __
3 Was the comparison group clinically meaningful? __
4 Was the treatment effect clinically meaningful? __
5 Were side effects adequately measured? __
6 Was approval from an institutional ethics committee explicitly reported? __
7 As far as could be determined from the article was the study ethical? __

CLINICAL Relevance score [TOTAL /14]: 0.______

It contains 7 questions relating to efficacy, generalizability and ethics (Table 11.2). A key was created to ensure consistency of scoring for the clinical relevance (CR) instrument, similar to that for the methodological tool.

11.8. Quality control and data integrity

The primary data extraction form was created in a computer database (FileMaker Pro), and was successfully piloted in a review of classical homeopathy only. The form allowed visual identity between the paper form used for the initial handwritten recording of the information for each trial and the subsequent on-screen data entry. After data entry the complete file was proof-checked by an experienced technical editor against the original handwritten forms. A random selection of 20 (9.8%) included trial reports were entered manually into the data extraction form twice, and there were no significant disagreements at this level.

The MQ and CR forms were again designed in FileMaker Pro and integrated with the data extraction file. Similar quality procedures to those for the primary data extraction form were followed. Additionally, before on-screen entry, each handwritten sheet for the two instruments was checked by the editor against the keys created for them, to ensure the rules had been observed consistently.

11.9. Sensitivity analysis and statistics

The review was not hypothesis-driven, and descriptive statistics, charts and d ata plots were the primary means used to explore data. Intrahomeopathic differences were looked for in many areas including trial design, clinical area, publication type or language, potency level and results. Adequacy of assignment and masking methods and attrition handling were looked at for effects on strength of results. Possible correlations with MQ scores were investigated in, e.g. publication type or language, type of homeopathic or control treatment, attrition handling, potency levels and adverse events reporting.

The MQ scale used here does not contain a high-quality cut point. Both Kleijnen et al. (1991) and Linde et al. (1997) independently stated that the best 10% of trials in their sets could be regarded as having good internal validity. In the context of the present review objectives, such a narrow band seemed unduly restrictive so the top 20% of scores were used as an objective standard for inclusion of trials in more detailed discussion.

Score totalling, rounding and conversion to percentages were automated in Filemaker Pro for both the MQ and CR instruments. Inferential statistics were used in some cases to test the strength of apparent relationships and trends, but are exploratory in nature. All analyses were performed in DataDesk.

The results of the analysis are presented in Ch. 12.

12. Results

Reports of 279 prospective controlled trials of homeopathy were found in 264 separate publications dating from 1941 to December 1998. The 74 excluded trials are tabulated in Appendix 1 (see CD), along with reasons for exclusion. 205 reports in 191 separate publications met the inclusion criteria, and details of each trial can be found in Appendix 2 (see CD) as follows:

App. 2.1	Classical homeopathy
App. 2.2	Clinical homeopathy
App. 2.3	Complex homeopathy
App. 2.4	Isopathy.

Basic characteristics of the set are shown in Table 12.1.

Table 12.1 Characteristics of 205 controlled clinical trials of homeopathy

Design	**n**	**Control treatment**	**n**	**Publication type**	**n**
Parallel	192	Placebo	153	Journal article	148
Crossover	11	Orthodox treatment	37	Thesis	25
Cohort control	1	No treatment	15	Conference proceedings	21
Historical control	1			Report	7
				Book section	3
				Book	1
Patients		**Disease level**		**Language**	
Sum	46 790	Acute	109	English	117
Mean	228	Chronic	87	French	38
Median	60	Subacute	8	German	36
SD	1704	Acute and chronic	1	Italian	5
• excluding Castro & Nogueira (1975):				Spanish	4
				Dutch	2
Sum	22 426			Portuguese	2
Mean	110			Norwegian	1
Median	60				
SD	189				

Table 12.1 Characteristics of 205 controlled clinical trials of homeopathy (cont.)

Attrition		**Clinical areas**		**Country**	
Sum	823	Respiratory infections & ENT	39	Germany	48
Mean (%)	4 (8)	Surgical trauma	30	France	37
Median	0	Musculoskeletal & rheumatology	21	UK	37
SD (%)	49 (13)	Neurology & psychiatry	21	Italy	14
Range (%)	813 (80)	Dermatology	17	India	13
Assignment		Gastroenterology	16	S. Africa	10
Random	153	Gynecology and obstetrics	16	Greece	7
Nonrandom	33	Infections (misc)	12	Brazil	6
Pseudorandom	9	Asthma & allergy	11	Austria, USA	4
Matched Pairs	6	Cardiovascular	7	Netherlands	3
Missing	4	Metabolic disorders	6	Israel, Mexico, Nicaragua, Norway, Poland, Romania	2
Masking		Oncology	4	Australia, Belgium, Chile, Cuba, Ghana, Iran, Nepal, Peru, Ukraine, Zaire	1
Double	145	Trauma	3		
Open	37	Ophthalmology	2		
Single	23	**Homeopathy type**			
		Clinical	88		
		Classical	54		
		Complex	37		
		Isopathy	26		
		Potency level			
		Molecular i.e. <C12, D24	93		
		Ultramolecular i.e. ≥C12, D24	70		
		Missing	42		

12.1. Design

Patients were assigned to parallel treatment groups in 94% of trials, and a further 5% also included a crossover, with only 2 (1%) historical or cohort control studies.[27] Methods of creating balanced comparison groups included randomization (75%), pseudorandomization (4%) and matched pairs (3%) in 82% of

[27] In the text of this chapter, all percentages are based on the set of 205 trials, and rounded to the nearest whole number.

trials, while 16% were nonrandom, and information was missing in the remaining 2%. Most trials were controlled by placebo or no treatment, although 18% compared homeopathy with orthodox treatments. Evaluation was double masked in 71% of trials, single masked in 11% and open in 18%. The total number of patients was 46 790, trial mean 228, although excluding a single outlier (Castro & Nogueira 1975) approximately halved those totals. The chronological distribution of trials found is shown in Figure 12.1.

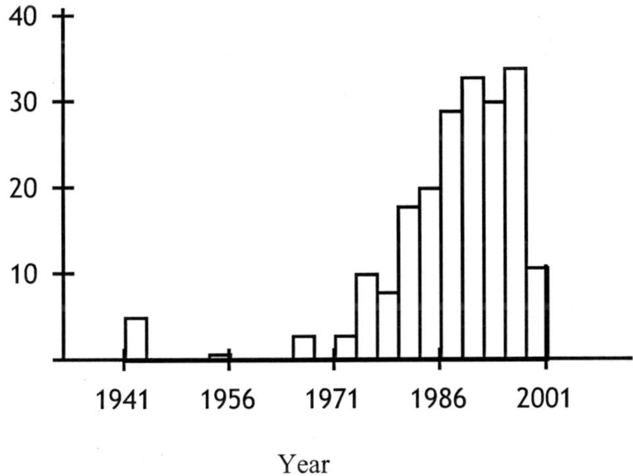

Figure 12.1 Distribution of trials by date

In all, 4 types of homeopathy were trialled: classical, clinical, complex and isopathy. Dilution data were missing from 20% of reports, but molecular potencies (i.e. those not diluted beyond N_A) were tested in 57% of the remainder. 120 separate conditions in 14 clinical areas were treated, the largest single group comprising ear, nose and throat (ENT) and general respiratory infections (19%). Acute ailments were treated in 53% of trials, chronic in 42%, with negligible numbers of sub-acute or mixed conditions.

Trials were conducted in 27 countries, with nearly 60% taking place in one of 3 countries: Germany (23%), France and the UK (18% each). They were reported in 8 different languages, but only 7% were in languages other than English (57%), French (18%) and German (18%). Journal articles accounted for 72% of reports.

12.2. Intrahomeopathic differences

Considerable differences of size and clinical objectives between the 4 different types of homeopathy on trial were visible. Even the median dates were different, indicative of changing research interests and prescribing trends. Classical homeopathy trials were the smallest on average despite accounting for more than 26% of the whole set. Conversely, even after excluding Castro & Nogueira (1975), the mean size of isopathic trials was more than twice that of the second most populous group, complex, although isopathy constituted fewer than 13% of the set (Table 12.2).

Table 12.2 Populations and median dates of homeopathy types

Homeopathy	Count	Median date	Sum	Mean	SD
Classical	54	1991	3706	68.62	54.89
Clinical	88	1986	8098	92.02	127.2
Complex	37	1992	4375	118.24	186.02
Isopathy	26	1988	30611	1177.35	4745.4
Isopathy excl. Castro & Nogueira (1975)	25		6247	249.88	400.57

There were notable differences in the disease level and clinical areas as well. Chronic diseases were treated in classical trials 3 times as often as acute disease, but less than half as often across the other 3 categories (Table 12.3).

Table 12.3 Homeopathy type and disease level

Disease level	Classical	Clinical	Complex	Isopathy
Acute	13	54	25	17
Acute + chronic	0	1	0	0
Chronic	39	29	10	9
Subacute	2	4	2	0
total	54	88	37	26

Striking differences were even reflected in publication language: 81% of classical trials were published in English, representing 38% of the English-language total, while they accounted for only 19% of German-language trials, and none at all were found in French (Table 12.4).

Table 12.4 Homeopathy type and publication language

Language	Classical	Clinical	Complex	Isopathy
Dutch	0	0	0	2
English	44	44	14	15
French	0	17	13	8
German	7	20	9	0
Italian	0	3	1	1
Norwegian	1	0	0	0
Portuguese	1	1	0	0
Spanish	1	3	0	0
total	54	88	37	26

There were also clear differences beween the clinical areas researched within each homeopathic category. For instance, the largest single group (20%) of classical trials accounted for more than half of all trials in neurology and psychiatry. This contrasted with more than one-third of complex and nearly one-half of isopathic treatments aimed at respiratory infections and ear, nose and throat problems. A predominance of trials for trauma and the sequelae of surgery was apparent in clinical homeopathy, accounting for 79% of all such trials.

Table 12.5 Homeopathy type and clinical areas

Clinical area	Classical	Clinical	Complex	Isopathy
Asthma & allergy	0	5	2	4
Cardiovascular	1	5	1	0
Dermatology	7	6	2	2
Gastroenterology	7	7	2	0
Gynecology and obstetrics	4	7	2	3
Infections (misc)	7	3	0	2
Metabolic disorders	1	4	0	1
Musculoskeletal & rheumatology	6	8	7	0
Neurology & psychiatry	11	4	6	0
Oncology	4	0	0	0
Ophthalmology	0	2	0	0
Respiratory infections & ENT	5	9	13	12
Surgical trauma	1	25	2	2
Trauma	0	3	0	0
total	54	88	37	26

Quantitative intrahomeopathic differences were reflected in the choice of controls: clinical homeopathy and isopathy were predominantly interested in the placebo question (which accounted for 86% and 77% of their respective totals), while classical and complex homeopathy comprised 70% of pragmatic or equivalence trials.

Table 12.6 Homeopathy type and control treatment

Homeopathy	No treatment	Orthodox	Placebo
Classical	5	14	35
Clinical	3	9	76
Complex	3	12	22
Isopathy	4	2	20
total	15	37	153

Category differences were also found when potency levels were compared. Leaving aside missing data, Table 12.7 shows that over three-quarters of classical homeopathy and isopathy trials reported the potency level tested as ultramolecular, in contrast to molecular dilutions only in complex homeopathy. Both levels were reported to be tested more often in clinical homeopathy. Underreporting of potency data was most prevalent in classical trials, accounting for 64% of all missing dilution data.

Table 12.7 Homeopathy type and potency level

Homeopathy	Molecular	Ultramolecular	No data
Classical	6	21	27
Clinical	48	32	8
Complex	34	0	3
Isopathy	5	17	4
total	93	70	42

Further evidence of intrahomeopathic category difference was found in attrition levels (Table 12.8). Since proportionally more clinical homeopathy trials were placebo-controlled than among other types, this may also help to account for the increased attrition found in placebo-controlled trials (Table 12.9).

Table 12.8 Homeopathy type and percent attrition

Homeopathy	Total	No data	Mean %	SD
Classical	53	1	7.79	10.86
Clinical	82	6	10.32	16.04
Complex	36	1	3.89	8.35
Isopathy	23	3	6.09	7.52

F-Test $p \leq 0.0001$

Table 12.9 Control type and percent attrition

Control	Total	No data	Mean %	SD
No treatment	15	0	5.63	7.68
Orthodox medicine	35	2	5.75	9.81
Placebo	144	9	8.70	13.83

F-Test $p \leq 0.0001$

12.3. Treatment effects

The majority of trials reported positive effects, either significant or strong trends, regardless of the type of control or homeopathy that was trialled. However, when stratified by homeopathy type and control, it was apparent that 28 (67%) of 42 negative results were reported in a single category: clinical homeopathy, including 25 placebo-controlled negative results (Table 12.10).

Table 12.10 Votes for homeopathy type by control

Homeopathy	No treatment				Placebo				Orthodox treatment		
	(-)	0	(+)	+	(-)	0	(+)	+	<	=	>
Classical	0	1	0	4	1	5	13	16	2	6	6
Clinical	0	0	0	3	1	24	13	37	3	3	3
Complex	0	1	0	2	0	2	4	17	1	8	3
Isopathy	0	0	0	4	0	1	6	13	0	2	0
total	0	2	0	13	2	32	36	83	6	19	12

No relationship between potency level and vote was apparent. Results were related to characteristic indicators of internal validity, such as concealment of randomization (Table 12.11) and levels of masking (Table 12.12), however. In both cases, placebo-controlled trials were more likely to include negative results the more rigorously randomized and masked they were.

Table 12.11 Assignment method and vote

Assignment	(-)	0	(+)	+	<	=	>	total
Matched pairs	0	0	1	2	0	1	2	6
Missing	0	1	0	2	0	1	0	4
Nonrandom	0	4	1	21	2	2	3	33
Pseudorandom	0	2	0	4	0	1	2	9
Random	2	27	34	67	4	14	5	153
total	2	34	36	96	6	19	12	205

Table 12.12 Masking and vote

Masking	(-)	0	(+)	+	<	=	>
None	0	2	0	14	2	12	7
Single	1	0	4	15	0	1	2
Double	1	32	32	67	4	6	3
total	2	34	36	96	6	19	12

In 74% of classical trials, therapists had a free choice of materia medica and results were largely positive (Table 12.13). Only 7 trials restricted therapists to a predefined selection of medicines, too few to observe a pattern, divided as they were between explanatory and pragmatic designs. However, 7 placebo-controlled trials that accepted only patients who firmly matched a preselected trial medicine reflected the direction of results in the open category.

Table 12.13 Classical group and vote

Prescribing	(-)	0	(+)	+	<	=	>	total
Open	1	3	11	14	1	5	5	40
Restricted	0	2	1	1	1	1	1	7
Selective	0	1	1	5	0	0	0	7

12.4. Adverse reactions

Adverse reactions were included as predefined outcomes in 15 trials, and were looked for in 97 (47%) trials altogether. The remainder either made no reference to them, or in a few cases included statements to the effect that homeopathy is free from risk per se. Side-effects, including initial aggravations, were reported in 41 homeopathy groups, while a further 15 trials found side-effects only in control groups. A clear trend for under-reporting in the clinical group compared with the other 3 categories can be seen in Table 12.14. The most fastidious category regarding reporting side-effects was complex homeopathy.

Table 12.14 Homeopathy type and adverse reactions reporting

	Classical	Clinical	Complex	Isopathy
Not reporting	29	56	9	14
Reporting	25	32	28	12
total	54	88	37	26

Chi-square = 16.21 with 3 df (p = 0.001)

Details of the 56 trials that reported side-effects are given in Appendix 3 (see CD). Such adverse reactions as were found were nearly all mild and transient and difficult to distinguish from reactions to placebo. Exceptions included one trial of palliative care for lung cancer in which initial aggravations of symptoms led to 2 dropouts (Hadjikostas & Diamantidis 1990b), and a large influenza prevention trial (n = 1573) where reactions to verum were clearly different in onset, intensity and prevalence (RR 4.7) from those in the placebo group (Attena, Toscano, Agozzino et al. 1995). The reporting of adverse events was also found to be related to the type of control treatment (Table 12.15), with only 27% of equivalence trials failing to mention the subject.

Table 12.15 Adverse events reporting and control treatments

	No treatment	Orthodox treatment	Placebo
Not reporting	9	9	90
Reporting	6	28	63
total	15	37	153

Chi-square = 14.57 with 2 df (p = 0.0007)

Occurrence of adverse events appeared not to be correlated to whether acute or chronic disease was treated (Chi-square = 6.808 with 6 df, p = 0.3389).

12.5. Holism, quality of life and economic evaluation

Only 8% of trials mentioned assessment of holistic effects of homeopathy, such as response of comorbidity to treatment, or improvements in general wellbeing. When stratified by homeopathy type it can be seen that the question was hardly considered outside classical homeopathy (Table 12.16).

Table 12.16 Holism and homeopathy type

Holism	Classical	Clinical	Complex	Isopathy	total
No	41	85	36	26	188
Yes	13	3	1	0	17
total	54	88	37	26	205

Even of classical trials mentioning the subject, most had low MQ scores making unquantified claims of improvements. Of better quality trials, only 3 included measures of general wellbeing as a predefined outcome – patient-rated scales in each case (Owen 1990; Brigo & Serpelloni 1991; Kuzeff 1998). Changes in baseline comorbidity were noted only in a trial for primary female infertility (Gerhard, Reimers, Keller et al. 1993).

A validated quality-of-life instrument (SF-36) was used in 1 trial only (Weiser, Strösser, Klein 1998).

Cost benefits of homeopathic medicines were referred to loosely in several reports, particularly those for diseases of poverty and malnutrition, but formal cost-benefit evaluation was included only in the infertility trial just mentioned (Gerhard, Reimers, Keller et al. 1993).

12.6. Methodological quality

It was possible to accept 197 trials for scoring with the methodological quality (MQ) instrument, mean 69.7, median 72 (SD 13.6). The full results for all trials are shown in Appendix 4 (see CD). The approximately normal distribution of MQ scores in the set can be seen in Figure 12.2.

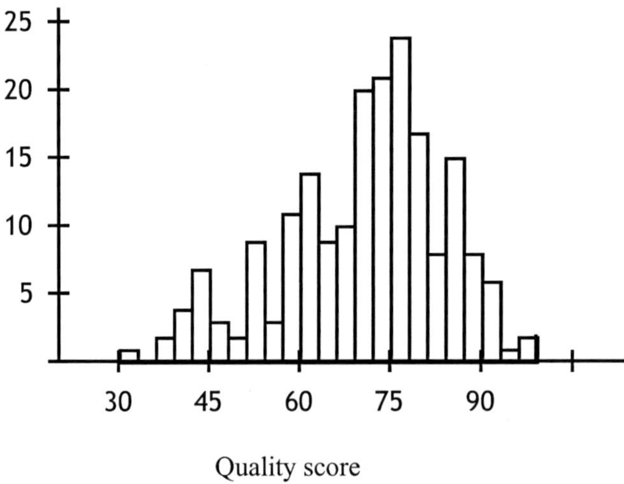

Figure 12.2 Distribution of methodological quality (MQ) scores

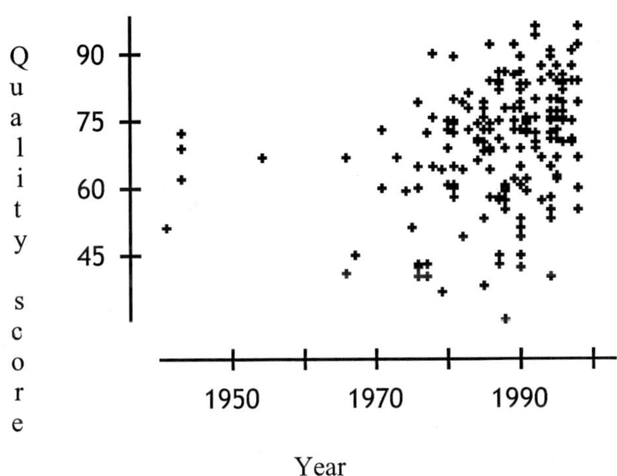

Figure 12.3 MQ scores by date

Figure 12.3 shows a scatterplot of the same scores and interestingly some of the earliest trials were near the mean for the whole set (British Homoeopathic Society 1943).

Table 12.17 MQ and publication type

Source	Included	Excluded	Mean	Median	SD
Book	1	0	67.0	67	•
Book section	3	0	63.3	58	10.12
Conference proceedings	18	3	55.3	55	14.30
Journal article	143	5	71.3	73	13.09
Report	7	0	61.8	61	9.42
Thesis	25	0	73.9	75	10.08

Publication type and MQ were related (Table 12.17), with theses at the top of the scale, slightly outperforming journal papers. Conference proceedings were likely to score poorly, even though conference abstracts were excluded from quality assessment.

Language of publication was not an indicator of quality as between English, German and French (93% of all sources), while sources in other languages were too few to generalize from.

Table 12.18 MQ and publication language

Language	Included	Excluded	Mean	Median	SD
Dutch	2	0	72.5	72	2.120
English	110	7	70.3	72	13.70
French	38	0	69.4	70	12.00
German	35	1	69.1	73	14.29
Italian	5	0	57.2	57	18.54
Norwegian	1	0	87.0	80	•
Portuguese	2	0	75.5	75	6.36
Spanish	4	0	66.0	71	14.63

Small differences in MQ score were apparent between homeopathic categories (Table 12.19), and much larger differences between control treatments (Table 12.20).

Table 12.19 MQ and homeopathy type

Homeopathy	Included	Excluded	Mean	Median	SD
Classical	50	4	68.56	71.0	13.74
Clinical	84	4	70.12	72.5	12.37
Complex	37	0	71.67	75.0	14.91
Isopathy	26	0	67.50	70.0	15.17

Table 12.20 MQ and control treatment

Control	Included	Excluded	Mean	Median	SD
No treatment	15	0	49.0	51.0	8.46
Orthodox treatment	36	1	67.9	69.5	13.77
Placebo	146	7	72.2	73.5	12.02

F-test $p \leq 0.0001$

Surprisingly, no relationship could be found between results and the scores for adequacy of handling exclusions and dropouts (Table 12.21).

Table 12.21 Adequacy of attrition handling

Attrition score	(-)	0	(+)	+	<	=	>
Inadequate	0	4	2	9	0	4	3
Partial	0	3	6	8	0	3	0
Adequate	1	17	19	33	3	7	4
No attrition	0	9	7	43	3	4	5
total	1	33	34	93	6	18	12

A scatterplot also shows no obvious relationship between percentage attrition and MQ scores (Figure 12.4).

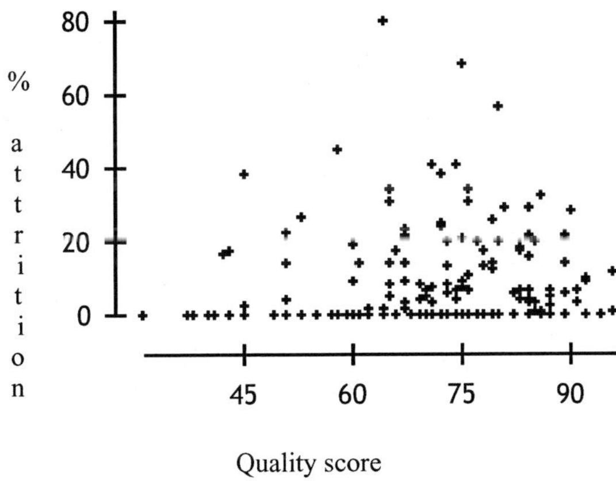

Figure 12.4 MQ and percentage attrition

The relationship between MQ scores and reported results was also problematic (Table 12.22). Except for a single trial which reported marginally better results in the placebo group (Walach, Haeusler, Lowes et al. 1997), only small MQ differences could be seen between negative and positive results in trials with no treatment or placebo controls, or between negative and equivalent results in pragmatic trials. The largest discrepancy came in trials reporting superiority of homeopathy to orthodox treatment.

Table 12.22 MQ and vote

Vote	Included	Excluded	Mean	Median	SD
(-)	2	0	84.5	84.5	9.19
0	34	0	69.4	73	14.32
(+)	32	3	72.0	73.5	10.90
+	93	3	69.3	72	14.05
<	6	0	69.3	71	10.97
=	18	1	69.1	72	14.15
>	12	0	65.4	63	15.11

Rigour of randomization was strongly related to results (Question 10), with nearly all null and marginal placebo-controlled votes for homeopathy occurring in trials with adequate concealment (Table 12.23).

Table 12.23 Concealment of randomization and vote

Concealment	(-)	0	(+)	+	<	=	>
None	0	5	9	24	2	9	3
Inadequate	1	2	2	8	1	1	0
Adequate	1	20	18	33	1	3	2
No data	0	7	3	28	2	5	7
total	2	34	33	93	6	18	12

Although the primary quality scale did not look for adverse reaction reporting, a statement that side-effects were sought – regardless of whether they were reported or not reported by participants – seemed to be a predictor of general trial quality. 108 trials (mean 66.7, SD 13.0) omitted to mention side-effects, and scored significantly worse than 97 that mentioned looking for adverse reactions (mean 72.7, SD 13.5) (2-Sample t-Test p = 0.0019).

12.6.1. Comparison with other quality scales

Table 12.24 compares the 197 trials in the set eligible for MQ scoring with 81 of these previously reviewed by Kleijnen et al. (1991), and 81 of those reviewed by Linde et al. (1997).

Table 12.24 Scores under 3 methodological quality instruments

MQ tool	Included	Excluded	Patients	Mean	Median	SD	r
Cho & Bero	197	8	13725	69.67	72	13.56	.985
Kleijnen et al.	81	124	3453	42.60	40	20.37	.988
Linde et al.	81	124	4848	59.85	57	21.21	.989

The two sets of 81 were not identical but came from a pool of 113 eligible for quality scoring in this review that had also been scored in either or both the other 2 reviews. The individual trial scores for the comparison scales were derived from the same publications. The mean scores under the 3 scales differ strongly.

Table 12.25 Rank correlations between methodological quality instruments

MQ tool	Cho	Kleijnen	Linde
Cho & Bero	1.000	•	•
Kleijnen et al.	0.743	1.000	•
Linde et al.	0.827	0.635	1.000

However, all 3 scales showed approximately normal distribution, and the rank correlation between the scale used for this review and the other 2 scales was good (Table 12.25). The correlation between the 2 comparison scales was somewhat less good, perhaps because of the smaller number of trials in common.

12.7. Highest quality trials

A sample was taken comprising 20% of trials with the highest scores (n = 40, score ≥ 81%) (Table 12.26).

Table 12.26 Vote by homeopathy type of top fifth of trials (MQ ≥81%)

Homeopathy	(-)	0	(+)	+	<	=	>	total
Classical	1	1	5	2	0	0	0	9
Clinical	0	5	0	6	0	1	1	13
Complex	0	2	2	7	0	2	1	14
Isopathy	0	0	0	4	0	0	0	4
total	1	8	7	19	0	3	2	40

Although the proportion of equivalence trials was similar to that in the whole set, the overall proportion occupied by 2 of the homeopathic types in the top fifth was clearly different, with clinical homeopathy relatively underrepresented and complex homeopathy more prevalent. Results were strongest for isopathy and complexes. Classical results were more equivocal, and clinical homeopathy posed the most problems. Trials in the sample are discussed in detail in Ch. 13.

12.8. Clinical relevance

Quality scoring of the 197 reports also included assessment with the clinical relevance (CR) tool (Cho & Bero 1994). Individual scores for each question appear in Appendix 4 (see CD), and showed approximately normal distribution (r = .988).

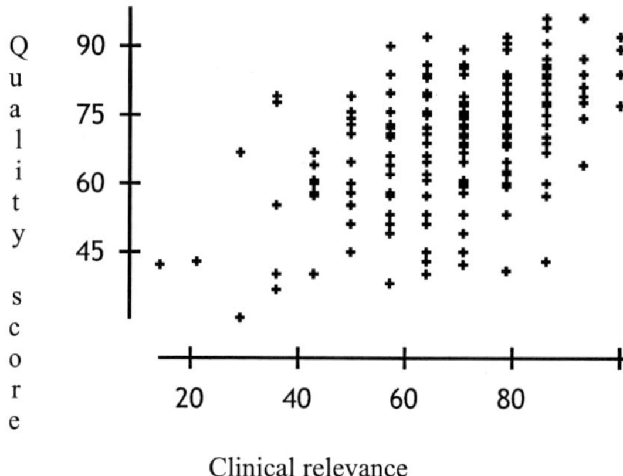

Figure 12.5 CR and MQ scores

All 197 trials were scored, including those with negative results, and a scatter-plot shows the direction of the relationship between CR and MQ scores (Figure 12.5). The distribution of CR scores is shown in Table 12.27, where considerable overlap between trials returning positive and negative results can be seen in the standard deviations of the adjacent groups.

Table 12.27 CR and votes

Vote	Included	Excluded	Mean	Median	SD
(-)	2	0	57.5	57.5	30.41
0	34	0	57.8	57	18.52
(+)	32	4	66.6	71	17.28
+	93	3	72.3	71	14.50
<	6	0	60.7	64	16.03
=	18	1	75.5	79	15.20
>	12	0	71.9	71	14.18

Less quantifiable aspects of clinical relevance are discussed in Ch. 13.

13. Discussion

Arguments included in this chapter have appeared in or as:

Dean M.E. (1998). Out of step with the *Lancet* homoeopathy meta-analysis. More objections than objectivity? *Journal of Alternative and Complementary Medicine.* 4 (4): 389–398.

Dean M.E. (2000). More trials, fewer placebos, please. *British Homoeopathic Journal.* 89 (4): 191–194.

Dean M.E. (2001). Study shows double standards in evaluation of homeopathy. *British Medical Journal.* 322 (20 January): 169–170.

13.1. Overview

Analysis of the trial set showed that intrahomeopathic differences were readily apparent in the choice of clinical areas and conditions, but also in choice of control treatments and in efficacy. Homeopathy was equivalent or superior to orthodox treatment in most cases where it was compared. Homeopathic medicines appeared to be relatively risk-free in terms of adverse reactions and unwanted effects. Global effects, e.g. on comorbidity, wellbeing and quality of life, were generally not included in outcomes, and neither was economic evaluation, but they tended to favour homeopathy when they were. The methodological quality (MQ) scale chosen appeared to function as well as others previously used to grade homeopathic trials, but was significantly more informative. Homeopathy's clinical relevance cannot be measured in the same way as treatments regarded as plausible in biomedicine – decisions to research or reject homeopathy remain as value-laden as in the nineteenth century. Each of these areas is now covered in more detail.

13.2. Efficacy

As mentioned in Ch. 11, the MQ scale used here does not have a cut point. A decision was made to base detailed discussion on the 20% of trials with the highest scores (n = 40, MQ = 81–96%), extended to include trials that were replicated in the highest quality group, or others that had particular clinical or methodological interest. Of the top 40, 27 were published after Kleijnen et al.'s review (1991), indicative of the chronological trend of improved methodological standards seen across the set. The proportional difference in styles of homeopathy from the set as a whole is interesting, and also noteworthy is the presence of 5 equivalence trials in which homeopathy was compared with orthodox treatment (Tables 13.1–4). The most problematic areas were classical and clinical homeopathy.

13.2.1. Classical

From a set of 40 trials just 4 classical studies were considered by Hill & Doyen (1990). Kleijnen et al. (1991) evaluated 105 trials comparing homeopathy with either placebo or orthodox treatment, but only 14 classical studies (13%) could be included. Linde et al. (1997) included 13 classical trials from a total of 89 (15%). By contrast, 54 of 205 trials (26%) in the present review could be described as classical homeopathy. The inclusion of orthodox treatment controls is partly responsible, since proportionally more classical trials used these. Important also is the increasing familiarity of therapists with research methods, and of researchers with homeopathy. Hill & Doyen (1990) presumed that researchers probably imagined controlled trials of homeopathy had to test a standard homeopathic treatment, but this limitation no longer holds. Chronologically, classical homeopathy has emerged since the 1980s as the preferred mode in many parts of the world, including those where clinical homeopathy was the norm previously (e.g. Rasky, Freidl, Haidvogl et al. 1994).

Table 13.1 Characteristics of 9 classical homeopathy trials MQ ≥81

First author, date	Condition	Control	Vote	MQ scores		
				Cho	Kleijnen	Linde
Jacobs 1994	Diarrhea (acute childhood)	P	+	91	ni	86
Walach 1997	Migraine	P	(-)	91	ni	ni
de Lange-de Klerk 1993	Upper respiratory infections (recurrent childhood)	P	(+)	87	ni	100
Lökken 1995	Post-extraction dental neuralgia	P	0	87	ni	86
Straumsheim 1997	Migraine	P	(+)	87	ni	ni
Whitmarsh 1997	Migraine	P	(+)	87	ni	ni
Brigo 1991	Migraine	P	+	86	68	79
Jacobs 1993	Diarrhea (acute childhood)	P	(+)	84	ni	64
Kuzeff 1998	Well-being	P	(+)	84	ni	ni

As shown in Table 13.1, the top fifth of this set included 9 (22%) classical trials, 2 of which were placebo-controlled studies in infantile diarrhea (Jacobs,

Jiménez, Gloyd et al. 1993; Jacobs, Jiménez, Gloyd et al. 1994). These belong to a series of trials of the ultramolecular potency C30 by the same team in different parts of the world where diseases of poverty and malnutrition are endemic, but the most recent replication was available only as a conference abstract and could not be evaluated (Jacobs, Malthouse, Chapman et al. 1997). All children in verum and placebo groups received oral rehydration therapy (ORT) at the same time, and it is impossible to say whether this affected the estimate of specific homeopathic effect in either direction. The difficulties of conducting ethical and valid trials of homeopathy in situations where an orthodox treatment exists and should not be withheld are obvious, and they are complicated further in this case by the fact that it is unusual for children to receive ORT in comparable regions. A survey of childhood dysentery in rural Bangladesh found only 25% of patients were treated with ORT (Ronsmans, Bennish, Chakraborty et al. 1991) and Jacobs et al. mention the prohibitive cost of ORT packs for the poor. These 3 trials can also be viewed as independent replications of an earlier Mexican trial for the same condition with acceptable methodology (MQ = 76%), just out of the top 20% (Villatoro Cadena & Luis Cuevas 1991). The same treatment model was used – ORT with either classical homeopathy or placebo – with the exception that a potency below N_A was used (C6). Inferential statistics were not presented, but the effect size seems comparable. In this trial parents prepared ORT at home, reducing costs, but their ability to read instructions and access to clean water would be questionable. In spite of problems, this group of 4 trials appears to demonstrate the superiority of single-medicine individualized homeopathy plus ORT to placebo plus ORT in an acute vector-borne illness.

Another high-quality placebo-controlled trial produced a positive result in chronic migraine (Brigo & Serpelloni 1991). However, 3 attempted replications in the top fifth produced negative or marginally positive results (Straumsheim, Borchgrevink, Mowinckel et al. 1997; Walach, Haeusler, Lowes et al. 1997; Whitmarsh, Coleston-Shields, Steiner 1997). There is clear evidence that the patients were atypical in each of the unsuccessful trials (Whitmarsh 2000), and the issue is complicated in terms of homeopathic theory since the epidemiology of migraine suggests the condition may reduce the risk of more serious cardiac disease (Waters, Campbell, Elwood 1988), thus requiring even more extended treatment than the longest follow-up periods of 4 months found in these trials. However, even though marginal evidence of efficacy was found in 2 trials, the results are disappointing for proponents of single high-potency medicines in the treatment of chronic disease (see Ch. 4). The director of the foundation that funded the least successful of the 3 has said that further similar research into classical homeopathy for migraine is not warranted (Albrecht 1999). The results of these failed replications have also been used to question the positive effects of homeopathy found in the meta-analysis by Linde et al. (Ernst & Barnes 1998). However, a more systematic literature search for randomized placebo-controlled trials that were published after Linde et al.'s cut-off date of October 1995 found this view had ignored many positive trials that met the meta-analysis criteria (Dean 1998). The risk of Type–1 error in premature and unsystematic updating of meta-analyses has been noted in Ch. 10 and elsewhere (Pogue & Yusuf 1998).

Two further classical trials in the highest 20% also failed to produce convincing advantages over placebo in recurrent upper respiratory tract infections (URTI) (de Lange-de Klerk 1993), or in postextraction dental neuralgia (Lökken, Straumsheim, Tveiten et al. 1995). The URTI comparison was complicated by the inclusion of 'careful dietary counselling' in both groups, not normally a feature of everyday general practice. The bilateral oral surgery prescriptions could only be made from a restricted predefined set of medicines, regardless of the presenting symptoms in any individual, and repetition of doses was based on a highly unusual and rigid scheme.

In keeping with classical theory, patients with many different conditions were accepted for an innovative trial in the top 20% in which the main outcome measure was mental-emotional and physical wellbeing (Kuzeff 1998). Patients rated their own progress on separate 10-point VAS, and although baseline measurements were missing, a trend for mental-emotional wellbeing and significant superiority for physical wellbeing were found in the verum group.

Another trial that probably did not contain serious threats to validity (MQ = 70%), but suffered from poor reporting, showed substantial patient-rated benefits from homeopathy in myalgic encephalitis/postviral fatigue syndrome (ME/PVFS) at 12 months in 33% of patients, with no corresponding benefit from placebo (Awdry 1996). The clinical relevance of this result in a neglected group of patients is discussed further in 13.6.5 (ME/PVFS) below.

All the classical trials in the top group were placebo-controlled, but it is worth mentioning a double dummy equivalence trial to compare classical homeopathy and chloroquine for treatment of malaria that took place in Ghana and also scored well (MQ = 79%) (Van Erp & Brands 1996). An 11% superiority of homeopathy over orthodox treatment was found. However, the generalizability of this comparison is problematic because although the checklist of signs, symptoms and modalities used to repertorize each patient appears rigorous, the outcome measure of improvement on ≥3 of 9 symptoms could have been more detailed.

13.2.2. Clinical

Although 88 clinical homeopathy trials constituted the largest single group (43%), only 13 (32%) appeared in the top 40 (Table 13.2).

The most successful subgroup in this category were the allergic rhinitis studies (Wiesenauer, Häussler, Gaus 1983; Wiesenauer, Gaus, Häussler 1990; Wiesenauer & Lüdtke 1995) that are part of a long-running series of replications using *Galphimia glauca* in very low potencies. The author's own meta-analysis was highly positive, showing success rates comparable with standard antihistamine therapy, but with no side-effects (Wiesenauer & Lüdtke 1996).

Table 13.2 Characteristics of 13 clinical homeopathy trials MQ ≥81

First author, date	Condition	Control	Vote	MQ scores		
				Cho	Kleijnen	Linde
Lievre 1992	Burns	OT	>	94	ni	ni
Grecho 1989	Postoperative ileus	P	0	92	90	86
Rahlfs 1978	Irritable bowel syndrome	P	+	90	50	79
Valero 1981(ii)	Postoperative ileus	P	+	89	70	64
Hofmeyr 1990	Childbirth	P	0	86	ni	100
Eid 1994	Childbirth	P	+	85	ni	ni
Friese 1997	Adenoidal growths	P	0	84	ni	ni
Hart 1997	Postoperative pain and infection	P	0	84	ni	ni
Wiesenauer 1995	Allergic rhinitis	P	+	84	ni	ni
Wiesenauer 1987	Hypotension	OT	=	83	58	ni
Wiesenauer 1990	Allergic rhinitis	P	+	83	ni	86
Bignamini 1987	Hypertension (essential)	P	0	82	58	ni
Wiesenauer 1983	Allergic rhinitis	P	+	81	75	79

Traditional homeopathic recommendations of *Opium* for constipation and *Raphanus* for abdominal bloating and pain were the subject of 2 trials in the top fifth for postoperative intestinal stasis (ileus) (Valero 1981; GRECHO, U292 Inserm, ARC et al. 1989). They were part of a series of replications (Castelain 1979; Estragnin 1979; Chevrel, Saglier, Destable 1984; Aulagnier 1985; Dorfman, Amodéo, Ricciotti et al. 1992), and all were positive except the large GRECHO trial (n = 600). A meta-analysis of the series found a positive effect for low potencies, and a negative one for ultramolecular potencies (Barnes, Resch, Ernst 1997).

Part of native North American herbal lore, *Caulophyllum thalictroides* has featured in homeopathic obstetrics since the nineteenth century largely on empirical grounds. The C7 potency was tested for prolonged labour in 2 trials, the one in the top fifth being a replication of a case-control pilot study (Eid, Felisi, Sideri 1993; Eid, Felisi, Sideri 1994). The randomized trial found mean duration of labour of 3.5 hours under verum vs almost 6 hours with placebo ($p = 0.0$). *Caulophyllum* C5 was also successful in a small trial for false labour and dystocia (MQ = 80%): favourable responses were observed in 13/17 vs 2/17 under placebo ($p < 0.005$) (Deguillaume 1981). Ultramolecular *Caulophyllum* was also given in a pragmatic comparison with standard obstetric preparation in the following sequence at 30-minute intervals: *Pulsatilla* M, *Secale* C50, *Caulophyllum* C50, *Actea racemosa* C200, *Arnica* M (Ventoskovskiy & Popov 1990) (MQ = 78%). Homeopathy was as or significantly more effective on each outcome, including uterine inertia (nsd), ineffective first stage ($p < 0.05$), false labour ($p < 0.05$), blood loss (nsd) and Apgar scores (nsd). A homeopathic complex containing *Caulophyllum* is discussed in 13.2.3.

There were only 2 equivalence trials of clinical homeopathy vs standard treatments in the top group. *Haplopappus* D2 was found to be equivalent, with a weak trend for slightly greater effectiveness, than etilefrin in raising low blood pressure (Wiesenauer & Gaus 1987). A standard homeopathic wound treatment, *Calendula*, yielded results in first- and second-degree burns superior to placebo or the orthodox proteolytic ointment (Lievre, Marichy, Baux et al. 1992). It is discussed further in 13.6.2.

A successful trial of *Asafoetida* D3 for irritable bowel syndrome (Rahlfs & Mössinger 1978), also in the top group, was conducted to validate a clinical *Asafoetida* subgroup found in the pilot study (Rahlfs & Mössinger 1976), and entry was restricted to patients who matched ≥3 of 9 *Asafoetida* symptoms. This trial was part of an interesting methodological subgroup on the borders of clinical and classical homeopathy, requiring very abbreviated symptom matching (Alibeu & Jobert 1990; Fisher 1986; Shipley, Berry, Broster et al. 1983).

Turning to the unsuccessful high-quality trials, another schematic sequence of clinical medicines was used in one, but had little influence on adenoidal growths (Friese, Feuchter, Moeller 1997). Another tested *Arnica* and showed little difference from placebo in post-partum recovery, although the D30 potency appeared to produce a worse outcome than D6 or placebo (Hofmeyr, Piccioni, Blauhof 1990). Although *Arnica* has rarely been recommended as an analgesic, the C30 potency was trialled for postoperative pain and again showed no difference from placebo (Hart, Mullee, Lewith et al. 1997). Based on the toxicology of soluble barium salts, a high-quality trial of *Baryta car-*

bonica C15 for essential hypertension showed no difference from placebo overall, although good reductions in arterial BP were found in all prescreened patients who matched *Baryta* symptomatology, while equivalent responders who received placebo experienced a net increase in BP (Bignamini, Bertoli, Consolandi et al. 1987).

The appearance in the clinical category of 65% of all failed trials in the whole set requires additional explanation, especially since it can no longer be assumed that homeopathic trials of high internal validity will automatically yield null results. As noted in Ch. 4, the earliest attempts to simplify the ideal of full individualization led in one direction to keynote prescribing and in another to nosological homeopathy. Keynotes are still patient-based rather than disease-based and do not belong in the clinical category. On the other hand, nosological prescriptions, often based on traditional empirical recommendations rather than fresh analysis of a prevalent condition, constitute the majority of trials in this sector. The attractions of the model for biomedically-orientated research, and the inherent problems of the model in a homeopathic framework, should be apparent by now, and need little further comment. As discussed in Chs 7 and 9, historical trials of *Belladonna* for scarlet fever, regardless of fluctuations in virulence and prevalent symptomatology, showed the limitations of this sort of nosological homeopathy (West 1854: 600; Wesselhoeft Jr 1917). Many trials here continued this line, often testing prescriptions of doubtful validity. For example, although empirically recommended for whooping cough, the provings of *Drosera* were shown long ago to bear little resemblance to the disease (Wesselhoeft Jr 1917), a finding apparently confirmed in an unsuccessful trial (Lewis 1984). Homeopaths in the nineteenth century were highly critical of the routine homeopathic use of *Colchicum* for gout (Kent 1911: 430), and a recent trial bore out their scepticism (Puterman 1994). *Blatta orientalis* was used empirically for asthma because a patient found relief after drinking tea in which the Indian cockroach had been accidentally infused (Clarke 1925). No proving data is available, and *Blatta* was not found to be significantly different from placebo in a randomized asthma trial (Freitas, Goldenstein, Sanna 1995). *Arnica* in particular was favoured in many of these trials, including some in the top 20%, probably because it is the best known medicine used in homeopathy, with a traditional reputation as a first-aid treatment for bruising and shock, and because researchers have often looked for a standard treatment model to test the ultramolecular hypothesis. However, it was adopted from folk medicine – Hahnemann (1828) recommending its use as an unpotentized lotion, even in his high-potency phase – and there is scant physiological evidence of its homeopathicity to trauma (Baillargeon, Drouin,

Desjardins et al. 1993). It is arguable that potentized medicines only, and not collective similia, were tested in many trials in this category.

In contrast to trials of traditional and essentially empirical clinical prescriptions, pathological homeopathy has received little attention since the reanalysis of mumps on a lesional basis (Wesselhoeft Jr 1924) (Ch. 9), and only a few contemporary trials took this approach. The trial of *Baryta* for hypertension has been mentioned above, and suggested further research with prescreened responders could be indicated. Based on the physiological action of physostigmine, which contracts the ciliary muscles and impairs accommodation, infrequent local application of an aqueous *Physostigma* solution in high potencies produced promising long-term results in 2 placebo-controlled trials for myopia (Basu 1980; 1981) (MQ = 61%). If genuine, these results are astonishing given current understanding of the cause and treatment of errors of accommodation, and it would be relatively easy to replicate the trials with greater rigour. Copper's toxicology includes muscular spasm, and a placebo-controlled trial of *Cuprum metallicum* C15 for hemodialysis-related cramps appeared to bear out the similia principle in this instance (Hariveau, Nolen, Holtzscherer 1991) (MQ = 75%). The similarity between phosphorus toxicology and the lesions seen in experimental liver disease induced by trichloroethylene has led to many in vitro and animal experiments (e.g. Bildet, Bonini, Gender et al. 1984), but the model was tested in only 1 human trial found here (Chirila 1990). This was a conference report of uncertain quality (MQ = 45%), but showed substantially reduced hospital stays for children with type-B hepatitis who received *Phosphorus* C7 compared with placebo (8 days vs 20 days). Repertorization of the common symptoms of acute hypertension led to a successful randomized trial of the snake venom *Lachesis mutus* C200 in a hospital A&E department (Ochoa-Bernal, Ruiz-Hernandez, Searcy Bernal 1995) (MQ = 76%). Interestingly, conventional renin-angiotensin inhibitors are based on a chance discovery of a bradykinin potentiating factor in the venom of *Bothrops jararaca* (Krieger, Salgado, Assan et al. 1971). However, the symptomatology of *Lachesis* has been well recognized in homeopathy since the mid nineteenth century – the repertory used by the authors may have been computerized but was actually Kent's – and suggests that the boundary zone between biomedicine and homeopathy could be fruitfully explored, not just by homeopathic researchers.

13.2.3. Complex

A completely different approach to improving the accuracy of nosological prescriptions is found in complex homeopathy, and there appear to be fewer problems with the design and conduct of trials in this category.

Table 13.3 Characteristics of 14 complex homeopathy trials MQ ≥81

First author, date	Condition	Control	Vote	MQ scores		
				Cho	Kleijnen	Linde
Böhmer 1992	Sprains and contusions	P	+	96	ni	100
Weiser 1998	Vertigo	OT	=	96	ni	ni
Weiser 1994	Sinusitis (chronic)	P	+	89	ni	79
Zell 1990	Sprains	P	+	89	80	100
Maiwald 1988	Influenza	OT	>	86	65	ni
Hill 1996	Mosquito bites (experimental)	P	(+)	85	ni	ni
Ferley 1987	Influenza	P	0	84	68	79
Hill 1995	Mosquito bites (experimental)	P	(+)	84	ni	ni
Lasserre 1986	Childbirth	P	+	84	80	71
Nahler 1996	Osteoarthrosis	OT	=	84	ni	ni
McCutcheon 1996	Anxiety	P	0	83	ni	ni
Wiesenauer 1991	Chronic polyarthritis	P	+	83	ni	79
Abelson 1996	Allergic conjunctivitis	P	+	82	ni	ni
Ernst 1990	Varicose veins	P	+	82	ni	71

One reason for this could be the heavy involvement of homeopathic pharmaceutical companies. Traditional single-medicine homeopathy is overwhelmingly based on freely available and unpatentable materia medica, and offers few obvious commercial opportunities. In contrast, unique proprietary combinations can be tested and marketed like conventional drugs, as is the case with all but 1 of the 14 complexes in the highest 40 (Table 13.3).

The relatively high MQ scores of complex trials compared with the other categories may also be related to the trend towards contracting out the design and running of trials of complexes to independent specialist clinical trial organizations (e.g. Weiser, Strösser, Klein 1998). Conditions showing homeopathic superiority to placebo in the top group include: allergic conjunctivitis (Abelson 1996); sprains and bruising (Zell, Connert, Mau et al. 1990; Böhmer & Ambrus 1992); chronic polyarthritis (Wiesenauer & Gaus 1991); chronic sinusitis (Weiser & Clasen 1994); mosquito bites (Hill, Stam, Tuinder et al. 1995; Hill, Stam, Haselen 1996); and varices (Ernst, Saradeth, Resch 1990).

Indicative of the high level of development of complex homeopathy, and the confidence of the manufacturers, were randomized trials of proprietary homeopathics vs biomedical treatments. Homeopathy was found to be equivalent to or better than standard treatments in vertigo (Weiser, Strösser, Klein 1998), influenza (Maiwald, Weinfurtner, Mau et al. 1988), and osteoarthritis (Nahler 1996).

Less successful was the placebo-controlled trial of another proprietary complex marketed as L.72 in France and Anti-anxiety in the USA (McCutcheon 1996). It showed no reduction in state or trait anxiety, but did show a significant reduction ($p = 0.05$) in another prespecified outcome: insomnia. This hypnotic effect supports the finding of an earlier randomized equivalence trial that compared L.72 with diazepam (Heulluy 1985), and suggests that L.72 may well be formulated and marketed inappropriately for its target condition (the 9 listed ingredients have stronger indications overall for insomnia than anxiety in the materia medica and repertory), but it does not follow that it is therefore pharmacologically inert. However, L.52 from the same manufacturer showed no significant difference from placebo in prevention of influenza (Ferley, Poutignat, Azzopardi et al. 1987).

The historical origins of the ideological objections of most classical homeopaths to polypharmacy are well-known (see Chs 3 and 4), but they have led to neglect of research into useful interactions and combinations of safe homeopathic medicines. Apart from the products of the pharmacies, there were few trials in this area altogether, and only 1 in the top group. A low-potency (C5) combination containing *Actaea racemosa*, *Arnica*, *Caulophyllum*, *Gelsemium* and *Pulsatilla* was compared with placebo in preparation for labour (Lasserre 1986). Highly significant ($p < 0.001$) reductions in both duration of labour (5.1 hours vs 8.5 hours) and incidence of dystocia (6/53 vs 16/40) were seen, comparable with similar obstetric trials in the single-medicine clinical group (13.2.2).

Also worth mentioning, for its methodology rather than results, is a factorial trial (MQ = 69%) for vaginal discharge that allowed the traditional clinical prescription *Borax* C30 to be compared and combined with the nosode *Candida* C30 (Carey 1986). The combination appeared to have a more powerful effect than its components individually. The trial was too small to be more than suggestive of a line for future research, but factorial designs are probably the best way of analysing combinations. Single medicine trials for post-surgical pain and recovery have often been unsuccessful, whether clinical using only *Arnica* (e.g. Hart, Mullee, Lewith et al. 1997), or classical (e.g. Lökken, Straumsheim, Tveiten et al. 1995). However, two clinical homeopathy trials which alternated *Arnica* with *Hypericum* (traditionally recommended for bruising and neuralgia respectively) were highly successful (Bendre & Dharmadhikari 1980; Albertini, Goldberg, Sanguy et al. 1985) (MQ = 69% and 68%). Another successful trial (MQ = 60%) alternated *Arnica* with *Apis* to treat edema following rhinoplasty (Michaud 1981). There is a case to be made for factorial trials in the area of homeopathic first-aid and traumatology, and other areas where individualization can be unfeasible.

13.2.4. Isopathy

Only 4 trials of isopathy were included in the top fifth, from 26 isopathy trials altogether. Because direct causal agents are unknown for so many contemporary patterns of illness, isopathy has clear limitations as therapy, although its similarity to biomedical areas such as immunology has attracted researchers interested primarily in the ultramolecular–placebo question. The trials by Reilly and colleagues for atopy, including hay fever and asthma, were designed and conducted for this purpose and produced their own highly positive meta-analysis, with 2 appearing in the highest-quality group (see Table 13.4) (Reilly & Taylor 1985; Reilly, McSharry, Taylor et al. 1986; Reilly, Taylor, Beattie et al. 1994). They are discussed further in 13.6.5 (Inhalant allergy).

Table 13.4 Characteristics of 4 isopathy trials MQ ≥81

First author, date	Condition	Control	Vote	MQ scores		
				Cho	Kleijnen	Linde
Papp 1998	Influenza	P	+	92	ni	ni
Reilly 1986	Allergic rhinitis	P	+	92	90	93
Reilly 1994	Allergic asthma	P	+	89	ni	93
Ferley 1989	Influenza	P	+	85	88	79

Two isopathic influenza trials in the top 40 used the ultramolecular nosode *Oscillococcinum*® C200, made from infected duck heart and liver (Ferley, Zmirou, D'Adhemar et al. 1989; Papp, Schuback, Beck et al. 1998). Altogether there have been 4 (n = 1250, mean n = 312) randomized placebo-controlled postexposure treatment trials in widely different influenza epidemics (Casanova 1984; Casanova & Gerard 1992). Unlike nosodes and vaccines derived from specific influenza strains, *Oscillococcinum*® is derived from a rich mixture of pathogens and antigens, probably providing nonspecific immune enhancement. All 4 trials showed significant reductions in symptoms, and illness duration, and are discussed further in 13.6.5 (Influenza treatment). Although prophylactic effects were claimed in a case-control study (Masciello & Felisi 1985) (MQ = 38%), a better-quality randomized trial (MQ = 62%) found no statistical difference from placebo (Attena, Toscano, Agozzino et al. 1995).

Isopathy seems to have been the most consistently successful homeopathic category reviewed here, and other isopathic trials investigated mostly similar conditions, with similar results. Different clinical areas included the 1941 mustard gas trials reviewed in Ch. 9, and 2 good quality placebo-controlled trials of potentized human ovarian hormone for premenstrual syndrome. Lepaisant (1995) (MQ = 77%) gave *Folliculinum* C5 to women showing marked premenstrual symptoms for more than 3 months. The apparent 20% attrition rate was due to the 1 month placebo run-in: 13/58 were not assigned because of positive responses – or natural remission – while on placebo. Masked evaluation of global success (including breast tension, pain, duration) favoured verum (p = 0.0159). In the other trial (Gillespie 1994) (MQ = 75%), patient-rated scores on validated scales showed ultramolecular *Folliculinum* C15 had been very much more effective than placebo (89% vs 7% of women recorded improvements), although significance tests were not given.

13.3. Safety

The search for evidence of adverse reactions found some authors claiming that homeopathy was risk free (e.g. Awdry 1996). A prior belief might of course make the search for evidence during a trial seem unnecessary. However, it would appear that homeopathy is not without side effects, although severe ones necessitating abandonment of therapy were hardly noticeable (see App. 3), since primary aggravations leading to 2 dropouts were found only in a single palliative trial for lung cancer (Hadjikostas 1990?b). A trial for primary female infertility reported transient skin symptoms in 10% of the homeopathically treated group, and explained these as a predictable and harmless eliminative response (Gerhard, Reimers, Keller et al. 1993). One trialist included aggravations and returns of old symptoms as a predefined outcome (Schwab 1990) – according to miasmatic theory, chronic illness proceeds from the suppression of skin diseases in the patient's (or the community's) past, and healing is believed to allow suppressed symptoms to surface. Intriguingly though, many initial aggravations were found in some placebo groups as well (e.g. Reilly, McSharry, Taylor et al. 1986), suggesting that some ostensibly homeopathic aggravations might be psychological reactions to medication per se. Unfortunately, no information was given on whether patients were primed with expectations of adverse events – as part of informed consent, in trial information leaflets, for instance.

Against the nocebo interpretation, the most convincing evidence of different unwanted reactions to verum and placebo was found in a large (n = 1573) influenza prevention trial (Attena, Toscano, Agozzino et al. 1995). Symptoms were reported by 10% of patients in the 24 hours after administration of the ultramolecular verum (*Oscillococcinum*® C200), and reactions such as myalgia, low grade fever and rhinorrhea predominated – as might be expected after conventional influenza vaccination (Govaert, Dinant, Aretz 1993). In contrast, only 2% of patients in the placebo group reported side-effects, and these were general symptoms such as dizziness, skin numbness and GI disturbance, as seen in other placebo groups in this review (see App. 3). Moreover, the incidence of responses to 3 subsequent doses of verum diminished over time, while placebo responses were more equally distributed.

That such a large trial was needed to to produce a statistically reliable comparison between unsought post-verum and post-placebo symptoms indicates a major difficulty of trying to evaluate homeopathic safety from reports of small clinical trials which for the most part did not prespecify adverse reactions as endpoints. It probably has even more serious implications for the validity of contemporary pathogenetic drug tests, most of which have been extremely small, and rarely include placebo washouts as used in the latter half of the nineteenth century (see Ch. 8 and: Dantas & Fisher 1998).

Notwithstanding the absence of reported adverse events in the trial set, there are a number of safety issues, directly and indirectly attributable to homeopathic treatment, that need to be addressed.

Toxicity: For the most part, serial dilution progressively removes directly toxic substances from the medicine. However, very low potencies may contain traces of the potentized substance. Low potency complex treatments under review appear to have been formulated knowledgeably and subject to prior safety testing, and were consequently well tolerated. This is not always the case, and complexes containing traces of heavy metals and other contaminants are sold over the counter in India and elsewhere, and have sometimes been imported into Europe and the US (Hentschel, Kohnen, Hahn 1998). Indian recommendations for the minimum safe potency for each substance have been published, although the extent to which such guidelines are currently observed is unknown (Varma & Indu 1992).

Interactions: In most cases, concurrent treatments were excluded from the protocols, preventing assessment of drug interaction. Homeopaths have traditionally conceptualized their medicines as acting non-materially, and certainly not according to orthodox mass action-receptor site theory. Accordingly, drug interactions are not seen by them as a problem. However, the tendency for patients to self-prescribe homeopathic medicines alongside orthodox drugs suggests this view may be complacent. Although the present review contained few trials for acute life-threatening conditions as grave as diphtheria, as seen in Ch. 9.4.4, combined serum plus homeopathy showed higher mortality than serum alone (Hess 1942). Disregarding possible allocation bias, the finding appeared to corroborate the homeopathic recommendation to halve serum doses when using it with homeopathy. This highlights an area of potential concern, that could be particularly relevant when prescribing tautopathic potencies of concurrently prescribed orthodox drugs.

Withholding treatment: An indirect effect of increasing patient reliance on private homeopathic treatment is the possibility that standard biomedical interventions may be foregone. This has been shown to be the case in the UK, where many non-doctor homeopaths advise parents against vaccinating their children, because of fears about vaccine safety and inutility (e.g. Moskowitz 1992), and in the belief that homeopathic prophylaxis or treatment is sufficient in diseases such as chicken pox, measles, mumps, rubella and whooping cough (Pinto & Feldman 2000: 133).

13.4. Holism, quality of life and economic evaluation

The poor quality of evidence relating to homeopathy's global effects, and the dearth of evidence relating to quality of life and economic evaluation has been noted in Ch. 12. This was particularly puzzling since, when these elements were incorporated into trial evaluation, they tended to favour homeopathy.

13.4.1. Comorbidity and wellbeing

In an equivalence trial for primary female infertility (Gerhard, Reimers, Keller et al. 1993), (MQ = 57%) improvements in baseline comorbidity were found in 19% of those receiving classical homeopathy (including: loss of libido; chronic headaches; chronic conjunctivitis and lymphadenitis; hay fever and headaches). The control treatments included hormone replacement and in-vitro fertilization, but no comparable improvements were noted, and 29% of patients in this group reported feeling worse than before the trial.

A 1987 randomized trial of classical homeopathy for migraine seems to have been the earliest in the set to measure a global outcome (Brigo and Serpelloni 1991). Patients were asked to rate their own general wellbeing (cenesthesia) on a 10-point visual analogue scale (VAS) on 3 occasions, and the verum group showed significant improvement, unlike placebo.

A VAS was again used to let patients rate changes in their sense of wellbeing in a trial comparing classical homeopathy with orthodox treatment in irritable bowel syndrome (Owen 1990) (MQ = 73%). The homeopathy group did not report as much benefit on this measure as the conventional group, but significant improvements were found in both groups when patients were asked to record improvements in their own worst-rated symptom on another VAS.

As mentioned in 13.2.1, mental-emotional and physical wellbeing, as rated by patients with many different presenting conditions, were the main outcomes in another classical trial also in the top 20% (Kuzeff 1998).

13.4.2. Quality of life

Unfortunately, only 1 trial used a validated QOL instrument (SF-36), and it may be significant that the trial was an equivalence study conducted by a specialist trial organization (Weiser, Strösser, Klein 1998). Patients treated for vertigo with the complex VertigoHeel or betahistine hydrochloride were tested 3 times, and no significant difference was found between the improvements recorded in both groups. The MRC will not fund clinical trials that do not measure QOL (unless its omission can be justified), and although there are some objections to this (The Lancet 1995), homeopaths in particular need not resist the requirement since it begins to quantify something they have used intuitively for 200 years as an index of the progress of treatment in chronic illness. The choice of QOL instrument needs consideration, however. The limitations and rigidities of off-the-shelf questionnaires have been recognized more generally, and the intuitively attractive idea of patient-generated measures has come to seem the most appropriate (Gill & Feinstein 1994; Ruta, Garratt, Leng et al. 1994).

13.4.3. Economic evaluation

The infertility trial mentioned in 13.4.1 above was the only one to include cost–benefit analysis (Gerhard, Reimers, Keller et al. 1993). The clinic costs (treatment and therapist time) per successful birth ('take home baby') were 335 DM for homeopathy vs 11 661.5 DM for orthodox treatment. Social costs were not included, but it was recorded that orthodox treatment required patients to attend hospital 6 times as often on average. It is particularly interesting that these figures should reflect so closely the cost comparisons made in pragmatic trials in the middle of the nineteenth century (Ch. 8). It would be unwise to extrapolate these results too far outside this immediate clinical situation however: orthodox infertility treatment is notoriously expensive at present, and NHS postcode rationing is common, while many orthodox drugs for many other conditions are comparatively cost-effective.

Several authors state that one of the reasons for employing homeopathy is the low cost of treatment, and this was particularly mentioned in those trials concerned with diseases of poverty. This seems borne out in a European context by a survey of costs in 1988 obtained from the North-Württemberg Kassenärztliche Vereinigung (a health insurance union). General practitioners in this area at that time were compared to an equivalently sized group of GPs who also practised naturopathy or homeopathy, and differences between the 2 groups were significant with respect to drug costs and sickness certificates, but not with respect to physician fees (Wiesenauer, Groh, Haussler 1992). However, in some clinical conditions, the increased cost of homeopathic practitioner time would undoubtedly offset the small savings on medication – e.g. the irritable bowel trial which found that classical homeopathy with extended interviews was no more effective than orthodox treatment involving dicyclomine hydrochloride, fecal bulking agents and a diet advice sheet (Owen 1990).

13.5. Methodological quality measurement

The MQ scale used here provided good comparability with scales devised by Kleijnen et al. (1991) and Linde et al. (1997) for systematic reviews of homeopathy trials, and appeared well-suited for its purpose of discriminating finely between studies of widely different conduct and reporting quality. It showed the same approximately normal distribution as the 2 comparison scales, but the floor and ceiling effect seen in the other scales were absent – the inclusion criteria used here meant no trial could score below 17%, and no trial scored more than 96%, almost certainly because of Questions 8 and 9 about random selection of patients from the target population.

A post hoc validation and justification for the choice of scale emerged after quality scoring had been completed. A comparison of 25 quality scales was made by rating 17 trials of low-molecular-weight heparin (LMWH) or standard heparin in prevention of deep vein thrombosis during surgery (Jüni, Witschi,

Bloch et al. 1999). The sample of 17 trials was taken from an earlier meta-analysis which recommended standard heparin (Nurmohamed, Rosendaal, Buller 1992). The reviewers demonstrated a wide spread of estimates of effect, from scales which appeared to replicate the findings of Nurmohamed et al. to scales such as Linde et al. (1997) which showed greater benefit from LMWH, reversing the original meta-analysis. Because of this variation, the reviewers questioned the function and reliability of quality scales per se. However, the reversal of results appears to correlate more with the level of high-quality cut points in the individual scales than with the scale components themselves (Dean 2001). Linde et al.'s scale in particular had an exceptionally high cut point of 70% relative to the mean score of 60% obtained with it, scoring only 3 trials from 17 as high-quality. By comparison, Jadad et al.'s (1996) scale contains highly similar components – but the cut point of 60% was identical with its mean, conferring high-quality status on 9 of 17 trials. The heparin meta-analysis obtained from Cho & Bero's MQ scale appeared among the least skewed in either direction in Jüni et al.'s review, along with Jadad et al.'s well-regarded but deliberately much less informative instrument.

The scale used here has the additional advantage that designs excluded from this review – such as intrahomeopathic comparison studies without external controls, or even prospective case-series – could be included in the database at a later date and evaluated to a common standard.

13.6. Clinical relevance

The results of evaluation with the CR instrument correlated well with MQ scores. However, since CR scores contain a maximum of 14% of points for efficacy, it is possible for an unsuccessful treatment to achieve a higher CR score than an effective treatment, simply because it was better reported. It follows that the tool as it stands should probably only be used to measure clinical relevance of treatments known to be effective, and may need modification. The instrument could be described as measuring clinical fitness in situations where health professionals need to make decisions about whether to offer treatments where there may be little independently evaluated evidence available.

In spite of the use here of a quantitative CR instrument, it must be acknowledged that the clinical relevance of homeopathy is a much more difficult problem to address than the placebo question. Put simply, at what point do the clinical, socioeconomic or psychological advantages of a novel treatment make its adoption desirable, inevitable or imperative? When the competing therapy is as challenging to biomedical assumptions as homeopathy, some would argue that it can never be clinically relevant – even when superiority to placebo has been demonstrated (Langman 1997). Since this is the case, how can homeopathy be expected to demonstrate clinical relevance in the face of institutional scepticism and the consequent withholding of research funding? This important question is too large to be considered fully here, but implications for trial design and conduct can at least be considered on the basis of the clinical trials in this review. The discussion looks in turn at the operational and ethical questions posed by different sorts of comparative trial, the inclusion of patient preferences, and the evaluation of intrahomeopathic heterogeneity.

13.6.1. Placebo problems

In response to the difficulties found in the 3 classical migraine trials that failed to replicate the positive results of an earlier one (13.2.1), it has been suggested that the days of randomized placebo-controlled trials of homeopathy might be numbered, to be replaced by observational studies, audit and quality-of-life assessment (Whitmarsh 2000). QOL assessment is not an alternative to trials, and has been discussed above (13.4.2). However, placebo controls themselves are problematic, to the extent that the validity of the construct faces serious challenge (Kaptchuk 1998b; Kienle & Kiene 1998). It is certainly arguable that placebos have been over-sold in clinical research, sometimes as a way of bringing new drugs to market that are less effective than those already available. It is also true that participants in randomized placebo-controlled trials, both patients and therapists, may differ systematically from those who would not give consent. And placebos are simply unethical in many contexts. In protracted trials patients cannot be denied a different treatment known to be effective just to suit the interests of the researchers.

Yet classical homeopaths have traditionally claimed they can successfully treat chronic disease when time is not a constraint, and there is good retrospective evidence to support this, e.g. in bronchial asthma (Eizayaga, Eizayaga, Eizayaga 1996). In the only prospective trial in this review to follow a severe debilitating relapsing chronic condition (ME/PVFS) for the sort of period homeopaths would normally recommend, it is reasonable to assume that patients only agreed to the possibility of being assigned to placebo over 12 months because of the absence of plausible biomedical treatments (Awdry 1996).

Although observation and audit are frequently proposed as an answer to the confusing state of placebo research and the need for realistic treatment times, the nonexperimental approach brings its own uncertainties. An audit cycle certainly allows therapists to find out what they are doing, and improve standards by feeding back the results of best practice. But what then? Observational studies, even of best practice, still have limited generalizabilty because of unknown biases (Sheldon 1995). And there are particular reasons why homeopathy may need to be cautious about a call for flexibility that originates from within biomedicine, and relates to competing but less controversial treatments (Black 1996). Because research into homeopathy's mechanisms has been so retarded, a retreat from experimental rigour – even in empirical outcomes research – would be seen as an admission of failure.

13.6.2. Pragmatic trials

However, the format of the clinical trial has evolved over the last 200 years to include not just placebos and double-blinding, but also randomization and statistical analysis (Lilienfeld 1982). There are good reasons for wanting to retain the advantages of the last two, and not throwing the baby out with the bathwater. Although some would dispense with randomization (Urbach 1985) they have not convinced many that observational studies and historical comparisons are an adequate substitute. This is the point at which pragmatic and equivalence trials become relevant (Schwarz & Lellouch 1967). To show simultaneously the possible advantages of these over the observational and placebo-controlled models, a simple clinical situation that can easily be double-masked and controlled by a orthodox treatment and placebo is useful.

The high-quality randomized three-armed trial (n = 156) mentioned in 13.2.2 found *Calendula* ointment for second and third degree burns marginally significantly better than the vaseline excipient alone for rate of healing (p = 0.05), and much better at pain relief (p = 0.002) (Lievre, Marichy, Baux et al. 1992). *Calendula* promoted healing as well as a proprietary proteolytic ointment, Elase® (nsd). Elase® was significantly more likely to cause pain, however, being poorly tolerated in 41 of 52 patients (p = 0.002). Audit or observation of calendula treatment alone would have shown little. Suspicion of selection bias would prevent any attempt to publish the results outside the internal literature. Meaningful historical comparisons could not be made, because although Elase® was used in burns units throughout France it had not been subjected to satisfactory trials. A simple placebo-controlled trial of calendula might have been published, but would tend to be dismissed because the primary outcome (rate of healing) could be found once in every 20 trials by chance.

Clearly, the inclusion of the orthodox treatment raised the information value of the trial, and such findings are relevant whether the evaluation concerns homeopathy vs placebo, adverse reactions, QOL, or costs. This is now realized more widely than was the case, and the high-quality trial of a complex versus betahistine hydrochloride for vertigo showed that it is no longer necessary to have a separate placebo arm to be published in mainstream journals (Weiser, Strösser, Klein 1998). There are occasions when orthodox treatments cannot be substituted for placebos (Tramèr, Reynolds, Moore et al. 1998), but this argument rarely applies to homeopathy.

13.6.3. Randomization and patient preferences

To allow valid comparisons between treatments believed to be equivalent in some respects, it is necessary to recruit enough patients to meet the increased statistical power requirement (Jones, Jarvis, Lewis et al. 1996), although the significantly lower levels of attrition in pragmatic trials found in this review (Table 12.9) might be indicative that placebo controls introduce other sorts of inefficiency. It also goes without saying that when treatment is given unblinded, independent masked assessment of outcomes is needed. However, the inclusion of classical homeopathy for chronic disease in a simple randomized comparison poses further problems. Similarly to therapists and patients who volunteer for double-blind placebo-controlled trials, patients who agree to be randomized to widely different open treatments may differ in important ways from the target population – an argument often put forward against randomization. This would be appear to be particularly true of treatments requiring a great deal of patient and therapist commitment, such as classical homeopathy. Also, patients informed of the risks and benefits found in previous trials might be expected in many situations to express a treatment preference at the outset.

Nevertheless, ways of retaining the benefits of randomization and analysis have been proposed. Brewin and Bradley (1989) suggested that trial patients could be assigned to their preferred treatment (arms A and B) or randomized to either if they were equipoised (arms C and D). Such a design can provide even more information than a preference-only or randomized-only trial. An integrated pluralist health service may think it important to find out not only how groups A and B respond to their preferred treatments, but also how C and D feel about the acceptability of treatments after random assignment. One such trial of two methods of termination of pregnancy found A and B were equally satisfied, unlike C and D, where far more women in one group said they would not choose the same method again (Henshaw, Naji, Russell et al. 1993). A trial with a similar design reviewed here has shown that classical homeopathy is an acceptable alternative for women who reject conventional treatment for unexplained infertility, and convincingly demonstrated homeopathy's minimal drug costs and beneficial effects on unrelated comorbidity (Tarne, Runnebaum, Roebruck et al. 1998, later published as Gerhard 1999). It also provided evidence of potential weaknesses in the Brewin–Bradley model: few with this condition were willing to be randomized; and sociodemographic analysis revealed that the homeopathy preference group was significantly better educated and had unsuccessfully tried significantly more therapies before the trial. One answer to the limited generalizability of results obtained from unbalanced preference groups is to ask patients their preference, but to retain it only as a prognostic variable for analysis rather than to determine assignment, which is randomized as usual (Torgerson, Klaber-Moffett, Russell 1996).

13.6.4. Intrahomeopathic comparisons

One of the advantages of pragmatic trials is that comparisons can be made between different homeopathic methods at the same time. Of the 4 migraine trials (13.2.1), 3 allowed single medicines only (Straumsheim, Borchgrevink, Mowinckel et al. 1997; Walach, Haeusler, Lowes et al. 1997; Whitmarsh, Coleston-Shields, Steiner 1997) while the fourth allowed 2 to be combined in any one prescription (Brigo & Serpelloni 1991). Although this trial took place before the IHS definitions were drawn up, the inclusion criteria suggest that the patients were not so different from the migraine and chronic headache patients of the other 3 that the successful result can be ignored. Trial quality is frequently a reason for suspecting positive results, but this review suggests all 4 trials were strictly comparable, with MQ scores clustered in a range of 86–91%. Given such a fundamental treatment difference, it is questionable whether the 3 later trials can be regarded as replications of the earlier one, and reasonable to ask whether unicist or pluralist treatment was a significant variable. The 4 unicist trials for childhood diarrhea (see 13.2.1) were more closely related, the main difference being the use of C30 and C6 potencies.

Answers are needed to many similar internal and traditionally divisive questions, and observational study followed by pragmatic trial (perhaps involving patient preferences for the type of homeopathy) can do this more quickly than separate placebo-controlled trials, which are often incommensurable because of differences in design, recruitment, ethos and so on. Preliminary outcomes research exists to suggest that some classical repertorization strategies may indeed be more widely applicable or effective than others (Frei 1999), but experimental testing is needed before valid conclusions can be drawn. In an interesting attempt to make just such an intrahomeopathic comparison (excluded from the review because it lacked external controls), a standardized complex preparation for primary female infertility was tested against classical homeopathy (Gerhard, Keller and Schmück 1993). An innovative trial design allowed an optional crossover from complex to classical treatment for women who were dissatisfied with treatment, but was unbalanced by the absence of opportunity for a reciprocal crossover from the classical arm. Conceptions after crossover were attributed to classical treatment when they might have been carryover effects of the complex. Nevertheless, the staffing difficulties encountered in the trial meant that many more women could be treated with the complex.

It is evident from the general literature that clinical and complex homeopathy and isopathy are often dismissed by the proponents of exclusively classical methodologies on theoretical grounds, and these attitudes could be detected in this review even in the face of evidence of efficacy and possible clinical relevance (e.g. the editorial comments accompanying Basu 1980; 1981). However, if trials show that changes in prescribing styles are indicated, then homeopaths have to be willing to adopt them. At the same time, health services need much better content-specific intrahomeopathic information than has been available hitherto. For example, classical homeopathy has been commissioned for atopy because successful high-quality isopathic trials have been conducted, even though classical homeopaths are unlikely to offer the same treatment (Reilly 1996).

13.6.5. Clinically relevant trial proposals

To sum up this discussion of clinical relevance, in situations where orthodox treatment is cost-effective, the question whether or not homeopathy is relevant by virtue of its supposed global effects cannot be answered on the basis of the trials in this review, and does not seem to have been formally tested. Probably the only feasible method of exploring the question would involve tracking sizeable and strictly comparable cohorts of patients receiving homeopathic and orthodox treatment over a considerable number of years.

However, a key question thrown up here is whether homeopathy should be actively considered in situations where biomedicine has current difficulties in understanding or targetting a condition or its etiology, or where treatments have not been developed because of differing research priorities and economic objectives, or where they create unacceptable side-effects, or are rationed because of costs. Evidence of homeopathic efficacy in each of these overlapping areas has been presented, as well as independent replication in some cases. Using these as clinical relevance criteria it is possible to envisage pragmatic trials comparing cost-effectiveness and patient acceptability of homeopathic and orthodox treatment within the UK health system in several conditions.

Unexplained female infertility

Standard treatments (including AI and IVF) for female infertility of unknown origin have only ≤20% efficacy on average, and are frequently invasive and expensive. Women trying to conceive for ≥2 years were treated with classical homeopathy or standard treatment in a trial where permission to randomize could not be obtained, but careful matching on 12 prognostic criteria was used (Gerhard, Reimers, Keller et al. 1993). The number of successful births in each group was equivalent, and the global and economic advantages of homeopathy found in this trial have been mentioned above (13.4.1, 13.4.3). An independent replication incorporating partial randomization and patient preferences again found equivalence in the primary outcome, as well as superiority of homeopathy's global effects and costs (Tarne, Runnebaum, Roebruck et al. 1998). A study group looking at infertility treatment has created an evidence-based hierarchy for treatment recommendations (Royal College of Obstetricians and Gynaecologists 2001). Grade A requires at least one randomized trial as part of a body of literature of overall good quality and consistency addressing the specific recommendation; Grade B requires availability of well-conducted clinical studies in the absence of randomized trials on the topic of recommendation; and Grade C includes expert evidence and clinical experience of respected authorities. The classical homeopathy trials undertaken in Germany are part of a growing body of research and evidence that currently falls between Grades A and B. A replication in the UK comparing homeopathy with RCOG's recommended treatment for unexplained infertility (ovarian stimulation with intrauterine insemination), and using local inclusion criteria such as trying to conceive for ≥3 years would seem to be justified. This is particularly relevant since RCOG stressed that the Department of Health's advice to NHS commissioners should provide evidence about cost-effectiveness as well as clinical efficacy.

ME/PVFS

Classical homeopathy showed significant benefits over placebo in patients meeting standard diagnostic criteria for this relapsing chronic condition (Awdry 1996), and a randomized placebo-controlled replication is under way. No somatic treatment has proved satisfactory, and treatment with antidepressants is common. However, a placebo-controlled trial of fluoxetine showed no difference from placebo after 8 weeks on any outcome measure including depression, and 15% of verum patients dropped out from side-effects (Vercoulen, Swanink, Zitman et al. 1996). A second trial randomized patients to fluoxetine plus a graded exercise programme, fluoxetine and appointments only, graded exercise only, or placebo, and after 6 months still found no difference from placebo, as well as 13% dropouts from side-effects (Wearden, Morris, Mullis et al. 1998). It would appear that biomedicine has little to offer patients, despite ME/PVFS having a greater impact on personal, physical and emotional disability than angina, hypertension, arthritis or chronic bronchitis (Wessely, Chalder, Hirsch et al. 1997). A cognitive behaviour therapy (CBT) package aimed to help patients cope better with the disease has shown significant benefits over ordinary medical care or relaxation therapy in 2 randomized trials (Sharpe, Hawton, Simkin et al. 1996). Although classical homeopathy aims to do more than help patients cope better, it could usefully be compared with CBT, possibly using a similar design to the unsuccessful fluoxetine plus graded exercise trial.

Influenza treatment

Biomedicine has had little success in targetting viral infections, and influenza treatment has traditionally consisted of advice to rest, maintain fluid intake and use antipyrexics or analgesics as needed. The recently-licensed zanamivir (Relenza) is supported by evidence from RCTs of symptom relief and reduction in time to recovery of 0.5 days. The R&D costs were enormous, leading to high prices, and the drug was subsequently not approved for NHS use, on the grounds that the trials showed insufficient evidence of effects. Outcry from practitioners and the manufacturer's economic threat to withdraw altogether from UK drug research were followed by limited approval for NHS use in at-risk groups (NICE 2000). *Oscillococcinum*'s superiority to placebo in treatment of influenza appears to have been established in the 4 trials reviewed here, and a systematic review showed a mean reduction in illness duration of 0.28 days (Vickers & Smith 2000). The clinical relevance of this reduction has been questioned (FACT 2001), but it is equally questionable whether this single outcome adequately summarized the evidence. *Oscillococcinum* also showed significant relief of influenza symptoms in each trial, but costs much less than zanamivir (and less still when sold as the generic *Anas barbarae*). Moreover, while zanamivir can only be dispensed on prescription, *Oscillococcinum* is available over the counter, with possible implications for reducing demand on health services. A randomized equivalence trial of these competing treatments would seem to be justified on economic grounds alone.

Inhalant allergy

Biomedical treatment of atopy, including hayfever and asthma, is principally confined to management, typically with corticosteroids. Hyposensitization with allergen extract vaccines has not proved effective in asthma. Vaccines have been more successful in allergic rhinitis when specific allergens are known but are little used because of the risks of anaphylactic shock. Homeopathic immunotherapy (HIT) with specific allergens in C30 potency proved safe and significantly superior to placebo on a range of outcome measures in the series of trials for hay fever and asthma mentioned in 13.2.4 above (Reilly & Taylor 1985; Reilly, McSharry, Taylor et al. 1986; Reilly, Taylor, Beattie et al. 1994). Although the trials were planned to test the ultramolecular-placebo hypothesis, and the authors said there were no implications for clinical practice, a recent independent multicentric replication studying the model in perennial allergic rhinitis showed an effect on nasal inspiratory peak flow comparable to that found with topical nasal steroids (Malmberg, Holopainen, Simola et al. 1991; Taylor, Reilly, Llewellyn-Jones et al. 2000). A pragmatic trial of HIT and steroidal treatment of atopy would now seem to be justified, and could make use of the results of a randomized placebo-controlled comparison of 2 different potencies in the same model (Kayne & Beattie 1996, interim report excluded from this review).

13.7. Limitations of the present review

Less space has been given to criticism of internal validity of trials than in most previous homeopathy reviews, and more consideration to homeopathic validity and generalizability. This could be seen as avoiding the placebo question which has driven earlier reviews. Single-reviewer evaluation is also problematic, and if more resources had been available, twin MQ and CR scoring with a test for inter-rater agreement might have been preferable. A validated MQ instrument was used, however, which showed good rank correlations with MQ scores from previous high-quality systematic reviews, and allowed discussion to be restricted to best evidence for the most part.

Although an advance on dichotomized results, the use of a stratified vote count is an imprecise measure of effect size. It was adopted because of the need to display and compare results from trials with more than 1 clinically relevant outcome. The development of meta-analytic techniques that are not limited to single outcomes – or alternatively, more frequent use of global outcomes such as QUALYs – ought to enable greater precision without sacrificing global effects.

13.8. Further recommendations

Suggestions concerning homeopathic trial design and conduct have been made throughout this chapter. Reviewers in all fields of healthcare are expected to urge researchers to improve reporting standards of clinical trials, and more help is available than ever before (CONSORT 2001; Moher, Schulz, Altman et al. 2001). On the basis of the reports reviewed here, areas specific to homeopathy where reporting (and probably trial planning) could be greatly improved without exceeding space restrictions in biomedical journals include the descriptions or identifications of:

- rationales for selection of test medicines, potencies and repetition in clinical and complex homeopathy and isopathy
- repertorization and prescribing strategies in classical homeopathy
- names, potencies and repetition of trial medicines in classical homeopathy, along with a frequency table of at least the principal medicines
- which pharmacopeia and laboratory were used to manufacture test medicines
- placebo details where used, e.g. unmedicated blanks, plain or serially diluted diluent, succussed or unsuccussed.

Space is less limited in homeopathic and complementary healthcare journals, and it has been suggested that classical trials could be reported in much greater detail there, in parallel with abbreviated but more prestigious reports of the same trials in the biomedical press (Linde & Melchart 1998). This advice should probably hold good for all types of homeopathy.

Further development and maintenance of an evaluated international trial database searchable by many variables, as used in the preparation of this review, should be a priority. It will allow efficient online systematic searches and reviews of clinical evidence, currently hampered by the grey literature and language problems, and enable rapid identification of significant similarities and differences between designs, inclusion and exclusion criteria, demographics, treatments and outcomes. Incorporating experimental and quasiexperimental designs not included here will be feasible, since the MQ instrument used is designed to allow such designs to be evaluated to a common standard, and will make studies that merit analysis and rigorous replication more readily available than hitherto.

If the database were to be further expanded to incorporate preregistration of homeopathy trials it would begin to address the problem of publication bias in homeopathy. If structured to correspond with the CONSORT recommendations for parallel group randomized trials, or similar recommendations for other designs, it could also benefit prospective researchers in homeopathy by demonstrating standards of trial design and reporting to aim at. For political reasons, such a database should probably not be held in an existing homeopathic or biomedical centre, but in an impartial evidence-based healthcare environment

Part IV: Conclusion

14. Retrospect and prospect

I: Homeopathy's place in the history of therapeutics

In spite of high ideals and eager observation, neither the French nor the German attempts to reconstitute medicine in the late eighteenth century had much to offer therapeutically. Inductive description of the processes and endstates of disease did not lead to relief for patients; and the basic sciences, which would later reveal 'causes' and the possibility of treatments aimed at them, did not yet exist to underpin the search for deductive principles.

Within both schools, the vacuum created by the abandonment of the apothecaries' concoctions was filled by increased reliance on blood-letting and a handful of drugs as the sole treatments. Therapeutic nonsense was replaced by therapeutic nihilism. Calomel, still in use today as a pesticide, continued as a mainstay of internal medicine throughout the nineteenth century, and was used into the 1920s as a purgative in the management of pneumonia (Porter 1997: 674). Likewise, blood-letting did not die out quickly after its inefficacy was timidly demonstrated in a single condition by Louis (1835). The retired British prime minister Sir Robert Peel was bled while dying – from concussion, multiple fractures and internal hemorrhaging, after falling from his horse – in central London in 1850. Most doctors in that year before the Great Exhibition complained that he should have been bled much more intensively – 20 leeches were just too few to save him (Youngson 1979: 18). And blood-letting was still advocated in pneumonia in the twentieth century at the highest levels of medical education (e.g. Osler 1912: 99).

Hahnemann's rejection of the therapeutic anarchy of the late eighteenth century came before his homeopathic research, and proceeded alongside the new therapy until the end of his career. He was a highly competent critic, and the accuracy and prescience of his rejection of blood-letting and rationalist medical theories, and his calls for reform of the abuses of the apothecaries and the treatment of the mentally ill, were subsequently confirmed historically and scientifically. His plea for humane treatment of suicides took longer to be heard (Hahnemann 1819b): they committed a criminal offence in the UK until 1961.

A century after his death, opponents were still trying to neutralize the critique, claiming that homeopathy was an involuntary reaction and medical reform really began with the French school (Osler 1941: 221). In spite of earlier reluctance to acknowledge him, medical historians have more recently given Hahnemann much of the credit for orthodoxy's gradual abandonment during the nineteenth century of bleeding, purging, polypharmacy and massive doses, as well as the belated adoption of the precautionary principle that medicines should be tested on the healthy before administering them to the sick (Shryock 1948: 139; Ackerknecht 1982b: 143f; Porter 1997: 390f). If he had done nothing else, Hahnemann's revival and continued aggressive advocacy of the forgotten principle of *primum non nocere* (first do no harm), from 1790 until his death in 1843, can still reasonably be said to have had as much practical influence on medicine as any other individual reformer's contribution. The author of the entry for homeopathy in the 10th edition of the *Encyclopaedia Britannica* remarked:

> Hahnemann undoubtedly deserves the credit of being the first to break decidedly with the old school of medical practice, in which, forgetful of the teachings of Hippocrates, nature was either overlooked or rudely opposed by wrong and ungentle methods. We can scarcely now estimate the force of character and of courage which was implied in his abandoning the common lines of medicine. (Helmuth 1911)

Hahnemann's commitment to Enlightenment ideals is hard to fault, and attempts to explain his critique away as a product of his personal inadequacies seem to have little basis in fact.

Turning to Hahnemann's therapeutics, in order to assess the validity of the arguments that it was merely invented, or derived from Paracelsus, the distinctive aspects of the Hahnemannian research programme must be described, and then placed in their historical context. It is possible to see that far from being unconnected to the acknowledged problems of eighteenth-century medicine – e.g.: its lack of any rational connection between materia medica and diseases; its dangerous therapies – Hahnemannian homeopathy built on critical ideas, experiments and therapeutic procedures already conjectured or in existence – particularly those of von Störck, Plenciz and John Hunter. Homeopathy began as a rational Enlightenment enterprise designed to fulfill the Kantian dream of a scientific medicine to match the other sciences, but with the added irony that it purported to be an unKantian science centred on aggregated human qualities and perceptions rather than measureable physical quantities. Homeopathy could be rejected because it was claimed that it was opposed to all scientific advances in medicine per se. Yet therapeutics was Hahnemann's primary target, not science:

> Without disparaging the services which many physicians have rendered to the sciences auxiliary to medicine, to natural philosophy [physics] and chemistry, to natural history [biology] in its various branches, and to that of man in par-

ticular, to anthropology, physiology and anatomy, etc., I shall occupy myself here with the practical part of medicine only, with therapeutics itself, in order to show how it is that diseases have hitherto been so imperfectly treated. (Hahnemann 1833c: Introduction)

Looking beyond the incompatible aspects of Kantian and Hahnemannian medical assumptions, there are interesting similarities in Hahnemann's and Hegel's programmes that undoubtedly warrant further study. Post-Kantians with ambitions to transform their disciplines, they both believed they had transcended the rationalism or empiricism of their medical and philosophical predecessors and contemporaries. Both rejected mind–body dualism, and created integrated systems that were phenomenologically and semantically based – possibly under Herder's influence – while asserting their scientific validity. There are ironic similarities in their reception as well. Both have frequently been derided as charlatans, or 'too difficult to understand', by practitioners and historians of medicine and philosophy, who have too often felt free to abandon academic objectivity when writing about them (for Hegel's reception, see: Cottingham 1984: 91ff). Both are often confused with the *Naturphilosophen*, despite their having taken care to distance themselves from biological and philosophical Romanticism. Both had immense influence on the subsequent development of their disciplines, that has often gone unacknowledged.

As scholars such as Pagel (1982a; 1982b) and Debus (1998) have pointed out in regard to their postpositivist reassessments of Paracelsus' and Van Helmont's significance, Hahnemann's synthesis ought really to be regarded as a sign of his great creativity and seminal importance. In view of Hahnemann's stature, during his life to some extent, and certainly after his death, homeopathy inevitably acquired many aspects of a personality cult. Attempts to prevent this were heard within homeopathy from the 1820s on – such as the German 'critical' homeopaths like Wolf, and independent medical thinkers like Tessier in France, or Dudgeon and Hughes in Britain – but their voices were lost as homeopathy and an infant biomedicine became increasingly divergent and antagonistic, rather than learning from each other.

External rejection and internal division have usually been presented as consequences of a one-sided failure of homeopathy to keep up with 'the progress of science' (Campbell 1978; Bellavite & Signorini 1995). Another view would construct the problem slightly differently, and say that the accelerating growth of mechanistic reductionism in the nineteenth century did not use postmortem lesions, laboratory parameters and germ theory to try to augment understanding of the patient's experience of illness, but as a replacement for understanding. A version of science intent on removing the human observer from the universe succeeded in relegating the perception and description of human sensation and emotion – proper subjects for medicine, not just homeopathy – to the arts. One could say the deliberate exclusion of homeopathy from biomedicine forced both streams into narrower channels. In homeopathy's case, clinical research gave way to scriptural exegesis of the canonical works (e.g. Kent 1900), and acausal phenomenology was sometimes lost in neorationalist backwaters of speculation about constitution, occult etiology and spiritized posology. This seems to have been more responsible for the objections of the clinical homeopaths than any objection to semiology on their part, and their contribution really comprises a self-correcting tendency within homeopathy, not a root-and-branch replacement. The later developments and ramifications of homeopathy are not invariably signs of 'confusion', but also point to an underlying reality: the belief in the biological activity and therapeutic efficacy of homeopathic serial agitated dilutions across wide domains of sickness.

II: Homeopathy and the development of clinical evaluation

An adaptation of the systematic review technique has allowed important historical questions about the reception of homeopathy by science and orthodox medicine, and the reciprocal relationship between homeopathy and allopathy in the development of clinical evaluation, to be posed and answered in terms of evidence from trials and clinical practice. This is in marked contrast to the debate about scientific rationality and the resistance to change within orthodox medicine (including the rejection of dissident or alien therapies such as mesmerism, homeopathy and acupuncture) in the first half of the nineteenth century – a debate that is as familiar as it is undecideable, when based mainly on theoretical considerations and epistemological hindsight.

This approach also allows an entirely different biographical perspective to emerge in which the key players are not the fabled elders and theoreticians of traditional and recent homeopathic historiography, hagiography and education, such as Hahnemann, Hering, Bönninghausen, Kent et al., who form the subject of Part I. Instead, names such as Marenzeller, Tessier, Casper and Wurmb, Wesselhoeft Senior and Junior, Boyd and Paterson occupy the stage – characters whose absence from homeopathic awareness in the present day ought to be a matter for concern.

It has been shown here that the very earliest external placebo-controlled trials of homeopathy to be discovered used placebos modelled on those already in use as part of Hahnemannian practice. Convinced of the fundamental soundness of their therapy, homeopaths seem to have been uninterested in placebo-controlled therapeutic trials, and insisted on pragmatic trials of homeopathy versus allopathy. Although the 1854 cholera treatment evaluation in London has been recognized as a defining moment in the evolution of the clinical trial (Lilienfeld 1982), the suppression and subsequent publication of the superior homeopathic results appears to be unknown outside homeopathic historiography. Medical historiography which continues to ignore large well-conducted comparative trials by experienced homeopaths such as Tessier's in favour of invalid earlier trials such as Andral's can no longer be seen as an impartial account of homeopathy's development. The main lesson from this period of clinical evaluation is that the opportunity was missed to research the possibilities of homeopathy as a distinct and useful approach within medicine, despite the attempts of homeopaths, hospital administrators and government officials. Only a Nobel laureate with no career at stake could risk saying:

> If I were confronted with a hitherto incurable disease and could see no way to treat it other than with homeopathy, I can assure you I would not be deterred from following this course by dogmatic considerations. (Behring 1905: xxvif)

Remarkably, there is no evidence that homeopaths used placebo before the twentieth century to disguise a lack of treatment possibilities (as allopathy traditionally did), but only ever as a control. Homeopathy clearly has a long-standing tradition of awareness of psychological factors that affect the way we react to treatment, and incorporated a sophisticated use of placebo very early on in order to minimize apparently veridical but actually misleading responses in everyday clinical practice. However, the adoption by homeopaths of an explanatory biomedical approach in the early part of the twentieth century performed a useful service in allowing traditional empirical treatments to be discarded. Once again homeopaths appear to have been quick to take advantage of methodological developments in clinical evaluation, in order to demonstrate the validity of their therapy.

III: Is homeopathy clinically relevant?

The most enthusiastic proponents of homeopathy have consistently claimed it is entirely safe and free from side effects, that it is designed to treat the person as well as disease narrowly defined, and that it is a complete medical system – i.e. to be used at any time, with any patient, and for almost any condition (even including many that would normally be regarded as requiring surgery). This point of view notwithstanding, common sense says that controlled trials are likely to show that some clinical areas and therapeutic avenues yield stronger evidence of efficacy than others. The evidence that it was possible to uncover in the review of contemporary trials suggests that:

- homeopathy appears mostly as safe as reputed, but far more rigorous data collection and evaluation is required;
- non-holistic clinical, complex and isopathic variants of homeopathy are possible, but require careful problem and treatment modelling;
- classical homeopathy does appear to be capable of influencing global outcomes such as wellbeing and comorbidity, but it is unlikely that all versions of classical homeopathy are equally valid;
- economic benefits are noticeable in the treatment of some conditions and not others.

It may be no accident that clinically relevant areas seem to have been uncovered in pragmatic comparisons with biomedical treatments as well as in explanatory placebo-controlled trials, particularly in cases where the efficacy or costs of orthodox treatment are problematic. This would seem to be an area that has been as overlooked in the current homeopathy–placebo debate as it was in the mid nineteenth century. It is worth recalling that the structure and extended format of individualized homeopathic treatment in chronic diseases such as migraine, bronchial asthma and ME/PVFS has much in common with complex interventions such as psychotherapy, multistage surgery, and social and educational programmes (Medical Research Council 2000). These are the disciplines where pragmatic trials were developed because of the obvious problems of applying the pharmacological gold standard. The similarity in appearance of homeopathic medicines and orthodox drugs may have blinded users and researchers to remarkable differences in the content and operation of the fundamental therapeutic model, when confronted by the need to evaluate the therapy to acceptable scientific standards.

There are further reasons for emphasizing pragmatic rather than placebo trials. Sceptics demand evidence from high-quality randomized placebo-controlled trials of homeopathy, only to reject it when it proves positive (e.g. Aulas, Bordelay, Royer 1991: 154ff; Sampson & London 1995; Meyer 1996: 99; Vandenbroucke 1997; 2000), even though large numbers of biomedical treatments have not been similarly validated (Bower 1998). Leaving aside a priorism, the question as always is: What is the question? If you want to know whether some or all homeopathic medicines are just sugar pills, then placebo trials may be appropriate. However, the fact that few patients would demand placebo rather than verum, given a choice, shows something may be wrong with making placebo controls the automatic research model outside the laboratory.

There are more urgent questions, though. Health services are desperately short of hard information on the comparative benefits of treatments. It is more useful for them to know if homeopathy – or which of its versions – can be appropriately offered to some or all patients, whether it makes sense to introduce it into primary, secondary or tertiary care, and what the costs and benefits of its processes and outcomes are. To answer this type of question, pragmatic trials are more informative, testing unblinded homeopathy against the best available biomedical or other complementary treatments. This shift in perspective also allows the need for larger trials – acutely problematic in homeopathy because of isolation and underfunding – to be reframed as an opportunity: pragmatic trials are by their very nature collaborative and orientated towards health services requirements, so funding and recruitment could prove less difficult than hitherto.

• • •

Philosophically, the late twentieth-century rediscovery of psychology's 'double ontology' – that personhood coexists with but is not necessarily reduceable to Cartesian co-ordinates or molecular activity (e.g. Harré 1998) – seems to have gone hand-in-hand with the realization that Hegel's 'hermeneutic circle' could well be a more productive model for current developmental theory than the accepted Cartesian–Kantian one (e.g. Marková 1982; Kelso 1995). Whether this reorientation will eventually encompass Hahnemann's medical personalism and what his expanded nondualistic notion of pharmacology might be able to tell us about ourselves remains to be seen. Certainly, the outlook for homeopathy will improve at all levels in proportion to the extent that it interests researchers in adjacent fields, such as immunology, toxicology, psychopharmacology and health psychology, so long as they do not feel intimidated by historic prejudice from entering a forbidden zone (e.g. Calabrese & Baldwin 1999). But as far as homeopathy's enigmatic biomedical status as an irrefutable but unassimilable therapy is concerned (Unschuld 1995), it cannot be denied that recent commitments to pragmatic evidence-based healthcare have allowed Hahnemann's *rationelle Heilkunst* to surface and be examined more impartially than at any time since its inception – not just for what it might 'be', but also for what value it might have to offer patients, therapists and society on its own terms.

Appendices

(see CD included)

App. 1	Details of excluded homeopathic trials
App. 2.1	Overview of controlled trials of classical homeopathy
App. 2.2	Overview of controlled trials of clinical homeopathy
App. 2.3	Overview of controlled trials of complex homeopathy
App. 2.4	Overview of controlled trials of isopathy
App. 3	Trials (n = 56) reporting adverse reactions in homeopathy or control groups
App. 4	Methodological quality (MQ) and clinical relevance (CR) scores of prospective controlled trials of homeopathy

Glossary

aggravation (initial) Temporary worsening of symptoms following treatment.

anthroposophical medicine Treatment according to the medical ideas of the German theosophist Rudolf Steiner (1861–1925). Anthroposophical doctors prescribe quasi-homeopathic (i.e. serially diluted but unsuccussed) medicines, according to psychospiritual theories that owe more to *Naturphilosophie* and Paracelsus than Hahnemann.

centesimal potency A *serial dilution* of 1 part in 100. Centesimal potencies are designated here by a number up to 200 preceded by the letter C, but in other systems the number may precede the letter. Thus C6 (or 6C or 6c) represents a 1 in 100 dilution carried out serially 6 times, each with a burst of *succussion*. The next potency used above C200 is 1M, where M = 1000. Therefore 1M = C1000, 10M = C10 000 etc.

chronic miasms Three infectious *miasms* – 'itch' (including scabies), gonorrhea and syphilis – eventually believed by Hahnemann (1828) to be responsible for all chronic disease. Modified by post-Hahnemannians to mean diathesis or dyscrasia, i.e. acquired or hereditary general traits and (pre)dispositions to illness.

classical homeopathy Treatment based on strict semiotic individualization of each case, including psychological symptoms, and usually using a single medicine in a single prescription. Associated with *symptom complex* and *unicist* homeopathy, qqv.

clinical homeopathy Treatment based mainly on nosological categories or *pathological* indications, without individualization.

complex homeopathy Treatment with a combination of two or more *clinical* homeopathic medicines incorporated into one dosage form.

concomitants Symptoms linked concurrently with other symptoms, constituting a clinical unit in the *materia medica* and *repertory*, e.g. stool accompanied by coryza.

constitution Originally a biomorphological category. More usually, essential characteristics of healthy individuals, rather than the same characteristics affected by illness or disease, in which case they form part of the *symptom complex*. Constitutional prescribing treats patients with medicines corresponding to their healthy constitutional state.

decimal potency A *serial dilution* in the proportion of 1 part in 10. Decimal potencies are designated here by a number with the letter D preceding it, but in other systems the number may precede the letter x. Thus D6 (or 6x) represents a 1 in 10 dilution carried out serially 6 times, each with a burst of *succussion*. Decimal potencies range from D1 to D200.

dynamization Release of therapeutic power of a substance by means of *trituration*, *serial dilution* and *succussion*. Also known as *potentization*, qv.

***genius epidemicus*, epidemic remedy** Medicine corresponding to, or that has proved curative in, a particular epidemic disease at the population level.

isopathy Treatment of a disease with medicines derived from the causative agent or organism of the disease (cf. *nosode*).

keynote symptom Symptom providing a leading indication for a particular medicine, e.g. worse for movement, *Bryonia*.

materia medica In homeopathy, a systematic register of symptoms produced in drug *provings*. Frequently augmented with symptoms or conditions cured in clinical practice not seen in provings.

miasm Traditionally a nonspecific noxious emanation, Hahnemann's preferred term for specific infectious agents including microorganisms. Now usually referring to a *chronic miasm*.

modality Of great importance in homeopathy, any factor modifying the quality of a symptom, or the patient as a whole.

mother tincture The standardized liquid preparation (symbol: Ø) derived from raw source materials before *potentization*. Different processes are used to make mother tinctures, depending on the nature of the source, e.g. expressed plant juices, fresh plant material, dried plant material, animal material, organ preparations, *nosodes* etc.

nosode Medicine derived from diseased organ, disease product or causative organism of disease (cf. *isopathy*).

pathological prescribing *Clinical* treatment based on the correspondence of the patient's lesional pathology with lesional toxicology described in the *materia medica*, with little reference to semiology or other individualizing characteristics.

pluralist homeopathy Treatment with more than one medicine representing different aspects of the illness given in a single prescription. The adjective 'pluralist' may describe the practitioner or the method. The instructions usually require the different medicines to be taken at different times, as distinct from complex homeopathy which uses fixed mixtures in a single dosage form.

plussing Further dilution of medicines with *succussion* before each dose or at intervals during regular repetition of the dose.

potency Therapeutic power released or developed by *dynamization*. The scalar degree to which a medicine has been potentized.

potency scale Scale denoting the potency degree. Three are in common use: *centesimal* (C), *decimal* (D) and *quinquagintamillesimal* (Q).

potentization The process developed by Hahnemann after 1816 by which medicinal power is released or increased, involving initial *trituration* followed by *serial dilution* with *succussion*.

proving Pathogenetic drug test (German *Prüfung*) involving administration of substances (in material dose, *mother tincture* or *potency*) to healthy volunteers, to elicit effects from which the therapeutic sphere of influence of the substance may be derived according to the *similia principle*.

Q (quinquagintamillesimal) potency A *serial dilution* of 1 part in 50 000. Q potencies are designated here by a number with the letter Q preceding it, although in other systems the number may be preceded by the Roman numerals LM. Thus Q6 (or LM6) represents a 1 in 50 000 dilution carried out serially 6 times, each with a burst of *succussion*. Q potencies range from Q1 to Q30.

radionics A twentieth-century development of medical dowsing or radiesthesia, involving remote transmission of therapeutic energies or information. Makes frequent use of conventional and simulated homeopathic medicines in diagnosis and treatment, but the principles underlying the therapy and the reasons for prescriptions are often entirely different.

repertory Symptomatic index to the homeopathic *materia medica*. Repertorization is the process of case analysis used to identify the medicine that best matches the patient's *symptom complex*.

serial dilution A component of the *potentization* process. The sequential addition of 1 part of the stock or of the previous dilution as a specified proportion of diluent: 1:9, 1:99 or 1:49 999 (see *centesimal*, *decimal* and *Q* potencies respectively). The number of dilutions defines the *potency*. The two methods principally used are: Hahnemannian, using a fresh flask or bottle for each dilution; and the more economical Korsakov or single flask method in which the container is emptied after *succussion* and refilled with diluent.

specific A homeopathic medicine specifically indicated for a particular clinical condition.

similia principle From '*similia similibus curentur*' (let like be cured by like) – the treatment of disease with substances that have induced similar symptoms in a healthy subject in a *proving*.

simillimum The most accurate match possible between the patient's *symptom complex* and the *materia medica*.

succussion Vigorous jolting given at each stage of *serial dilution* during *potency* preparation.

symptom complex The aggregate of the patient's symptoms considered as a meaningful whole or essence (German *Symptomeninbegriff*). Sometimes translated as 'totality of symptoms', although this misses *Inbegriff*'s dual meaning of epitome.

tautopathy *Isopathic* treatment with a *potentized* preparation of a chemical substance, especially a conventional drug, that has had or is having some adverse effect on the patient.

trituration Initial preparation and *potentization* from solid and insoluble source material, and in some cases from fresh plants, by grinding 1 part together with 99 parts of lactose as a diluent.

unicist homeopathy Treatment with one medicine, ideally representing the *symptom complex* in a single prescription. The adjective 'unicist' may describe the practitioner or the method.

Abbreviations and symbols used in tables

Ø	mother tincture
C	centesimal potency, range C1–C200
D	decimal potency, range D1–D200
K	Korsakov single-flask centesimal potency
1M, 10M	centesimal potency degrees corresponding to C1000, C10 000
Q	quinquagintamillesimal potency, range Q1–Q30
OT	orthodox (biomedical) treatment
P	placebo
TAU	(biomedical) treatment as usual

References

Trial reports 1821–1954 (Part II)

Académie de Médecine (1835). Séance du 17 mars. Discussion sur l'homoeopathie. *Gazette Médicale de Paris*. 3(12): 189–191.

Ameke W. (1885). *History of Homoeopathy: Its Origin, its Conflicts*. Ed. R.E. Dudgeon. Trans. A.E. Drysdale. London, E. Gould & Son.

Anon (1834). Expériences homéopathiques faites par M. Andral, à l'hôpital de la Pitié. *Bulletin Général de Thérapeutique Médicale et Chirurgicale*. 6(Sept.): 318–321.

Attomyr J. (1832). Homöopathische Heilversuche, angestellt im allgemeinen Krankenhause zu München. *Archiv für die homöopathische Heilkunst*. 11(2): 100–120.

Bellows H.P. (1906). *The Test Drug-Proving of the "O. O. & L. Society": A Re-Proving of Belladonna*. Boston, O. O. & L. Society.

Bier A. (1925). Wie sollen wir uns zu der Homoeopathie stellen? *Münchener Medizinische Wochenschrift*. 72(1): 713–717, 773–776.

Boyanus C. (1882). *Gomeopatija v Rossii. Istoriceskiij ocerk*. Moskva.

British Homoeopathic Society (1943). Report on mustard gas experiments (Glasgow and London). *British Homoeopathic Journal*. 33(Suppl.): 1–12.

Burnett J.C. (1888). *Fifty Reasons for Being a Homoeopath*. London, Homoeopathic Publishing Company.

Chargé A. (1855). *L'Homéopathie et ses détracteurs à l'occasion de l'épidémie de choléra qui a régné à Marseille en 1854*. Paris, Baillière.

Chicago Herald (1881). [Cook County]. *Chicago Herald*. Nov. 29: 1, col. 7.

Chicago Medical Society (1922). *History of Medicine and Surgery in Chicago*. Chicago.

Cook County Board of Commissioners (n.d.). *Proceedings, 1881–1882*. Chicago.

Cook County Hospital (1885). *Annual Report, 1884*. Chicago.

Cook County Hospital (1888). *Annual Report, 1887*. Chicago.

de Horatiis C. (1829). *Saggio di clinico omiopatica, la prima volta publicamente tentata in Napoli, nell' ospedale generale della Trinità*. Naples.

Donner F. (1948). *Zwölf Vorlesungen über Homöopathie*. Berlin, Haug.

Editorial (1849). Homéopathie dans les hôpitaux de Paris. *L'Union Médicale*. 3(146, 8 decembre): 581.

Eidherr M. (1862). Erfahrungen über die Heilwirkungen der 6., 15. und 30. Arzneiverdünnung auf die entzündete Lunge. *Zeitschrift des Vereines der homöopathischen Aertze Oesterreichs*. 1 n.s. (1): 1–165.

Esquirol E. (1835). [Review of] Panvini, P. I quaranta giorni …, etc.; c'est-à-dire Les Quarante Jours de la Clinique Homoeopathique établie à l'hôpital militaire de Naples, sous la direction du chevalier Cosme de Horatiis et d'une commission de médecins; exposés avec des réflexions; par le chevalier Pasquale Panvini, médecin de l'hôpital Della Pace, etc.; ouvrage dédié à Hippocrate. Naples, 1829. *Gazette Médicale de Paris*. 3(12): 191–192.

Forbes J. (1846). Homoeopathy, Allopathy and 'Young Physic'. *British & Foreign Medical Review*. 21: 225–65.

Gallavardin J.-P. (1860). *Projet d'hôpitaux mixtes allopathiques et homoeopathiques: projet de dispensaires mixtes. Mémoire adressée à MM. les administrateurs des hôpitaux*. Paris, Baillière.

General Board of Health (1854–55). *Letter of the President of the General Board of Health accompanying a Report from Dr Sutherland on epidemic cholera in the Metropolis in 1854*. Parliamentary Papers, no. 1893, xlv.

Guéyrard D.-M. (1833a). [Letter]. *Bulletin Général de Thérapeutique Médicale et Chirurgicale*. 5: 291–292.

Guéyrard D.-M. (1833b). [Letter]. *Gazette Médicale de Paris*. 1 n.s.(72): 776.

Herrmann D. (1831). Amtlicher Bericht des Herrn D. Herrmann über die homöopathische Behandlung im Militärhospitale zu Tulzyn in Podolien, welche er auf Befehl Sr. Maj. des Kaisers Nicolaus I. unternommen; nebst einer Abhandlung über die Kur der Wechselfieber. *Annalen der homöopathischen Klinik*. 2: 380–399.

Hess F.O. (1942). Nützt uns die Homöopathie bei der Diphtherie-Behandlung? *Münchener Medizinische Wochenschrift* (13): 296.

House of Commons (1854–55). *Return to an Address of the Honourable House of Commons*. Sessional Papers, no. 255. xlv: 189–226.

Irvine F.W. (1844). M. Andral's homoeopathic experiments at la Pitié. *British Journal of Homoeopathy*. 2(1): 49–64.

Johannsen (1848). Ueber den Gegenwärtigen Stand der Homöopathie in Russland. *Hygea*. 1 n.s.: 44–50.

Jousset P. (1862). *De l'expectation et du traitement homéopathique dans la pneumonie*. Paris, Baillière.

Ledermann E.K., Sutherland I., Lunt R. (1954). Homoeopathy tested against controls in surgical tuberculosis. *British Homoeopathic Journal*. 44: 83–97.

Lichtenstädt J. (1832). Beschluss des Kaiserl. Russ. Menicinalraths [sic] in Beziehung auf die homöopathische Heilmethode. *Litterarische Annalen der gesammten Heilkunde*. 24(4, December): 412–420.

Lisle E. (1861). Feuilleton de l'homoeopathie orthodoxe. *L'Union Médicale*. (128): 11–72.

Löhner G. (1835). *Die homöopathischen Kochsalzversuche zu Nürnberg, Mit einem Anhang: Ein Beispiel homöopathischer Heilart*. Nuremberg.

Medical Council (1854–55a). *Appendix to the Report of the Committee for Scientific Inquiries in relation to the cholera epidemic of 1854*. Parliamentary Papers, no. 1996, xxi.

Medical Council (1854–55b). *Report of the Committee for Scientific Inquiries in relation to the cholera epidemic of 1854*. Parliamentary Papers, no. 1980, xxi.

Medical Council (1854–55c). *Report of the Medical Council in relation to the cholera-epidemic of 1854*. Parliamentary Papers, no. 1989, xlv.

Medical Council (1854–55d). *Report on the results of the different methods of treatment pursued in epidemic cholera*. Parliamentary Papers, no. 1901, xlv.

Ozanne J. (1850). Homoeopathy in Paris. *Homoeopathic Times*. 1: 695–9, 709–13, 723–7.

Ozanne J. (1853). Homoeopathy tested by statistics. *Homoeopathic Times*. 4(182): 372–375.

Ozanne J. (1857). The general mortality of hospitals. The hopital Ste.-Marguerite, of Paris. *Monthly Homoeopathic Review*. I: 533–539.

Panvini P. (1829). *I quaranta giorni della clinica omiopatica stabilita nell'ospedale militare di Napoli*. Naples, Trani.

Paterson J., Boyd W.E. (1941). A preliminary study of the alteration of the Schick test by a homoeopathic potency. *British Homoeopathic Journal*. 31: 301–9.

Peschier G. (1835). Mélanges. *Bibliothèque Homoeopathique*. 4: 122–126.

Pigeaux D.M.P. (1834). Étonnantes vertus homoeopathiques de la mie de pain: Expériences faites à l'Hôtel-Dieu. *Bulletin Général de Thérapeutique Médicale et Chirurgicale*. 6: 128–131.

Pointe (1833). Compte-rendu des expériences homoeopathiques faites a l'Hôtel-Dieu de Lyon, par M. Guérard. *Gazette Médicale de Paris*. 1 n.s.(68): 708–9.

Potter S., Storke E.F. (1880). Final report of the Milwaukee test of the 30th dilution. *Homoeopathic Times: A Monthly Journal of Medicine, Surgery and the Collateral Sciences*. 7(12): 280–281.

Rapou P.A. (1847). *Histoire de la doctrine homéopathique, son état actuel dans les principales contrées de l'Europe: application pratique des principes et moyens de cette doctrine au traitement des malades*. 2 vols. Paris, Baillière.

Schilsky B., Bayer W. (1941). Vergleich der Keuchhustendauer bei allgemeiner und bei homöopathischer Behandlung. *Hippokrates*. 12: 545–548.

Schmit J. (1831). Auszug eines Schreibens des Herrn Hofrath Sam. Hahnemann in Köthen vom 14. März, an den Herausgeber, betreffend Mittheilungen über die im Jahre 1828 von Dr. Marenzeller zu Wien angestellten homöopathischen Heilversuche. *Archiv für die homöopathische Heilkunst*. 10(2): 73–85.

Seidlitz C.v. (1833). Ueber die auf Allerhöchste Befehl im St. Petersburger Militärhospitale angestellten homöopathischen Heilversuche. *Wissenschaftliche Annalen der gesammten Heilkunde*. 27(3): 257–333.

Seidlitz C.v. (1834). Homöopathische Versuche. *Wissenschaftliche Annalen der gesammten Heilkunde*. 29(2): 161–179.

Simon L., Curie P. (1835). Renseignement sur la présence de MM. Léon Simon et Curie a l'hôtel-Dieu, dans le service de M. Le Docteur Bally. *Archive de la Médicine Homoeopathique*. 3: 31–39.

Sirus-Pirondi (1859). *Relation historique et médicale de l'épidémie cholérique qui a régné à Marseille en 1854*. Marseille.

Stern L. (1845). Entstehung, Dauer und Auflösung eines homöopathischen Spitals in Miskolz, nebst den Leistungen daselbst. *Allgemeine Homöopathische Zeitung*. 29(7): 97–108.

Tessier J.-P. (1850). *Recherches cliniques sur le traitement de la pneumonie et du choléra suivant la méthode de Hahnemann, précédées d'une introduction sur l'abus de la statistique en médecine*. Paris, Baillière.

Tessier J.-P. (1852). *De la médication homoeopathique*. Paris, Baillière.

Trousseau A., Gouraud H. (1834). Expériences homéopathiques tentées à l'Hôtel-Dieu de Paris. *Journal des Connaissances Médico-Chirurgicales*. 8(April): 238–241.

Wesselhoeft Sr C. (1877). A reproving of Carbo vegetabilis. Made for the purpose of demonstrating the necessity of countertests in drug-proving. In: *Transactions of the Thirtieth Session of the American Institute of Homoeopathy*. Philadelphia, Shermann: 184–280.

Wesselhoeft Jr C. (1917). Homoeopathy in the prophylaxis and treatment of scarlet fever. New England Medical Gazette. 52 (9): 461–475.

Wesselhoeft Jr C. (1924). The scope and limitations of homeopathy in the treatment of the common contagious diseases. Journal of the American Institute of Homeopathy. 16: 488–501.

Wesselhoeft Jr C. (1925). The sphere of homeopathic treatment in diphtheria. *Journal of the American Institute of Homeopathy*. 18: 103–131.

West C. (1854). *Lectures on the Diseases of Infancy and Childhood*. 3rd edn. London, Longman, Brown, Green, and Longmans.

Trial reports 1941–98 (Part III)

Excluded

Baillargeon L., Drouin J., Desjardins L., Leroux D., Audet D. (1993). Les effets de l'Arnica Montana sur la coagulation sanguine. *Le Médecin de Famille Canadien*. 39: 2362–2367.

Balachandran V.A. (1977). Effect of treatment with Hyoscyamus and Stramonium in potencies on schizophrenia. *Hahnemannian Gleanings*. 6: 42–45.

Barrois D. (1988). Entraînement du sportif en homéopathie. *Homéopathie française*. 76: 315–318.

Barros Camargo L.A., Bechara Ventriglia C.R. (1988a). Estudo piloto comparativo dos efeitos Placebo e medição homeopática, sobre os níveis pressóricos de pacientes hipertensos. *Revista homeopatica*. 53 (4): 132–134.

Barros Camargo L.A., Bechara Ventriglia C.R. (1988b). Estudo comparativo dos efeitos Placebo x medicamento homeopática, na totalidade sintomática característica, em hipertensos. *Revista homeopatica*. 53 (4): 135–137.

Barry R., Collins M., Machin D., Smith M., Hazleman B., Barry M. (1995). Feasibility study of homoeopathic remedy in rheumatoid arthritis. *British Journal of Rheumatology*. 34 (Suppl. 2): 17.

Bekkering G.M., Bosch W.J.v.d., Hoogen H.J.v.d. (1993). Bedriegt schone schijn? Een onderzoek om de gerapporteerde werking van een homeopathisch middel te objectiveren. *Huisarts en Wetenschap*. 36: 414–415.

Benzécri J.P., Maïti G.D., Belon P., Questel R. (1991). Comparaison entre quatre méthodes de sevrage après une thérapeutique anxiolytique (comp. sevrage). *Les Cahiers de l'Analyse des Données*. 16 (4): 389–402.

Berthier P. (1985). Etude sur 80 cas en patientele privée d'unc prémédication homéopathique pour les extractions et la chirugie buccale. *Proceedings of the 40th LMHI Congress*, Lyons: 79–82.

Bornoroni C. (1997). Trial clinico. Diatesi linfatico-essudativa in trattamento con Timosina a dosi omeopatiche. *TMA*. 11 (June): 3–9.

Brewitt B., Standish L.J. (1996). Positive outcomes in treating human immuno-deficiency viral (HIV) disease with high dilution growth factors (abstract). *Alternative Therapies in Health and Medicine*. 2 (4): 90.

Bruseth S., Tveiten D. (1992). Effekt av Arnica D30 ved hard fysisk anstrengelse. [Del II] En dobbeltblind randomisert undersøkelse under Oslo Maraton 1991. *Dynamis*. 2: 17.

Campbell A. (1976). Two pilot controlled trials of Arnica montana. *British Homoeopathic Journal*. 65: 154–158.

Carne K. (1996). A clinical trial of homoeopathy and autism. *British Homoeopathic Research Group Communications*. 24: 14–17.

Chapman E.H., Angelica J., Spitalny G., Strauss M. (1994). Results of a study of the homeopathic treatment of PMS. *Journal of the American Institute of Homeopathy*. 87 (1): 14–21.

da Silva P.V. (1986). Prova terapéutica com Haldol dinamizado em pacientes psiquiátricos internados — método triplo cego. *Revista homeopatica*. 170: 18–28.

Damien P. (1986). *Cobaltum metallicum: essai clinique de chélation du cobalt radioactif en centrale nucléaire* (Thesis), Université de Lille.

Danner D. (1998). Homeopathic treatment of premenstrual syndrome (abstract). *Alternative Therapies in Health and Medicine*. 4 (2): 92.

Davies A.E. (1988). A pilot study to measure Aluminium levels in hair samples of patients with dementia and the influence of Aluminium 30c compared with placebo. *Communications of the British Homoeopathic Research Group*. 18: 42–46.

Delaunay M. (1985). Homéopathie à la maternelle. *Médecines Douces* (September): 35–37.

Dorfman P., Tetau M. (1985). Homéopathie et pathologie du sportif. Deux exemples de double aveugle: marathon de New York et haltérophilie. *Cahiers de Biothérapie*. 86 (June, Suppl.): 77–89.

English J.M. (1986). Pertussin 30c: preventive for whooping cough? *British Homoeopathic Research Group Communications*. 16: 3–13.

Estragnin J. (1979). *Essai d'approche expérimentale de la thérapeutique homéopathique* (Thesis), Université de Grenoble.

Garrett B., Harrison P.V., Stewart T., Porter I. (1997). A trial of homoeopathic treatment of leg ulcers. *Journal of Dermatological Treatment*. 8: 115–117.

Gaucher C., Jeulin D., Peycru P., Pla A., Amengual C. (1993). Cholera and homoeopathic medicine: the Peruvian experience. *British Homoeopathic Journal*. 82: 155–163.

Geiger G. (1968). Klinische Erfahrungen mit Traumeel bei Weichteilkontusionen und Frakturen und mit Vertigoheel bei der Commotio cerebri acuta. *Medizinische Welt* (18, 4 May): 1203–1204.

Gerhard I., Keller C., Schmück M. (1993). Wirksamkeit homöopathischer Einzel- und Komplexmittel bei Frauen mit unerfülltem Kinderwunsch. *Erfahrungsheilkunde*. 42 (3): 132–137.

Grau W. (1992). Eine sinnvolle Alternative für die Behandlung von Magen-Darm-Beschwerden mit einem homöopathischen Kombinationspräparat. *Biologische Medizin*. 21 (3): 233–234.

Greenfield S. (1996). The Cantharis trial. *British Homoeopathic Research Group Communications*. 24: 30–32.

Guillemain J., Jessenne M.G., Pariente J., Renauld D., Alleaume B., Tetau M. (1983). Homéopathie: tentative d'essai clinique en double aveugle dans une épreuve sportive: le rallye Paris-Dakar 1983. *Cahiers de Biothérapie* (78, June): 35–40.

Hardy J. (1984). A double-blind, placebo controlled trial of house dust potencies in the treatment of house dust allergy. *Communications of the British Homoeopathic Research Group*. 11: 75–76.

Heidl R., Kastner H.-G., Lämmlein M.M. (1992). Organserum Lunge bei chronisch obstruktiven Lungenerkrankungen: Ergebnisse einer randomisierten, multizentrischen Doppelblindstudie. *Erfahrungsheilkunde*. 41 (5): 362–366.

Hess F.O. (1942). Nütz uns die Homöopathie bei der Diphtherie-Behandlung? *Münchener Medizinische Wochenschrift* (13, 27 March): 296.

Hildebrandt G., Eltze C. (1983a). Über die Wirksamkeit einer Behandlung des Muskelkaters mit Rhus toxicodendron D4. Ein Beitrag zur Pharmakologie adaptiver Prozesse. *Erfahrungsheilkunde*. 32 (6): 358–364.

Hildebrandt G., Eltze C. (1983b). Über die Wirksamkeit verschiedener Dosen und Potenzen (Verdünnungen) von Rhus toxicodendron beim experimentell ausgelösten Muskelkater. Ein Beitrag zur Pharmakologie adaptiver Prozesse (II Mitteilung). *Erfahrungsheilkunde*. 32 (11): 743–750.

Hildebrandt G., Eltze C. (1984). Über die Wirksamkeit verschiedener Potenzen (Verdünnungen) von Arnica beim experimentell erzeugten Muskelkater. Ein Beitrag zur Pharmakologie adaptiver Prozesse (III Mitteilung). *Erfahrungsheilkunde*. 33 (7): 430–435.

Hill N., Haselen R.v. (1993). Clinical trial of a homoeopathic insect after-bite treatment. *Homeopathy International R&D Newsletter* (3 April).

Jäckel W.H., Schirmer P. (1996). Wirksamkeit von Formica rufa und Eigenblut bei Patienten mit Spondylitis ankylosans (Morbus Bechterew). In: H. Albrecht, M. Frühwald, eds *Jahrbuch Band 2 (1995) Karl und Veronica Carstens-Stiftung*. Stuttgart, Hippokrates Verlag: 48–53.

Jansen G.R.H.L., Veer A.L.J.v.d., Hagenaars J., Kuy A.v.d. (1992). Lessons learnt from an unsuccessful clinical trial of homoeopathy: results of a small-scale, double-blind trial in proctocolitis. *British Homoeopathic Journal*. 81 (3): 132–138.

Jawara N., Lewith G.T., Vickers A.J., Mullee M.A., Smith C. (1997). Homoeopathic Arnica and Rhus toxicodendron for delayed onset muscle soreness: a pilot for a ranomized, double-blind, placebo-controlled trial. *British Homoeopathic Journal*. 86: 10–15.

Kayne S., Beattie N. (1996). Preliminary results from an investigation of three different isopathic dose regimes used in the treatment of allergy. *British Homoeopathic Research Group Communications*. 24: 26–29.

Kienle G. (1973). Wirkung von Carbo Betulae D6 bei respiratorischer Partialinsuffizienz. *Arzneimittel Forschung/Drug Research*. 23 (6): 840–842.

Kirchhoff E., Niehaus V., Schnitzlein U., Schulte H. (1989). Therapieerfolg bei degenerativen Gelenk- und Wirbelsäulenleiden: Dokumentation über eine kontrollierte Praxisstudie. *Natura Med.* 4 (9): 506–516.

Kubista E., Müller G., Spona J. (1986). Behandlung der Mastopathie mit zyklischer Mastodynie: Klinische Ergebnisse und Hormonprofile. *Gynäkologische Rundschau*. 26: 65–79.

Kurz C., Nagele F., Zorzi M., Karras H., Enzelsberger H. (1993). Bewirkt Homöopathie eine Verbesserung der Reizblasensymptomatik? *Gynäkologische Geburtshilfliche Rundschau*. 33 (Suppl. 1): 330–331.

Lara-Marquez M.L., Pocino M., Rodriguez F., Carvallo G.E., Ortega C.F., Rodriguez C. (1997). Homeopathic treatment for atopic asthma lung function and immunological outcomes in a randomized clinical trial in Venezuela [abstract]. *Proceedings of the 52nd LMHI Congress*, Seattle: 73.

Lewith G., Brown P.K., Tyrell D.A.J. (1989). Controlled study of the effects of a homoeopathic dilution of influenza vaccine on antibody titres in man. *Complementary Medical Research*. 3 (3): 22–24.

Manchanda R.K., Mehan N., Bahl R., Atey R. (1997). Double blind placebo controlled clinical trials of homoeopathic medicines in warts and molluscum contagiosum. *CCRH Quarterly Bulletin*. 19 (3/4): 25–29.

Mastromattei F. (1995). Mamme sprint con l'omeopatica. *Medicina Naturale* (3, May): 62–64.

Matusiewicz R. (1997). The homeopathic treatment of corticosteroid-dependent asthma. A double-blind, placebo-controlled study. *Biomedical Therapy*. 15 (4): 117–122.

Melchart D., Linde K., Worku F., Sarkady L., Holzmann M., Jurcic K., Wagner H. (1995). Results of five randomized studies on the immunomodulatory activity of preparations of Echinacea. *Journal of Alternative & Complementary Medicine*. 1 (2): 145–60.

Mergen H. (1969). Therapie postträumatischer Schwellungen mit Traumeel. Beitrag zur Relation 'Dosis : Wirkung' eines Kombinationspräparates. *Münchener Medizinische Wochenschrift*. 111: 298–300.

Mitchell G.R. (1975). *Homoeopathy*. London, WH Allen.

Mohan G.R., Jayalakshmi C., Devi A.L.M. (1996). Cervical spondylosis – a clinical study. *British Homoeopathic Journal*. 85: 131–133.

Mössinger P. (1984). *Homöopathie und naturwissenschaftliche Medizin: zur Überwindung d. Gegensätze*. Stuttgart, Hippokrates-Verlag.

Padamprakash B. (1979). The efficacy of Tuberculinum bovinum in urinary tract infections. *Proceedings of the 34th LMHI Congress*, Hamburg: 1–6.

Pallasser H. (1994). Die Beeinflussbarkeit des Icterus neonatorum durch Phosphorus C30. *Documenta Homoeopatica*. 14: 299–303.

Paterson J., Boyd W.E. (1941). A preliminary study of the alteration of the Schick test by a homoeopathic potency. *British Homoeopathic Journal*. 31: 301–9.

Reitzner T.B. (1987). *Explorative Studie über die Wirksamkeit von Arnica in den homöopathischen Dezimalpotenzen D2, D3, D4, D5, D6 und D8 beim experimentell ausgelösten Muskelkater* (Thesis). Marburg, Philipps-Universität.

Rost A. (1986). *Wirkungsnachweis homöopathischer Arzneien durch thermographische Messungen*. Karlsruhe, Deutsche Homöopathie-Union.

Ruff F. (1992). Homeopathische repliek op de stuifmeeltijd. *Arts en Alternatief*. 6: 9–10.

Schmidt C. (1996). A double-blind, placebo-controlled trial: Arnica montana applied topically to subcutaneous mechanical injuries. *Journal of the American Institute of Homeopathy*. 89 (4): 186–193.

Schreier T., Hartmann M., Petzoldt D., B. M., Roebruck P., Runnebaum B., Gerhard I. (1997). Homöopathie versus konventionelle Therapie bei männlicher Unfruchtbarkeit — Zwischenbericht einer randomisierten Studie. *Forschende Komplementärmedizin*. 4: 325–331.

Skaliodas S., Kivelou P., Kiriakopou E., Diamantidis S. (1988). Using tissue salts as a support of the similimum effect. *Proceedings of the 43rd LMHI Congress*, Athens: 572–575.

Sudan B.J.L. (1993). Abrogation of facial seborrhoeic dermatitis with homoeopathic high dilutions of tobacco: a new visible model for Benveniste's theory of 'memory of water'. *Medical Hypotheses*. 41: 440–444.

Sudan B.J.L. (1997). Total abrogation of facial seborrhoeic dermatitis with extremely low-frequency (1–1.1 Hz) 'imprinted water' is not allergen or hapten dependent: a new visible model for homoeopathy. *Medical Hypotheses*. 48: 477–479.

Tveiten D., Bruset S., Borchgrevink C.F., Norseth J. (1998). Effects of the homoeopathic remedy Arnica D30 on marathon runners: a randomized, double-blind study during the 1995 Oslo Marathon. *Complementary Therapies in Medicine*. 6: 71–74.

Tveiten D., Bruseth S., Borchgrevink C.F., Løhne K. (1991). Effekt av Arnica D30 ved hard fysisk anstrengelse: en dobbeltblind randomisert undersøkelse under Oslo Maraton 1990. *Tidsskrift Norske Lægeforen*. 111 (30): 3630–3631.

Vickers A.J., Fisher P., Smith C., Wyllie S.E., Lewith G.T. (1997). Homoeopathy for delayed onset muscle soreness: a randomised double blind placebo controlled trial. *British Journal of Sports Medicine*. 31: 304–307.

Vickers A.J., Fisher P., Smith C., Wyllie S.E., Rees R. (1998). Homoeopathic Arnica 30x is ineffective for muscle soreness after long-distance running: a randomized, double-blind, placebo-controlled trial. *Clinical Journal of Pain*. 14: 227–231.

Vu Dinh S., Delaunay M. (1983). Médicine douce et sport dur: un mariage heureux. *Homéopathie française*. 71: 147–149.

Wiesenauer M., Gaus W. (1986). Wirkamkeitsvergleich verschniedener Potenzierungen des homöopathischen Arzneimittels Galphimia glauca beim Heuschnupfen-Syndrom: eine multizentrische, kontrollierte, randomisierte Doppelblindstudie. *Deutsche Apotheker Zeitung*. 126 (40): 37–43.

Wolf J. (1992). Schlafstörungen ohne Hang-over behandeln: Ergebnisse einer klinischen Studie mit einem pflanzlich-homöopathischen Mittel. *Natura-Medizin*. 7 (9): 586–9.

Included

Abelson M.B., George M.A., Garofalo C., Weintraub D. (1996). An effective treatment for allergy sufferers. *Biological Therapy*. 14 (1): 161–164.

Albertini H., Goldberg W., Sanguy B.B., Toulza C. (1985). Homeopathic treatment of dental neuralgia using arnica and hypericum: a summary of 60 observations. *Journal of the American Institute of Homeopathy*. 78 (3): 126–128.

Alibeu J.P., Jobert J. (1990). Aconit en dilution homéopathique et agitation post-opératoire de l'enfant. *Pédiatrie-Bucur*. 45: 465–466.

Amodeo C., Musso R., Missiato A., Caglià P., Veroux P.F., Ricciotti F. (1987). Il ruolo dell'arnica nella prevenzione della patologia venosa da terapia infusionale protratta. Valutazione della aggregabilità piastrinica. *9 Congresso Nazionale della Società Italiana di Patologia Vascolare*, Copanetto: 1533–1543.

Andrade L.E., Ferraz M.B., Atra E., Castro A., Silva M.S. (1991). A randomized controlled trial to evaluate the effectiveness of homeopathy in rheumatoid arthritis. *Scandinavian Journal of Rheumatology*. 20 (3): 204–208.

Anonymous (1980). The Cantharis study. *Midlands Homoeopathic Research Group Newsletter*. 3: 19–20.

Atmadjian A., Jeanvoine C., Hariveau E. (1988). Analyse de l'étude d'Arnica dans l'accouchement. *Les Dossiers de l'Obstetrique*. 149: 17–18.

Attena F., Toscano G., Agozzino E., Del Giudice N. (1995). A randomized trial in the prevention of influenza-like syndromes by homoeopathic management. *Revue Epidémiologique et Santé Publique*. 43: 380–382.

Aulagnier G. (1985). Action d'un traitement homéopathique sur la reprise du transit post opératoire. *Homéopathie*. 2 (6): 42–5.

Awdry R. (1996). Homoeopathy and chronic fatigue: the search for proof. *International Journal of Alternative and Complementary Medicine*. 14 (2): 12–16.

Bakshi J.P. (1990). Homoeopathy: a new approach to detoxification. *Proceedings of the National Congress on Homeopathy & Drug Abuse and Current Medical Update*, New Delhi: 20–28.

Basu T.K. (1980). Studies on the role of Physostigma venenosum in the improvement of simple myopia. *Hahnemannian Gleanings*. 47 (6): 224–231.

Basu T.K. (1981). A clinical study of Physostigma venenosum in the improvement of progressive myopia. *Hahnemannian Gleanings*. 48 (4): 161–169.

Beer A.-M., Sturm R., Küpper F. (1995). Der Einsatz eines homöopathischen Komplexmittels beim klimakterischen Syndrom im Vergleich zur Hormonsubstitution. *Erfahrungsheilkunde*. 44 (5): 336–40.

Bendre V.V., Dharmadhikari S.D. (1980). Arnica montana and Hypericum in dental practice. *Hahnemannian Gleanings*. 47 (2): 70–72.

Bignamini M., Bertoli A., Consolandi A.M., Dovera N., Saruggia M., Taino S., Tubertini A. (1987). Controlled double-blind trial with Baryta carbonica 15CH versus placebo in a group of hypertensive subjects confined to bed in two old people's homes. *British Homoeopathic Journal*. 76 (3): 114–119.

Bignamini M., Saruggia M., Sansonetti G. (1991). Homeopathic treatment of anal fissures using nitricum acidum. *Berlin Journal of Research on Homoeopathy*. 1 (4/5): 286–287.

Böhmer D., Ambrus P. (1992). Treatment of sports injuries with Traumeel ointment: a controlled double-blind study. *Biological Therapy*. 10 (4): 290–300.

Bordes L.R., Dorfman P. (1986). Evaluation de l'activité antitussive du sirop Drosetux: étude en double aveugle versus placebo. *Les Cahiers d'Otorhinolaryngologie*. 21 (9): 731–734.

Bordes L.R., Soudant J., Dorfman P. (1988). Drosetux, un médicament homéopathique à l'épreuve du double insu. *Médecine & Enfance*. 8 (7): Suppl.

Bouchez D. (1988). *De l'évaluation de l'activité thérapeutique de l'homéopathie. A propos d'un essai thérapeutique d'une dilution homéopathique d'Arnica dans l'oedème post-traumatique du nouveau-né* (Thesis), Université Scientifique et Médicale de Grenoble.

Boucinhas J.C., de Medeiros Boucinhas I.D. (1990). Prophylaxie des crises d'asthme bronchique chez l'enfant par l'usage de Poumon histamine 5 CH. *Homéopathie française*. 78: 35–39.

Bourgois J.C. (1984). *Protection du capital veineux chez les perfusées au long cours dans le cancer du sein. Essai clinique en double aveugle: Arnica contre placebo* (Thesis), Université Paris Nord.

Brigo B., Serpelloni G. (1991). Homeopathic treatment of migraines: a randomized double-blind controlled study of sixty cases (homeopathic remedy versus placebo). *Berlin Journal of Research in Homoeopathy*. 1 (2): 98–106.

British Homoeopathic Society (1943). Report on mustard gas experiments (Glasgow and London): British Homoeopathic Society/Ministry of Home Security Report. *British Homoeopathic Journal*. 33 (Suppl.): 1–12.

Bungetzianu G. (1988). The results obtained by the homeopathical dilution (15CH) of antiinfluenzal (anti-flu) vaccine [abstract]. *Proceedings of the 43rd LMHI Congress*, Athens: 143.

Carey H. (1986). Double blind clinical trial of Borax and Candida in the treatment of vaginal discharge. *Communications of the British Homoeopathic Research Group*. 15: 12–14.

Carlini E.A., Braz S., Troncone L.R., Tufik S., Romanach A.K., Pustiglione M., Sposati M.C., Cudizio F.O., Prado M.I. (1987). Efeito hipnótico de medicação homeopática e do placebo. Avaliação pela técnica de 'duplo-cego' c 'cruzamento'. *Revista da Associação Medica Brasileira*. 33 (5/6): 83–88.

Casanova P., Gerard R. (1992). Bilan de 3 années d'études randomisées multicentriques oscillococcinum/placebo. In: P. Casanova, R. Gerard, eds *Oscillococcinum – Rassegna della Letteratura Internazionale*. Milan, Boiron: 13–16.

Casanova P.A. (1981). *Essai clinique d'un produit appelé 'Urarthone'*. Metz, Laboratoires Lehning.

Casanova P.A. (1984). Homéopathie, syndrome grippal et double insu. *Tonus*. 814 (21): 8.

Casper J., Foerstel G. (1967). Traumeel® bei traumatischen Weichteilschwellungen. *Therapiewoche*. 26: 892–895.

Castelain T. (1979). *Etude de l'action homéopathique de Raphanus sativus niger 5CH et d'Opium 15CH sur la reprise du transit en chirurgie digestive postopératoire* (Thesis), Université de Bordeaux II.

Castro D., Nogueira G.G. (1975). Use of the nosode Meningococcinum as a preventive against meningitis. *Journal of the American Institute of Homeopathy*. 74: 211–219.

Chakravarty B.N., Sen J.P., Mitra S.K., Pal D. (1977). The effect of homeopathy drugs in tonsillitis. *Proceedings of the 32nd LMHI Congress (Suppl.)*, New Delhi: 41–48.

Chapman E., Woo E., Weintraub R., Milburn M., O'Neil Pirozzi T., Lee R. (1997). The homeopathic treatment of mild traumatic brain injury [abstract]. *Proceedings of the 52nd LMHI Congress*, Seattle: 66.

Chevrel J.P., Saglier J., Destable M.D. (1984). Reprise du transit intestinal en chirurgie digestive. Action homéopathique de l'opium. *Presse Medicale*. 13 (14): 883.

Chirila P. (1990). Estudio clinico de los efectos del phosphorus triiodatus 7cH en hepatitis. *Proceedings of the OMHI International Congress*, Mexico: 209–211.

Davies A.E. (1971). Clinical investigations into the action of potencies. *British Homoeopathic Journal*. 60: 36–41.

de Lange-de Klerk E. (1993). *Effects of homeopathic medicines on children with recurrent upper respiratory tract infections* (Thesis), Vrije Universiteit te Amsterdam.

Deguillaume M. (1981). *Etude expérimentale de l'action du Caulophyllum dans le faux travail et la dystocie de démarrage* (Thesis), Université de Limoges.

Demonceaux A. (1990). Le rhume de cerveau. *Médecines Nouvelles*. 1 (1): 64–67.

Dexpert M. (1987). Prévention des naupathies par Cocculine®. *Homéopathie française*. 75: 353–355.

Diefenbach M., Schilken J., Steiner G., Becker H.J. (1997). Homöopathische Therapie bei Erkrankungen der Atemwege. Auswertung einer klinischen Studie bei 258 Patienten. *Zeitschrift für Allgemeine Medizin*. 73: 308–314.

Dorfman P., Amodéo C., Ricciotti F., Tétau M., Véroux G. (1992). Iléus post-opératoire et homéopathie: bilan d'une évaluation clinique. *Cahiers de Biothérapie*. 114: 33–36.

Eid P., Felisi E., Sideri M. (1993). Applicability of homoeopathic Caulophyllum thalictroides during labour. *British Homoeopathic Journal*. 82: 245–248.

Eid P., Felisi E., Sideri M. (1994). Super-placébo ou action pharmacologique? Une étude en double aveugle randomisé avec un remède homéopathique Caulophyllum thalicroides dans le travail. *Proceedings of the OMHI International Congress*, location unknown.

Ernst E., Saradeth T., Resch K.L. (1990). Complementary treatment of varicose veins: a randomized, placebo-controlled, double-blind trial. *Phlebology*. 5 (3): 157–163.

Felisi E., Saruggia M., Russo G., Balzarini A. (1994). Lésions cutanées précoces relevées au cours de radiothérapie misant au traitement du cancer du sein: l'efficacité d'une thérapie homéopathique. *Proceedings of the OMHI International Congress*, location unknown.

Ferley J.P., Poutignat N., Azzopardi Y., Charrel M., Zmirou D. (1987). Evaluation en médecine ambulatoire de l'activité d'un complexe homéopathique dans la prévention de la grippe et des syndromes grippaux. *Immunologie Médicale*. 20: 22–28.

Ferley J.P., Zmirou D., D'Adhemar D., Balducci F. (1989). A controlled evaluation of a homoeopathic preparation in the treatment of influenza-like syndromes. *British Journal of Clinical Pharmacology*. 27 (3): 329–335.

Fisher P. (1986). An experimental double-blind clinical trial method in homoeopathy: use of a limited range of remedies to treat fibrositis. *British Homoeopathic Journal*. 75 (3): 142–147.

Fisher P., Greenwood A., Huskisson E.C., Turner P., Belon P. (1989). Effect of homeopathic treatment on fibrositis (primary fibromyalgia). *British Medical Journal*. 299 (6695): 365–366.

Freitas L.A.S., Goldenstein E., Sanna O.M. (1995). A relação médico–paciente indireta e o tratamento homeopático na asma infantil. *Revista de Homeopatía*. 60 (2): 26–31.

Friese K.H., Feuchter U., Moeller H. (1997). Die homöopathische Behandlung von adenoiden Vegetationen. Ergebnisse einer prospektiven, randomisierten Doppelblindstudie. *HNO*. 45: 618–624.

Friese K.H., Kruse S., Lüdtke R., Moeller H. (1997). The homoeopathic treatment of otitis media in children — comparisons with conventional therapy. *International Journal of Clinical Pharmacological Therapy*. 35 (7): 296–301.

Gassinger C.A., Wünstel G., Netter P. (1981). Klinische Prüfung zum Nachweis der therapeutischen Wirksamkeit des homöopathischen Arzneimittels Eupatorium perfoliatum D2 (Wasserhanf composite) bei der Diagnose 'Grippaler Infekt'. *Arzneimittel Forschung/Drug Research*. 31 (I): 732–736.

Gaucher C., Jeulin D., Peycru P., Amengual C. (1994). A double blind randomised placebo controlled study of cholera treatment with highly diluted and succussed solutions. *British Homoeopathic Journal*. 83 (3): 132–134.

Gauthier J.E. (1983). *Essai thérapeutique comparatif de l'action de la clonidine et du Lachesis mutus dans le traitement des bouffées de chaleur de la ménopause* (Thesis), Université de Bordeaux II.

Gerhard I., Reimers G., Keller C., Schmück M. (1993). Vergleich homöopathischer Einzelmittel – mit konventioneller Hormontherapie. *therapeutikon*. 7 (7/8): 309–315.

Gibson J., Haslam Y., Laurenson L., Newman P., Pitt R., Robins M., Pitt E.M. (1991). Double blind trial of Arnica in acute trauma patients. *Homoeopathy*. 41 (3): 54–55.

Gibson R.G., Gibson S.L., MacNeill A.D., Buchanan W.W. (1980). Homoeopathic therapy in rheumatoid arthritis: evaluation by double-blind clinical therapeutic trial. *British Journal of Clinical Pharmacology*. 9: 453–459.

Gibson R.G., Gibson S.L., MacNeill A.D., Gray G.H., Dick W.C., Buchanan W.W. (1978). Salicylates and homoeopathy in rheumatoid arthritis: preliminary observations. *British Journal of Clinical Pharmacology*. 6: 391–395.

Gillespie N.B. (1994). *Hypercholesterolaemia and homoeopathy* (Thesis). Durban, Technikon Natal.

GRECHO, U292 Inserm, ARC, GREPA (1989). Evaluation de deux produits homéopathiques sur la reprise du transit après chirurgie digestive. Un essai contrôlé multicentrique. *La Presse Médicale*. 18 (2): 59–62.

Hadjikostas C., Diamantidis S. (1990a). *Comparative clinical study of parallel allopathic and homoeopathic treatment to allopathic treatment in cancer of the large intestine*. Athens, Researches of MIHRA.

Hadjikostas C., Diamantidis S. (1990b). *Comparative clinical study of parallel homoeopathic and allopathic treatment to allopathic treatment in cancer of the lung*. Athens, Researches of MIHRA.

Hadjikostas C., Paizis A., Drossou P., Papaconstantinou G., Diamantidis S. (1988). Comparative clinical study of homoeopathic and allopathic treatment of haemorrhage of the upper digestive tract. *Proceedings of the 43rd LMHI Congress*, Athens: 536–541.

Hariveau E. (1992). Comparaison de Cocculine® au placebo et à un produit de référence dans le traitement de la naupathie. *Homéopathie française*. 8 (2): 17–20.

Hariveau E., Nolen P., Holtzscherer A. (1991). A study of the effectiveness of ultra low doses of copper in the treatment of hemodialysis-related muscle cramps. In: C. Doutremepuich, ed. *Ultra Low Doses*. London, Taylor & Francis: 145–149.

Hart O., Mullee M.A., Lewith G., Miller J. (1997). Double-blind, placebo-controlled, randomized clinical trial of homoeopathic arnica C30 for pain and infection after total abdominal hysterectomy. *Journal of the Royal Society of Medicine*. 90: 73–78.

Heilmann A. (1994). A combination injection preparation as a prophylactic for flu and common colds. *Biological Therapy*. 12 (4): 249–253.

Heulluy B. (1985). *Essai randomisé ouvert de L.72 (specialité homéopathique) contre diazepam 2 dans les états anxio-depressifs*. Metz, Laboratoires Lehning.

Hill N., Stam C., Haselen R.A.v. (1996). The efficacy of Prrrikweg® gel in the treatment of insect bites: a double-blind, placebo-controlled clinical trial. *Pharmacy World & Science*. 18 (1): 35–41.

Hill N., Stam C., Tuinder S., Haselen R.A.v. (1995). A placebo-controlled clinical trial investigating the efficacy of a homoeopathic after-bite gel in reducing mosquito bite induced erythema. *European Journal of Clinical Pharmacology*. 49: 103–108.

Hitzenberger G., Korn A., Dorsci M., Bauer P., Wohlzogen F.X. (1982). Kontrollierte randomisierte doppelblinde Studie zum Vergleich einer Behandlung von Patienten mit essentieller Hypertonie mit homöopathischen und pharmakologisch wirksamen Medikamenten. *Wiener Klinische Wochenzeitschrift*. 94: 665–670.

Hochstetter K. (1966). Mercurius solubilis: a report on its action in gingivitis gravidica. *British Homoeopathic Journal*. 55: 84–85.

Hofmeyr G.J., Piccioni V., Blauhof P. (1990). Postpartum homoeopathic Arnica montana: a potency-finding pilot study. *British Journal of Clinical Practice*. 44 (12): 619–621.

Hourst P. (1981). *Tentative d'appréciation de l'efficacité de l'homéopathie* (Thesis). Paris, Université Pierre et Marie Curie.

Hunin M., Tisserand G., Dorfman P., Tétau M. (1991). Intérêt de la thymuline dans le traitement préventif des pathologies ORL récidivantes de l'enfant. *Schweize Zeitschrift für GanzheitsMedizin*. 6: 298–304.

Jacobs J., Jiménez L.M., Gloyd S.S., Carares F.E., Gaitan M.P., Crothers D. (1993). Homoeopathic treatment of acute childhood diarrhea: a randomized clinical trial in Nicaragua. *British Homoeopathic Journal*. 82 (2): 83–86.

Jacobs J., Jiménez L.M., Gloyd S.S., Gale J.L., Crothers D. (1994). Treatment of acute childhood diarrhea with homeopathic medicine: a randomized clinical trial in Nicaragua. *Pediatrics*. 93 (5): 719–725.

Jacobs J., Malthouse S., Chapman E., Jiménez L.M., Crothers D. (1997). Childhood diarrhea: results from Nepal and combined analysis [abstract]. *Proceedings of the 52nd LMHI Congress*, Seattle: 81–83.

Jenaer M.C., Marichal B.J., Doppagne A. (1990). Preliminary clinical study concerning the efficacy of an immunotherapeutic treatment in the AIDS-Syndrome. *Proceedings of the 45th LMHI Congress*, Barcelona: 207–217.

Joseph J.D. (1994). *Homoeopathy in hypercholesterolaemia* (Thesis). Durban, Technikon Natal.

Kainz J.T., Kozel G., Haidvogl M., Smolle J. (1996). Homoeopathic versus placebo therapy of children with warts on their hands: a randomized, double-blind clinical trial. *Dermatology*. 193: 318–320.

Kaziro G.S.N. (1984). Metronidazole (flagyl) and Arnica montana in the prevention of post-surgical complications: a comparative placebo controlled clinical trial. *British Journal of Oral and Maxillofacial Surgery*. 22: 42–49.

Kennedy C.O. (1971). A controlled trial. *British Homoeopathic Journal*. 60: 120–127.

Khan M.T. (1985). Clinical trials for the hallux valgus with the marigold preparations. *Proceedings of the 40th LMHI Congress*, Lyons: 232–235.

Khan M.T. (1986). Report on the clinical trials for Tagetes erecta sp. (Marigold) in the treatment of hallux valgus (bunions). *Journal of the British Association of Homoeopathic Chiropodists*. 2 (2): 4–23.

Khan M.T. (1996). The podiatric treatment of hallux abducto valgus and its associated condition, bunion, with Tagetes patula. *Journal of Pharmaceutical Pharmacology*. 48: 768–770.

Khan M.T., Potter M., Birch I. (1996). Podiatric treatment of hyperkeratotic plantar lesions with Marigold Tagetes erecta. *Phytotherapy Research*. 10: 211–214.

Khan M.T., Rawal R.S. (1976). Comparative treatments of verruca plantaris. *Proceedings of the 31st LMHI Congress*, Athens: 265–269.

Kirchhoff H.W. (1982). Ein Beitrag zur Behandlung des Lymphödems. *Der Praktische Arzt*. 21 (6): 621–633.

Kirtland K.A. (1994). *The efficacy of Folliculinum in the treatment of premenstrual tension* (Thesis). Durban, Technikon Natal.

Kivelou P., Diamantidis S. (1990). *Comparative clinical study of parallel homoeopathic and allopathic treatment to allopathic treatment in breast cancer*. Athens, Researches of MIHRA.

Kulkarni A., Nagarkar B.M., Burde G.S. (1988). Radiation protection by use of homoeopathic medicines. *Hahnemann Homoeopathic Sandesh*. 12 (1): 20–23.

Kumar A., Mishra N. (1994). Effect of homoeopathic treatment on filariasis. *British Homoeopathic Journal*. 83: 216–219.

Kumta P.S. (1977). Effectiveness of homoeopathic medicines in epidemic acute viral conjunctivitis, 1975 (acute haemorrhagic conjunctivitis). *Hahnemannian Gleanings*. 44 (6): 272–276.

Kuzeff R.M. (1998). Homeopathy, sensation of well-being and CD4 levels: a placebo-controlled, randomized trial. *Complementary Therapies in Medicine*. 6: 4–9.

Labrecque M., Audet D., Latulippe L.G., Drouin J. (1992). Homeopathic treatment of plantar warts. *Canadian Medical Association Journal*. 146 (10): 1749–1754.

Lamont J. (1997). Homoeopathic treatment of attention deficit hyperactivity disorder. *British Homoeopathic Journal*. 86: 196–200.

Lasserre M.N. (1986). *Préparation à l'accouchement par homéopathie: expérimentation en double insu versus placebo* (Thesis), Université Paris-Ouest.

Leaman A.M., Gorman D. (1989). Cantharis in the early treatment of minor burns. *Archives of Emergency Medicine*. 6: 259–261.

Lecocq P. (1985). L.52. Les voies thérapeutiques des syndromes grippaux. *Cahiers de Biothérapie*. 87: 65–73.

Ledermann E.K., Sutherland I., Lunt R. (1954). Homoeopathy tested against controls in cases of surgical tuberculosis. *British Homoeopathic Journal*. 44: 83–97.

Lepaisant C. (1995). Essai thérapeutique en homéopathie: traitement des tensions mammaires et mastodynies du syndrome prémenstruel. *Revue Française Gynécologique et Obstétrique*. 90 (2): 94–97.

Lewis D. (1984). Double-blind controlled trial in the treatment of whooping cough using Drosera. *Midlands Homoeopathic Research Group Newsletter*. 11: 49–58.

Lievre M., Marichy J., Baux S., Foyatier J.L., Perrot J., Boissel J.P. (1992). Controlled study of three ointments for the local management of 2nd and 3rd degree burns. *Clinical Trials and Meta Analysis*. 28: 9–12.

Lökken P., Straumsheim P.A., Tveiten D., Skjelbred P., Borchgrevink C.F. (1995). Effect of homoeopathy on pain and other events after acute trauma: placebo controlled trial with bilateral oral surgery. *British Medical Journal*. 310: 1439–1442.

Lüdtke R., Wilkens J. (1998). Arnica 30DH after knee surgery: three randomised double-blind clinical trials. (Presented at the 5th Annual Symposium on Complementary Healthcare, 10–12 December 1998, Exeter) [abstract]. *FACT: Focus on Alternative and Complementary Therapies*. 3 (4): 190.

Macchi C. (1984). L'omeopatia nell'ipertensione arteriosa essenziale del paziente anziano. *Cahiers de Biothérapie*. 81 (April, Suppl.): 83–86.

Maiwald L., Weinfurtner T., Mau J., Connert W.D. (1988). Therapie des grippalen Infekts mit einem homöopathischen Kombinationspräparat im Vergleich zu Acetylsalicylsäure. Kontrollierte, randomisierte Einfachblindstudie. *Arzneimittel Forschung/Drug Research*. 38 (4): 578–582.

Marrey L. (1989). Arnica, remède homoeopathique en stomatologie. *Recueil des interventions du Séminaire de l'EHHDS*, St-Jorioz (Haute-Savoie) les 20 et 21 mai 1989. Grenoble: 163–175.

Martel J.F., Hariveau E. (1985). Etude clinique d'une pâte gingivodentaire homéopathique dans les gingivites. *Le Chirurgien Dentiste de France*. 55 (302): 39–40.

Masciello E., Felisi E. (1985). Dilutions de materiel, à pourcentage élevé de ADN et ARN, dans la prévention des viroses epidémiques. *Proceedings of the 40th LMHI Congress*, Lyons: 271–274.

Master F.J. (1987a). A study of homoeopathic drugs in essential hypertension. *British Homoeopathic Journal*. 76: 120–121.

Master F.J. (1987b). Scope of homeopathic drugs in treatment of Broca's aphasia: a double-blind trial. *Proceedings of the 42nd LMHI Congress*, Arlington: 330–334.

Matusiewicz R. (1997). The effect of a homeopathic preparation on the clinical condition of patients with corticosteroid-dependent bronchial asthma. *Biomedical Therapy*. 15 (3): 70–74.

McCutcheon L.E. (1996). Treatment of anxiety with a homeopathic remedy. *Journal of Applied Nutrition*. 48 (1/2): 2–6.

McDavid G.M. (1994). *The homoeopathic treatment of acne* (Thesis). Durban, Technikon Natal.

Mesquita L.P. (1987). Homoeopathy and physiotherapy, with special reference to osteoarthropathy. *British Homoeopathic Journal*. 76 (1): 16–18.

Michaud J. (1981). *Action d'Apis mellifica et d'Arnica montana dans la prévention des oedèmes post-opératoires en chirurgie maxillo-faciale à propos d'une expérimentation clinique sur 60 observations* (Thesis), Université de Nantes.

Mokkapatti R. (1992). An experimental double-blind study to evaluate the use of Euphrasia in preventing conjunctivitis. *British Homoeopathic Journal*. 81 (1): 22–24.

Mössinger P. (1973). Die Behandlung der Pharyngitis mit Phytolacca. Ergebnis einer Fragebogenaktion der Forschungsgemeinschaft für Homöopathie. *Allgemeine Homöopathische Zeitung*. 218: 111–121.

Mössinger P. (1976a). Misslungene Wirksamkeitsnachweise. *Allgemeine Homöopathische Zeitung*. 221: 26–31.

Mössinger P. (1976b). Untersuchung über die Behandlung der akuten Pharyngitis mit Phytolacca D2. *Allgemeine Homöopathische Zeitung*. 221: 177–183.

Mössinger P. (1980). Zur therapeutischen Wirksamkeit von Hepar sulfuris calcareum D4 bei Pyodermien und Furunkeln. *Allgemeine Homöopathische Zeitung*. 225: 22–27.

Mössinger P. (1982). Untersuchung zur Behandlung des akuten Fliessschnupfens mit Euphorbium D3. *Allgemeine Homöopathische Zeitung*. 227: 89–95.

Mössinger P. (1985). Zur Behandlung der Otitis media mit Pulsatilla. *Der Kinderarzt*. 16: 581–582.

Nahler G., Metelmann H., Sperber H. (1996). Behandlung der Gonarthrose mit Zeel comp. Ergebnisse einer randomisierten, kontrollierten klinischen Prüfung im Vergleich zu Hyaluronsäure. *Orthopädische Praxis*. 32: 354–359.

Nollevaux M.A., Danhier P., Fagard H. (1991). *Klinische studie van Mucococcinum 200K als preventieve behandeling van griepachtige aandoeningen: een dubbelblinde test tegenover placebo*, Altermedica.

Nusche M. (1998). *Homöopathische Behandlung der GABHS-Tonsillitis im Kindesalter*. Stuttgart, Karl und Veronica Carstens-Stiftung und Hippokrates Verlag.

Oberbaum M. (1998). Experimental treatment of chemotherapy-induced stomatitis using a homeopathic complex preparation: a preliminary study. *Biomedical Therapy*. 16 (4): 261–265.

Ochoa-Bernal F., Ruiz-Hernandez A., Searcy Bernal R. (1995). Disminución de la tension arterial elevada con Lachesis muta 200cH. en el servicio de urgencias del Hospital Nacional Homeopático. *Boletin Mexicano de Homeopatía*. 28 (2): 48–53.

Owen D. (1990). An investigation into the homoeopathic treatment of patients with irritable bowel syndrome. *British Homoeopathic Congress*, 1–4 February, Windermere, UK.

Papp R., Schuback G., Beck E., Burkard G., Bengel J., Lehrl S., Belon P. (1998). Oscillococcinum in patients with influenza-like syndromes. *British Homoeopathic Journal*. 87: 69–76.

Pinsent R.J., Baker G.P., Ives G., Davey R.W., Jonas S. (1986). Does Arnica reduce pain and bleeding after dental extraction? *Communications of the British Homoeopathic Research Group*. 15: 3–11.

Polychronopoulou Z., Diamantidis S. (1990). *Comparative clinical study of parallel homoeopathic and allopathic treatment to allopathic treatment in cancer of the pancreas*. Athens, Researches of MIHRA.

Ponti M. (1986). Evaluation d'un traitement homéopathique du mal des transports: Bilan de 93 observations. In: J.B. Boiron, P; Hariveau, E, ed. *Recherches en Homéopathie*. Lyons, Fondation Française pour la Recherche en Homéopathie: 71–74.

Puterman D.J. (1994). *The treatment of gout using homoeopathy* (Thesis). Durban, Technikon Natal.

Rahlfs V.W., Mössinger P. (1976). Zur Behandlung des Colon irritabile: ein multizentrischer plazebo-kontrollierter Doppelblindversuch in der Allgemeinen Praxis. *Arzneimittel Forschung/Drug Research*. 26 (12): 2230–2234.

Rahlfs V.W., Mössinger P. (1978). Asa foetida bei Colon irritabile: Doppelblindversuch. *Deutsche Medizinische Wochenschrift*. 104: 140–143.

Rastogi D.P., Singh V.P., Singh V., Dey S.K., Rao K. (1998). Double blind placebo controlled clinical trial of homoeopathic medicines in HIV infection. *British Homoeopathic Journal*. 87: 86–88.

Reilly D., Taylor M.A., Beattie N.G., Campbell J.H., McSharry C., Aitchison T.C., Carter R., Stevenson R.D. (1994). Is evidence for homoeopathy reproducible? *The Lancet*. 344: 1601–1606.

Reilly D.T., McSharry C., Taylor M.A., Aitchison T. (1986). Is homoeopathy a placebo response? Controlled trial of homoeopathic potency, with pollen in hayfever as model. *The Lancet*. 8512: 881–886.

Reilly D.T., Taylor M.A. (1985). Potent placebo or potency? A proposed study model with initial findings using homoeopathically prepared pollens in hayfever. *British Homoeopathic Journal*. 74: 65–75.

Ríos Varela J.M., Calderón Rodríguez M., Torres Díaz J.H., Corrales Díaz O., Vega Palau M., Fernández Argüelles R. (1995). Terapéutica homeopática en la queratoconjuntivitis epidémica. *La Homeopatía de México*. 64 (574): 2–9.

Ritter H. (1966). Ein homöotherapeutischer doppelter Blindversuch und seine Problematik. *Hippokrates*. 37 (12): 472–476.

Rottey E.E., Verleye G.B., Liagre R.L. (1995). Het effect van een homeopathische bereiding van micro-organismen bij de preventie van griepsymptomen. Een gerandomiseerd dubbel-blind onderzoek in de huisartspraktijk. *Tijdschrift Integrerend Geneeskunde*. 11 (1): 54–58.

Saruggia M., Corghi E. (1992). Effects of homoeopathic dilutions of China rubra on intradialytic symptomatology in patients treated with chronic haemodialysis. *British Homoeopathic Journal*. 81 (2): 86–88.

Savage R.H., Roe P.F. (1977). A double blind trial to assess the benefit of Arnica montana in acute stroke illness. *British Homoeopathic Journal*. 66: 207–220.

Savage R.H., Roe P.F. (1978). A further double blind trial to assess the benefit of Arnica montana in acute stroke illness. *British Homoeopathic Journal*. 67: 210–222.

Schilsky B., Bayer W. (1941). Vergleich der Keuchhustendauer bei allgemeiner und bei homöopathischer Behandlung. *Hippokrates*. 12: 545–548.

Schmidt W. (1987). Zur Therapie der chronischen Bronchitis. Randomisierte Doppelblindstudie mit Asthmakhell®. *Therapiewoche*. 37: 2803–2809.

Schultz M. (1994). *The homoeopathic treatment of warts* (Thesis). Durban, Technikon Natal.

Schwab G. (1990). *Läßt sich eine Wirkung homöopathischer Hochpotenzen nachweisen?* (Thesis). Freiburg, Albert-Ludwigs Universität.

Shipley M., Berry H., Broster G., Jenkins M., Clover A., Williams I. (1983). Controlled trial of homoeopathic treatment of osteoarthritis. *The Lancet*. i (January 15): 97–98.

Singh V. (1994). *The use of Pilocarpus jaborandi in the treatment of emotional palmar hyperhidrosis* (Thesis). Durban, Technikon Natal.

Skaliodas S., Hatzicostas H., Lamropoulou N., Othonos A., Diamantidis S. (1988). Comparative clinical study of homoeopathic and allopathic treatment in diabetes mellitus type II. *Proceedings of the 43rd LMHI Congress*, Athens: 549–556.

Solanki M., Gandhi P.M. (1995). Is homoeopathy only a placebo therapy? Effect of homoeopathic treatment in amoebiasis and giardiasis. *Homoeopathic Heritage*. 20: 707–713.

Spitze B.H. (1995). *The treatment of cellulite using Natrum sulphuricum* (Thesis). Durban, Technikon Natal.

Stippig S.G. (1996). Homöopathische und konventionelle Behandlung gleich gut. *Der Allgemeinarzt*. 18: 2–8.

Straumsheim P.A., Borchgrevink C., Mowinckel P., Kierulf H.H.Ø. (1997). Homeopatisk behandling av migrene. En dobbelt-blind, placebokontrollert studie av 68 pasienter. *Dynamis*. 2: 18–22.

Tarne P.P., Runnebaum B., Roebruck P., Monga B., Gerhard I. (1998). Homoeopathy vs conventional therapy for female infertility. *Archives of Gynecology & Obstetrics*. 261 (Suppl. 1): 193–195.

Thiel W., Borho B. (1994). The treatment of recent traumatic blood effusions of the knee joint. *Biological Therapy*. 12 (4): 242–248.

Torbicka E., Brzozowska-Binda A., Wilczynski J., Uzarowicz A. (1998). RSV infections in infants: therapy with a homeopathic preparation. *Biomedical Therapy*. 16: 256–260.

Trapani G., Legnante G. (1994). Studio preliminare sull'attività di Dolisobios 15. *Medicina Naturale*. 4: 84–87.

Tsiakopoulos I., Labropoulo N., Hadjicostas C., Skaliodas S., Diamantidis S. (1988). Comparative study of homoeopathic and allopathic treatment of benign paroxysmal positional vertigo. *Proceedings of the 43rd LMHI Congress*, Athens: 94–97.

Tsolakis N. (1995). *The homeopathic treatment of primary dysmenorrhoea* (Thesis). Durban, Technikon Natal.

Ustianowski P.A. (1974). A clinical trial of Staphysagria in postcoital cystitis. *British Homoeopathic Journal*. 63: 276–277.

Valero E.M. (1981). *Etude de l'action préventive de: Raphanus sativus 7CH, sur le temps de reprise du transit intestinal post-opératoire (à propos de 80 cas); Pyrogenium 7CH sur les infections post-opératoires (à propos de 128 cas)* (Thesis). Grenoble, Université Scientifique et Médicale.

Van Erp V.M.A., Brands M. (1996). Homoeopathic treatment of malaria in Ghana: open study and clinical trial. *British Homoeopathic Journal.* 85: 66–70.

van't Riet A., de Lange-de Klerk E.S.M. (1985). An attempt to evaluate homoeotherapy in patients with constitutional eczema: a pilot experiment at the Vrije Universiteit Amsterdam. *Proceedings of the 40th LMHI Congress*, Lyons: 422–425.

Ventoskovskiy B.M., Popov A.V. (1990). Homoeopathy as a practical alternative to traditional obstetric methods. *British Homoeopathic Journal.* 79: 201–205.

Villatoro Cadena C.R., Luis Cuevas J. (1991). Tratamiento del síndrome diarreico agudo (SDA) con homeopatía. *La Homeopatía de México.* 550 / 551: 16–25 / 6–11.

Walach H., Haeusler W., Lowes T., Mussbach D., Schamell U., Springer W., Stritzl G., Gaus W., Haag G. (1997). Classical homeopathic treatment of chronic headaches. *Cephalalgia.* 17: 119–126.

Weiser M., Clasen B.P. (1994). Controlled double-blind study of a homeopathic sinusitis medication. *Biological Therapy.* 13 (1): 4–11.

Weiser M., Strösser W., P. K. (1998). Homeopathic vs conventional treatment of vertigo: a randomized double-blind controlled clinical study. *Archives of Otolaryngology – Head & Neck Surgery.* 124: 879–885.

Werk W., Galland F. (1994). Helianthus-tuberosus-Therapie bei Übergewicht: Gewichtsreduktion langfristig stabilisieren. *Therapiewoche.* 44 (1): 34–39.

Whitmarsh T.E., Coleston-Shields D.M., Steiner T.J. (1997). Double-blind randomized placebo-controlled study of homoeopathic prophylaxis of migraine. *Cephalalgia.* 17: 600–604.

Wiesenauer M., Gaus W. (1985). Double-blind trial comparing the effectiveness of the homeopathic preparation Galphimia potentisation D6, Galphimia dilution 10^{-6} and placebo on pollinosis. *Arzneimittel Forschung/Drug Research.* 35 (11): 1745–1747.

Wiesenauer M., Gaus W. (1987). Orthostatische Dysregulation - kontrollierter Wirkungsvergleich zwischen Etilefrin 5 mg und dem homöopathischen Arzneimittel Haplopappus D2. *Zeitschrift für Allgemeine Medizin.* 63: 18–23.

Wiesenauer M., Gaus W. (1991). Wirksamkeitsnachweis eines Homöopathikums bei chronischer Polyarthritis. Eine randomisierte Doppelblindstudie bei niedergelassenen Ärzten. *Aktuelle Rheumatologika.* 16: 1–9.

Wiesenauer M., Gaus W., Bohnacker U., Häussler S. (1989). Wirksamkeitsprüfung von homöopathischen Kombinationspräparaten bei Sinusitis. *Arzneimittel Forschung/Drug Research.* 39: 620–625.

Wiesenauer M., Gaus W., Häussler S. (1990). Behandlung der Pollinosis mit Galphimia glauca. Eine doppelblindstudie unter Praxisbedingungen. *Allergologie.* 13 (10): 359–363.

Wiesenauer M., Häussler S., Gaus W. (1983). Pollinosis-Therapie mit Galphimia glauca. *Fortschritte der Medizin.* 101: 811–814.

Wiesenauer M., Lüdtke R. (1995). The treatment of pollinosis with Galphimia glauca D4: a randomized placebo-controlled double-blind clinical trial. *Phytomedicine.* 2 (1): 3–6.

Yakir M., Kreitler S., Oberbaum M., Bzizinsky A., Vithoulkas G., Bentwich Z. (1994). Homeopathic treatment of premenstrual syndrome: a pilot study. *8th GIRI Meeting (International Research Group on Very Low Dose and High Dilution Effects)*, Jerusalem: 49–50.

Zell J., Connert W.D., Mau J., Feuerstake G. (1990). Treatment of acute sprains of the ankle: a controlled double-blind trial to test the effectiveness of a homoeopathic ointment. *Homeopathy International.* 4 (1): 8–11.

Zicari D., Ricciotti F., Vingolo E.M., Zicari N. (1992). Valutazione dell'azione angioprotettiva di preparati di Arnica nel trattamento della retinopatia diabetica. *Bollettino di Oculistica.* 71 (5): 841–848

General references

Abrams A. (1916). *New Concepts in Diagnosis and Treatment.* San Francisco, Philopolis Press.

Académie de Médecine (1835a). Séance du 17 mars. Discussion sur l'homoeopathie. *Gazette Médicale de Paris.* 3 (12): 189–191.

Académie de Médecine (1835b). Séance du 24 mars. Fin de la discussion sur l'homoeopathie. *Gazette Médicale de Paris.* 3 (13): 202–204.

Ackerknecht E.A. (1967). *Medicine at the Paris Hospital 1794–1848.* Baltimore, Johns Hopkins University Press.

Ackerknecht E.A. (1982a). Diathesis: the word and the concept in medical history. *Bulletin of the History of Medicine.* 56: 317–325.

Ackerknecht E.A. (1982b). *A Short History of Medicine.* 2nd edn. Baltimore, Johns Hopkins University Press.

Aegidi J. (1834). Vorschläge zur Erweiterung der homöopathischen Technik. *Archiv für die homöopathische Heilkunst.* 14 (3).

Albrecht H. (1999). Klinische Forschung zur Homöopathie: eine kritische Bewertung. *Allgemeine Homöopathische Zeitung*. 244 (2): 47–55.

Albury W.R. (1977). French nosologies around 1800 and their relationship with chemistry. In: Forbes E. G., ed. *Proceedings of the XVth International Congress of the History of Science*. Edinburgh, Edinburgh University Press: 502–517.

Alderson W. (1811). *An Essay on the Rhus toxicodendron, with Cases of its Efficacy in the Cure of Palsy and Disorders of the Stomach*. 4th edn. Hull / London, Longman, Hurst, Rees, Orme & Brown.

Alexander W. (1768). *Experimental Essays on the Following Subjects: i. On the External Application of Antiseptics in Putrid Disease; ii. On the Doses and Effects of Medicines; iii. On Diuretics and Sudorifics*. London, Edward and Charles Dilly.

Allen H.C. (1910). *The Materia Medica of the Nosodes with Provings of the X-Ray*. Philadelphia, Boericke & Tafel.

Allen T.F. (1874–80). *The Encyclopaedia of Pure Materia Medica*. 11 vols. Philadelphia, Boericke & Tafel.

Allen T.F. (1936). *A Primer of Materia Medica for Practitioners of Homoeopathy*. Philadelphia, Boericke & Tafel.

Ameke W. (1885). *History of Homoeopathy: Its Origin, its Conflicts*. Ed. Dudgeon R. E. Transl. A.E. Drysdale. London, E. Gould & Son.

Anon (1834). Expériences homéopathiques faites par M. Andral, à l'hôpital de la Pitié. *Bulletin Général de Thérapeutique Médicale et Chirurgicale*. 6 (Sept.): 318–321.

Anon (1852). Review of: The Fallacies of Homoeopathy, by C. H. F. Routh. *British Journal of Homoeopathy*. 10: 342–351.

Askenstedt F.C. (1915). Comparative statistics from the Louisville City Hospital. *Journal of the American Institute of Homeopathy*. 8 (4): 452–456.

Atran S. (1990). *Cognitive Foundations of Natural History. Towards an Anthropology of Science*. Cambridge, Cambridge University Press.

Aulas J.J., Bordelay G., Royer J.F. (1991). *Homéopathie – état actuel de l'évaluation clinique*. Paris, Frison Roche.

Autenrieth J.H.F. (1807–08). *Versuche fuer die praktische Heilkunde aus den clinischen Anstalten von Tuebingen*. Tübingen, Cotta.

Avicenna (1473). *Liber canonis*. Mediolani, P. de Lavagna.

Avicenna (1564). *Libri in re medica omnes*. Venice, V. Valgrisius.

Bacon F. (1620). *Novum Organum*. London, John Bill.

Barnes J., Resch K.-L., Ernst E. (1997). Homeopathy for postoperative ileus? *Journal of Clinical Gastroenterology*. 25 (4): 628–633.

Barrow L. (1986). *Independent Spirits: Spiritualism and English Plebians, 1850–1910*. History Workshop. Ed. Samuel R. London, Routledge & Kegan Paul.

Barrow L. (1988). An imponderable liberator: J.J. Garth Wilkinson. In: Cooter R., ed. *Studies in the History of Alternative Medicine*. Basingstoke, Macmillan.

Bassi A. (1835–36). *Del mal del segno calcinaccio o muscardino, malattia che afflige i bachi da seta e sul modo di liberarne le bigattaje anche le più infestate*. 2 vols. Lodi, Orcesi.

Baumes J.B. (1798). *Essai d'un système chimique de la science de l'homme*. Nîmes.

Baumes J.B. (1801–02). *Fondemens de la science méthodique des maladies*. 4 vols. Montpellier.

Bayes W. (1856). *Truth in Medicine; or, A Few Words on Homoeopathy*. London, W. & F.G. Cash.

Behring E.A. (1893). *Gesammelte Abhandlungen zur ätiologischen Therapie von austeckenden Krankheiten*. Leipzig, G. Thieme.

Behring E.A. (1898). Ueber Heilprinzipien, insbesondere ueber das aetiologische und das isopathische Heilprinzip. *Deutsche medicinische Wochenschrift* (5): 65–69.

Behring E.A. (1905). *Moderne phthisiogenetische und phthisiotherapeutische Probleme in historischer Beleuchtung*. Marburg.

Behring E.A. (1915). *Gesammelte Abhandlungen. Neue Folge*. Bonn, A. Marcus & E. Weber.

Bell B. (1793). *A Treatise on Gonorrhoea Virulenta and Lues Venerea*. 2 vols. Edinburgh, J. Watson & G. Mudie.

Bellavite P., Signorini A. (1995). *Homoeopathy: A Frontier in Medical Science*. Transl. Anthony Steele. Berkeley, CA, North Atlantic Books.

Berkowitz C.D. (1994). Homoeopathy: keeping an open mind. *Lancet*. 344: 701–702.

Berlin I. (1978). *Russian Thinkers*. Eds. Hardy H. & Kelly A. London, Hogarth Press.

Berliner H. (1982). Medical modes of production. In: Wright P. & Treacher A., eds *The problem of medical knowledge: Examining the social construction of medicine*. Edinburgh, Edinburgh University Press: 162–173.

Berliner H.S. (1977). New light on the Flexner Report: notes on the A.M.A.–Carnegie Foundation background. *Bulletin of the History of Medicine*. 51: 601–609.

Bier A. (1925). Wie sollen wir uns zu der Homoeopathie stellen? *Münchener Medizinische Wochenschrift*. 72: 713–717, 773–776.

Bildet J., Bonini F., Gender P., Aubin M., Demarque D., Quilichini R. (1984). Etude au microscope électronique de l'action de dilutions de phosphorus 15 CH sur l'hépatite toxique du rat. *Homéopathie française*. 72: 211.

Black N. (1996). Why we need observational studies to evaluate the effectiveness of health care. *British Medical Journal*. 312: 1215–1218.

Blackley C.H. (1873). *Experimental Researches on the Causes and Nature of Catarrhus Aestivus (Hay-Fever or Hay-Asthma)*. London, Baillière, Tindall & Cox.

Boas M. (1958). *Robert Boyle and Seventeenth-Century Chemistry*. Cambridge, Cambridge University Press.

Bolron C., Remy J. (1990). *Homéopathie: un combat scientifique*. Paris, Albin Michel.

Boissel J.-P., Cucherat M., Haugh M., Gauthier E. (1996). Critical literature review on the effectiveness of homoeopathy: overview of data from homoeopathic medicine trials. In: *Homoeopathic Medicine Research Group: report to the European Commission Directorate General XII: science, research and development*. Brussels: 195–210.

Bönninghausen C.M. (1832). *Systematisch-alphabetischen Repertorium der antipsorischen Arzneien, nebst einem Vorworte des Herrn Hofraths Dr. S. Hahnemanns, über Wiederholung der Gabe eines homöopathischen Heilmittels*. Münster, Coppenrath.

Bönninghausen C.M.F.v. (1908). A contribution to the judgement concerning the characteristic value of symptoms. In: Bradford T. L., ed. *The Lesser Writings*. Philadelphia, Boericke & Tafel.

Bower H. (1998). Double standards exist in judging traditional and alternative medicine. *British Medical Journal*. 316: 1694.

Boyanus C. (1882). *Gomeopatija v Rossii. Istoriceskiij ocerk*. Moskva.

Boyd W.E. (1936). Potency variation. *Transactions of the 11th Congress Liga Homoeopatica Internationalis*, 24–29 August, Glasgow: 364–371.

Bradford T.L. (1900). *The Logic of Figures: or Comparative Results of Homoeopathic and Other Treatments*. Philadelphia, Boericke & Tafel.

Brewin C.R., Bradley C. (1989). Patient preferences and randomised trials. *British Medical Journal*. 299: 313–315.

Brock W.H. (1992). *The Fontana History of Chemistry*. London, Fontana Press.

Brown J. (1780). *Elementa medicinae*. Edinburgh.

Brown J. (1791). *The Elements of Medicine, or, A Translation of the Elementa Medicinae Brunonis, with Large Notes, Illustrations, and Comments*. 2 vols. Philadelphia, William Spotswood.

Brown P.S. (1987). Social context and medical theory in the demarcation of nineteenth-century boundaries. In: Bynum W. F. & Porter R., eds *Medical Fringe and Medical Orthodoxy 1750–1850*. London, Croom Helm: 216–233.

Buckle G.E. (1920). *The Life of Benjamin Disraeli, Earl of Beaconsfield*. Vol 6: 1876–1881. London, John Murray.

Bull J.P. (1951). *A Study of the History and Principles of Clinical Therapeutic Trials* (Thesis). Medicine. Cambridge, Cambridge.

Bull J.P. (1959). The historical development of clinical therapeutic trials. *Journal of Chronic Disease*. 10 (3): 218–248.

Burnett J.C. (1879). *Gold as a Remedy in Disease*. London, Homoeopathic Publishing Company.

Burnett J.C. (1887). *Diseases of the Spleen*. London, Homoeopathic Publishing Company.

Burnett J.C. (1896). *Organ Diseases of Women, Notably Enlargements and Displacements of the Uterus, and Sterility, Considered as Curable by Medicine*. London, Homoeopathic Publishing Company.

Cabot R.C. (1909). Veracity and psychotherapy. In: Parker W. B., ed. *Psychotherapy, A Course of Reading in Sound Psychology, Sound Medicine, and Sound Religion*. 3 vols. New York.

Calabrese E., Baldwin L. (1999). The marginalization of hormesis. *Toxicologic Pathology*. 27 (2): 187–194.

Campbell A.C.H. (1978). Is homoeopathy scientific? A reassessment in the light of Karl Popper's theory of scientific knowledge. *British Homoeopathic Journal*. 67: 77–85.

Campbell A.C.H. (1984). *The Two Faces of Homoeopathy*. London, Jill Norman, Robert Hale.

Candegabe E.F. (1996). *Comparative Materia Medica*. Beaconsfield, Beaconsfield Publishers.

Canghuilhem G. (1991). *The Normal and the Pathological*. Transl. C.R. Fawcett & R.S. Cohen. New York, Zone Books.

Cassedy J.H. (1984). *American Medicine and Statistical Thinking, 1800–1860*. Cambridge, Mass., Harvard University Press.

Castiglioni A. (1941). *History of Medicine*. New York, Alfred A. Knopf.

Chalmers I., Altman D.G., eds. (1995). *Systematic Reviews*. London, BMJ Publishing Group.

Chalmers T.C., Smith Jr H., Blackburn B., Silverman B., Schroeder B., Reitman D., Ambroz A. (1981). A method for assessing the quality of a randomized control trial. *Controlled Clinical Trials*. 2: 31–49.

Cho N., Bero L. (1994). Instruments for assessing the quality of drug studies published in the medical literature. *Journal of the American Medical Association*. 272: 101–104.

Chrestien J.A. (1811). *Observations sur un nouveau remède dans le traitement des maladies vénériennes et lymphatiques*. Paris.

Cioffi F. (1970). Freud and the idea of a pseudo-science. In: Borger R. & Cioffi F., eds *Explanation in the Behavioural Sciences*. Cambridge, Cambridge University Press: 471–515.

Clarke J.H. (1900). *A Dictionary of Practical Materia Medica*. 2 vols. London, Homoeopathic Publishing Company.

Clarke J.H. (1911). *The Prescriber*. 7th edn, Homoeopathic Publishing Company.

Clarke J.H. (1923). *Hahnemann and Paracelsus*. London, Homoeopathic Publishing Company.

Clarke J.H. (1925). *A Dictionary of Practical Materia Medica*. 3 vols. 2nd edn. London, Homoeopathic Publishing Company.

Cochrane Collaboration, Royal College of Physicians of Edinburgh (1998). *Controlled Trials from History*. http://www.rcpe.ac.uk/controlled_trials/

Comrie J.D. (1932). *History of Scottish Medicine*. 2 vols. London, The Wellcome Historical Medical Museum; Baillière, Tindall & Cox.

CONSORT (2001). *www.consort-statement.org*.

Cook T.D., Leviton L.C. (1980). Reviewing the literature: a comparison of traditional methods with meta-analysis. *Journal of Personality*. 48: 449–472.

Cooter R. (1988). Alternative medicine, alternative cosmology. In: Cooter R., ed. *Studies in the History of Alternative Medicine*. Basingstoke, Macmillan.

Cottingham J. (1984). *Rationalism*. London, Paladin.

Coulter C. (1986). *Portraits of Homeopathic Medicines: Psychophysical Analyses of Selected Constitutional Types*. Washington, DC, Wehawken Books.

Coulter H. (1973). *Divided Legacy (III) Science and Ethics in American Medicine*. Washington, DC, Wehawken Book Company.

Coulter H. (1977). *Divided Legacy (II) The Origins of Modern Western Medicine: J.B. Van Helmont to Claude Bernard*. Washington, DC, Wehawken Book Company.

Coulter H. (1981). *Homoeopathic Science and Modern Medicine: The Physics of Healing with Microdoses*. Richmond, CA, North Atlantic Books.

Coulter H. (1994). *Divided Legacy (IV) Twentieth-Century Medicine: The Bacteriological Era*. Washington, DC, Center for Empirical Medicine.

Cox-Maksimov D.C.T. (1998). *The Making of the Clinical Trial in Britain: Expertise, the State and the Public* (Thesis), Cambridge University.

Creighton C. (1891–94). *History of Epidemics in Britain*. 2 vols. Cambridge, Cambridge University Press.

Crellin J. (1997). Herbalism. In: Porter R., ed. *Medicine, A History of Healing: Ancient Traditions to Modern Practices*. London, Michael O'Mara: 68–93.

Crombie A.C. (1953). *Robert Grosseteste and the Origins of the Experimental Science 1100–1700*. Oxford, Oxford University Press.

Crookshank F.G. (1923 [1946]). The importance of a theory of signs and a critique of language in the study of medicine. In: Ogden C. K. & Richards I. A., eds *The Meaning of Meaning*. 8th edn. Cambridge, Cambridge University Press: 337–355.

Crosland M.P. (1962). *Historical Studies in the Language of Chemistry*. 2 vols. London, Heinemann.

Cruikshank R. (1942). The pneumonias. In: Morland, ed. *Control of the Common Fevers*. London, The Lancet: 201–215.

Crumpe S. (1793). *Inquiry into the Nature and Properties of Opium*. London, J. Robinson.

Cullen W. (1789). *A Treatise of Materia Medica*. 2 vols. Edinburgh, C. Elliot.

Cullen W. (1790). *Abhandlung über die Materia medika*. 2 vols. Transl. S. Hahnemann. Leipzig, Schwickert.

Daniels G.H. (1971). *Science in American Society: A Social History*. New York, Knopf.

Dantas F., Fisher P. (1998). A systematic review of homoeopathic pathogenetic trials ('provings') published in the United Kingdom from 1945 to 1995. In: Ernst E. & Hahn E. G., eds *Homoeopathy: A Critical Appraisal*. Oxford, Butterworth Heinemann: 69–97.

Davies R.J. (1990). Respiratory disease. In: Kumar P. J. & Clark M. L., eds *Clinical Medicine*. London, Baillière Tindall: 627–704.

Dean M.E. (1998). Out of step with the *Lancet* homoeopathy meta-analysis. More objections than objectivity? *Journal of Alternative and Complementary Medicine*. 4 (4): 389–398.

Dean M.E. (2000). A homeopathic origin for placebo controls: 'An invaluable gift of God'. *Alternative Therapies in Health and Medicine*. 6 (2): 58–66.

Dean M.E. (2001). Study shows double standards in evaluation of homeopathy. *British Medical Journal*. 322 (20 January): 169–170.

Debus A.G. (1998). Chemists, physicians, and changing perspectives on the Scientific Revolution. *Isis*. 89: 66–81.

Dellmour F. (1997). Homöopathie und Lebenskraft. Begriffe bei Samuel Hahnemann. In: Swoboda F., ed. *Documenta Homoeopathica*. vol. 17. Vienna, W. Maudrich: 63–103.

Demachy J.F. (1784). *Laborant im Großen, oder Kunst die chemischen Produkte fabrikmäßig zu verfertigen*. 2 vols. Transl. S. Hahnemann. Leipzig, Crusius.

Demarque D. (1981). *L'Homéopathie — médecine de l'expérience*. 2nd edn. Metz, Maisonneuve.

Dhawale M.L. (1985). *Principles and Practice of Homoeopathy*. 2nd edn. Bombay, Institute of Clinical Research.

Dietl J. (1845). Praktische Wahrnehmungen nach den Ergebnissen im Wiednerbezirkskrankenhause. *Zeitschrift der k.u.k. Gesellschaft der Aertze zu Wien*. 1 (2): 9.

Dittmann J., Kanapin H., Harisch G. (1999). Biochemische Wirkung von hömöopathischer und elektronischer D8 von Kalium cyanatum. *Forschende Komplementärmedizin*. 6 (1): 15–18.

Donner F. (1942). Über vergleichende homöotherapeutische Untersuchungen bei Infektionskrankheiten. *Deutsche Zeitschrift für Homöopathie*. 58: 257–278.

Donner F. (1948). *Zwölf Vorlesungen über Homöopathie*. Berlin, Haug.

Donner F. (1969). Observations faites lors des vérifications relatives aux méthodes de l'homéopathie. *Les Cahiers de Biothérapie*. 21 (janvier): 5–26.

Dudgeon R.E. (1853). *Lectures on the Theory and Practice of Homoeopathy*. London, Leath & Ross.

Dunham C. (1852). The homoeopathic experiments of M. Andral, and his past and present opinion of them. *North American Journal of Homoeopathy*. 2: 263–268.

E. E. (1833). Lettre sur le progrès de la médecine homoeopathique en Allemagne, en Russie et la France. *Gazette Médicale de Paris*. 1: 567–574.

Editorial (1834). *Bulletin Général de Thérapeutique Médicale et Chirurgicale*. 7: 5–6.

Editorial (1849). Homéopathie dans les hôpitaux de Paris. *L'Union Médicale*. 3 (146, 8 December): 581.

Editorial (1857). Return of cases treated at the London Homoeopathic Hospital, from April 10, 1850, to December 31, 1855. *Monthly Homoeopathic Review*. 1: 42–50.

Eidherr M. (1862). Erfahrungen über die Heilwirkungen der 6., 15. und 30. Arzneiverdünnung auf die entzündete Lunge. *Zeitschrift des Vereines der homöopathischen Aertze Oesterreichs*. 1 n.s. (1): 1–165.

Eizayaga F.X. (1991). *Treatise on Homoeopathic Medicine*. Buenos Aires, Ediciones Marecel.

Eizayaga F.X., Eizayaga J., Eizayaga F.X. (1996). Homoeopathic treatment of bronchial asthma. *British Homoeopathic Journal*. 85: 28–33.

Eizayaga J. (1989). El pensamiento y la práctica de J.T. Kent. *Homeopatía*. 54: 29–50.

Elmiger J. (1998). *Rediscovering Real Medicine: The New Horizons of Homoeopathy*. Shaftesbury, Element.

Emerson R.W. (1850). Swedenborg. In: *Representative Men*. Boston.

Ernst E. (1995a). Evaluation of homoeopathy in Nazi Germany. *British Homoeopathic Journal*. 84: 229.

Ernst E. (1995b). The heresy of homoeopathy: a brief history of 200 years of criticism. *British Homoeopathic Journal*. 87: 28–32.

Ernst E., Barnes J. (1998). Meta-analysis of homoeopathy trials [letter]. *Lancet*. 351: 366.

Evans M. (2000). *Meditative Provings: Notes on the Meditative Provings of New Remedies*. York, The Rose Press.

Faber K. (1921). Nosography in modern internal medicine. *Annals of Medical History*. 4 (1): 1–63.

FACT (2001). A homoeopathic remedy to prevent influenza? *Focus on Alternative and Complementary Therapies*. 6: 41.

Farr W. (1852). *Report on the Mortality of Cholera in England, 1848–49*. London, Her Majesty's Stationery Office.

Fastner Z. (1980). Metals. In: Dukes M., ed. *Meyler's Side Effects of Drugs*. 9th edn. Amsterdam, Excerpta Medica: 368–382.

Faure O. (1992a). *Le Débat autour de l'homéopathie en France 1830–1870: évidences et arrières-plans*. Lyon, Boiron.

Faure O., ed. (1992b). *Practiciens, patients et militants de l'homéopathie aux XIXe et XXe siècles (1800–1940)*. Lyons, Boiron, Presses Universitaires de Lyon.

Fernando D. (1998). *Alchemy: An Illustrated A to Z*. London, Blandford.

Fisher P., Huskisson E.C., Scott D.L., Turner P. (1991). Trials of homoeopathy [letter]. *British Medical Journal*. 302: 727.

Fisken R.A. (1996). Complementary medicine must be based on sound science and well conducted research [letter]. *British Medical Journal*. 313: 882.

Flaherty G. (1995). The non-normal sciences: survivals of renaissance thought in the eighteenth century. In: Fox C. & Porter R. & Wokler R., eds *Inventing Human Science: Eighteenth Century Domains*. Berkeley, University of California Press: 271–291.

Flexner A. (1910). *Medical education in the United States and Canada*. New York, Carnegie Foundation for the Advancement of Teaching: Bulletin No. 4.

Foubister D. (1989). *Tutorials on Homoeopathy*. Beaconsfield, Beaconsfield Publishers.

Foucault M. (1963). *La Naissance du clinique*. Paris, Presses Universitaires de France.

Fracastoro G. (1546). *De sympathia et antipathia rerum liber unus. De contagione et contagiosis morbis et eorum curatione*. Venice, L. Giunti.

Frank J.P. (1779–1819). *System einer vollständigen medizinischen Polizey*. Mannheim, Tübingen and Vienna.

Frei H. (1999). Die Rangordnungen der Symptome von Hahnemann, Bönninghausen, Hering und Kent, evaluiert anhand von 175 Kasuistiken. *Zeitschrift für klassischen Homöopathie*. 43 (4): 131–142.

Fye W.B. (1990). Vasodilator therapy for angina pectoris: the intersection of homeopathy and scientific medicine. *Journal of the History of Medicine and Allied Sciences*. 45: 317–340.

Gale A.H. (1959). *Epidemic Diseases*. Harmondsworth, Penguin.

Gallavardin J.-P. (1860). *Projet d'hôpitaux mixtes allopathiques et homoeopathiques: projet de dispensaires mixtes. Mémoire adressée à MM. les administrateurs des hôpitaux*. Paris, Baillière.

Garden M. (1992). L'histoire de l'homéopathie en France — 1830–1940. In: Faure O., ed. *Practiciens, patients et militants de l'homéopathie aux XIXe et XXe siècles (1800–1940)*. Lyons, Boiron, Presses Universitaires de Lyon: 59–82.

Garrison F.H. (1917). *An Introdution to the History of Medicine*. Philadelphia, W.B. Saunders. 4th edn 1929.

Gay P. (1970). *The Enlightenment: An Interpretation (II) The Science of Freedom*. London, Weidenfeld and Nicholson.

Geber (1598). *De alchemia: Traditio summae perfectionis in duos libros divisa: item, Liber investigationis magisterii*. Strassburg, L. Zetzner.

Gerhard I. (1999). Homöopathie versus konventionelle Therapie bei weiblichen Fertilitätsstörungen: ein monozentrische, prospektive, offene und teilrandomisierte Therapievergleichsstudie. *Erfahrungsheilkunde*. 49 (9): 527–541.

Gevitz N. (1994). Unorthodox medical theories. In: Bynum W. F. & Porter R., eds *Companion Encyclopaedia of the History of Medicine*. vol. 1. London, Routledge: 603–633.

Gigerenzer G., Swijtink Z., Porter T., Daston L., Beatty J., Krüger L. (1989). *The Empire of Chance. How Probability Changed Science and Everyday Life*. Cambridge, Cambridge University Press.

Gijswijt-Hofstra M. (1996). Homeopathy's early Dutch conquests: the Rotterdam clientele of Clemens von Bönninghausen in the 1840s and 1850s. *Journal of the History of Medicine and Allied Sciences*. 51: 155–183.

Gill T.M., Feinstein A.R. (1994). A critical appraisal of the quality of quality-of-life measurements. *Journal of the American Medical Association*. 272: 619–626.

Goodwin J.S., Goodwin J.M. (1984). The tomato effect: the rejection of highly efficacious therapies. *Journal of the American Medical Association*. 251 (18): 2387–2390.

Govaert T.M.E., Dinant G.J., Aretz K. (1993). Adverse reactions to influenza vaccine in elderly people: randomised double blind placebo controlled trial. *British Medical Journal*. 307: 988–990.

Grauvogl E.v. (1860). *Die Grundsetze der Physiologie, Pathologie und homöopathischen Therapie*. Nuremberg, Erlangen.

Grauvogl E.v. (1866). *Lehrbuch der Homöopathie*. Nuremberg.

Griesselich L. (1848). *Handbuch zur Kenntniss der homöopathischen oder specifischen Heilkunst*. Carlsruhe, Malsch und Vogel.

Grieve M. (1931). *A Modern Herbal*. Ed. Leyel C. F. London, Jonathan Cape.

Grimm J., Grimm W. (1862). *Deutsches Wörterbuch*. Vol 4. Ed. Heyne M. Leipzig, S. Hirzel.

Gross G.W. (1822). Noch etwas über Pendelschwingungen. *Archiv für den Thierischen Magnetismus*. 10 (1): 168–172.

Gross G.W. (1837). Die Versammlung des homoeopathischen Zentralvereins am 10. August 1836 zu Magdeburg. *Archiv für die homöopathische Heilkunst*. 16: 169–174.

Guthrie D. (1945). *A History of Medicine*. London, Thomas Nelson.

Gutman W. (1978). *Homoeopathy: the Fundamentals of its Philosophy, the Essence of its Remedies*. Bombay, Homoeopathic Medical Publishers.

Guttentag O.E. (1940). Trends toward homeopathy: present and past. *Bulletin of the History of Medicine*. 8: 1172–1193.

Guttentag O.E. (1966). Homeopathy in the light of modern pharmacology. *Clinical Pharmacology and Therapeutics*. 7: 425–428.

Guy W.A. (1860). Croonian Lectures on the numerical method, and its application to the science and art of medicine. v. *British Medical Journal*. n.s. (186, July 21): 553–555.

Haas H., Fink H., Härtfelder G. (1959). Das Placeboproblem. *Fortschritte der Arzneimittelforschung / Progress in Drug Research*. 1: 279–454.

Haas W.S. (1956). *The Destiny of the Mind, East and West*. London, Faber and Faber.

Habrich C. (1991). Characteristic features of eighteenth-century therapeutics in Germany. In: Bynum W. F. & Nutton V., eds *Essays in the History of Therapeutics*. Amsterdam, Rodopi: 39–49.

Hacking I. (1990). *The Taming of Chance*. Cambridge, Cambridge University Press.

Haehl R. (1927). *Samuel Hahnemann, His Life and Work.* 2 vols. Transl. Marie M. Wheeler & W.H.R. Grundy. London, Homoeopathic Publishing Company.

Hahnemann S. (1784). *Anleitung alte Schaeden und faeule Geschwuere gruendlich zu heilen.* Leipzig.

Hahnemann S. (1789). *Unterricht für Wundärtze über die venerischen Krankheiten, nebst einem neuen Queksilberpräparate.* Leipzig.

Hahnemann S. (1792 / 1795). *Freund der Gesundheit.* 2 vols. Frankfurt am Main / Leipzig, Fleischer / Crusius.

Hahnemann S. (1793–99). *Apotheker Lexikon.* 4 vols. Leipzig, Crusius.

Hahnemann S. (1796a). Striche zur Schilderung Klockenbrings während seines Trübsinns. *Deutsche Monatsschrift.* 1 (Febr): 147–159.

Hahnemann S. (1796b). Versuch über ein neues Prinzip zur Auffindung der Heilkrafte der Arzneisubstanzen, nebst einigen Blicken auf die bisherigen. *Journal der practischen Arzneykunde und Wundarzneykunst.* 2: 391–439, 465–561.

Hahnemann S. (1801a). Fragmentarische Bemerkungen zu Brown's Elements of Medicine. *Neues Journal der practischen Arzneykunde und Wundarzneykunst.* 12 (2): 52–76.

Hahnemann S. (1801b). *Heilung und Verhütung des Scharlach-Fiebers.* Gotha, Becker.

Hahnemann S. (1801c). Monita über die drey gangbaren Kurarten. *Neues Journal der practischen Arzneykunde und Wundarzneykunst.* 11 (4): 3–64.

Hahnemann S. (1801d). Ueber die Kraft kleiner Gaben der Arzneien überhaupt und der Belladonna insbesondre. *Neues Journal der practischen Arzneykunde und Wundarzneykunst.* 13 (2): 152–159.

Hahnemann S. (1805a). *Aeskulap auf der Wagschale.* Leipzig, Steinacker.

Hahnemann S. (1805b). *Fragmenta de viribus medicamentorum positivis sive in sano corpore humano observatis. Pars prima: Textus. Pars secunda: Index.* 2 vols. Leipzig, J.A. Barth.

Hahnemann S. (1805c). Heilkunde der Erfahrung. *Neues Journal der practischen Arzneykunde und Wundarzneykunst.* 22 (3): 5–99.

Hahnemann S. (1806). Was sind Gifte? Was sind Arzneien? *Neues Journal der practischen Arzneykunde und Wundarzneykunst.* 24 (3): 40–57.

Hahnemann S. (1807). Fingerzeige auf den homöopathischen Gebrauch der Arzneien in der bisherigen Praxis. *Neues Journal der practischen Arzneykunde und Wundarzneykunst.* 26 (2): 5–43.

Hahnemann S. (1808a). Auszug eines Briefs an einen Arzt von hohem Range, über die höchst nöthige Wiedergeburt der Heilkunde. *Allgemeiner Anzeiger der Deutschen.* 2 (343): 3729–3741.

Hahnemann S. (1808b). Bemerkungen über das Scharlachfieber. *Allgemeiner Anzeiger der Deutschen.* 1 (160): 1745–1752.

Hahnemann S. (1808c). Ueber den Werth der speculativen Arzneysysteme, besonders im Gegenhalt der mit ihnen gepaarten, gewöhnlichen Praxis. *Allgemeiner Anzeiger der Deutschen.* 2 (263–64): 2841–2852, 2857–2868.

Hahnemann S. (1810). *Organon der rationellen Heilkunde.* Dresden, Arnold.

Hahnemann S. (1811–21). *Reine Arzneimittellehre.* 6 vols. Dresden, Arnold.

Hahnemann S. (1812). *Dissertatio historico-medica de helleborismo veterum [Habilitation].* Leipzig, Tauchnitz.

Hahnemann S. (1814). Heilart des jetzt herrschenden Nerven- oder Spitalfiebers. *Allgemeiner Anzeiger der Deutschen.* 1 (6): 49–54.

Hahnemann S. (1816). Belehrung über die venerische Krankheit und ihre gewöhnlich unrechte Behandlung. *Allgemeiner Anzeiger der Deutschen.* 2 (211): 2189–2201, (212): 2205–2211.

Hahnemann S. (1817). *Reine Arzneimittellehre.* Vol 3. Dresden, Arnold.

Hahnemann S. (1818). *Reine Arzneimittellehre.* Vol 4. Dresden, Arnold.

Hahnemann S. (1819a). *Organon der Heilkunst.* 2nd edn. Dresden and Leipzig, Arnold.

Hahnemann S. (1819b). Ueber die liebeslosigkeit gegen Selbstmörder. *Allgemeiner Anzeiger der Deutschen.* 1 (144): 1537.

Hahnemann S. (1822–27). *Reine Arzneimittellehre.* 6 vols. 2nd edn. Dresden, Arnold.

Hahnemann S. (1828–30). *Die chronischen Krankheiten, ihre eigenthümliche Natur und homöopathische Heilung.* 4 vols. Dresden and Leipzig, Arnold.

Hahnemann S. (1829). *Kleine medicinische Schriften.* 2 vols. Ed. Stapf E. Dresden und Leipzig, Arnold.

Hahnemann S. (1831). *Aufruf an denkende Menschenfreunde über die Ansteckungsart der asiatischen Cholera.* Leipzig, Berger.

Hahnemann S. (1832). *Doctrine et traitement homoeopathique des maladies chroniques.* 2 vols. Transl. A-J-L Jourdan from the 1st German edn. Paris, Baillière.

Hahnemann S. (1833a). *The Homoeopathic Medical Doctrine, or, 'Organon of the Healing Art;' A New System of Physic.* Transl. Charles H. Devrient from the 4th German edn of 1829 with notes by Samuel Stratten. Dublin, W.F. Wakeman.

Hahnemann S. (1833b). Magnes. In: *Reine Arzneimittellehre.* vol. 1. 3rd edn. Dresden, Arnold.

Hahnemann S. (1833c). *Organon der Heilkunst.* 5th edn. Dresden and Leipzig, Arnold.

Hahnemann S. (1833–37). *Reine Arzneimittellehre*. 3rd edn. Dresden, Arnold.

Hahnemann S. (1835). *Die chronischen Krankheiten, ihre eigenthümliche Natur und homöopathische Heilung*. Vol 1. 2nd edn. Dresden and Leipzig, Arnold.

Hahnemann S. (1837). *Die chronischen Krankheiten, ihre eigenthümliche Natur und homöopathische Heilung. Antipsorische Arzneien*. Vol 3. 2nd edn. Düsseldorf, Schaub.

Hahnemann S. (1845). *The Chronic Diseases*. Transl. C. Hempel. Boston, William Radde.

Hahnemann S. (1852a). How can small doses of such very attenuated medicine as homoeopathy employs still possess great power? In: Dudgeon R. E., ed. *The Lesser Writings*. London, Headland: 728–734.

Hahnemann S. (1852b). *The Lesser Writings*. Transl. and ed. R.E. Dudgeon. London, Headland.

Hahnemann S. (1865). *Organon der Heilkunst*. 6th edn. Ed. Lutze A. Coethen, Lutze'schen Klinik.

Hahnemann S. (1880). *Materia Medica Pura*. 2 vols. Transl. R.E. Dudgeon. London, Hahnemann Publishing Society.

Hahnemann S. (1889). Letters. *The Homoeopathic World*. 24: 200–209.

Hahnemann S. (1893). *Organon of Medicine*. Transl. and ed. R.E. Dudgeon from the 5th German edn of 1833. Calcutta, Roy, [1961].

Hahnemann S. (1896). *The Chronic Diseases: Their Peculiar Nature and their Homoeopathic Cure*. 2 vols. Transl. L. Tafel from the 2nd German edn. Philadelphia, Boericke & Tafel.

Hahnemann S. (1913). *Organon of the Rational Healing Art*. Transl. Charles Edwin Wheeler from the 1st German edn of 1810. London, J.M. Dent, Everyman's Library.

Hahnemann S. (1921). *Organon der Heilkunst*. 6th edn. Ed. Haehl R. Leipzig, Willmar Schwabe.

Hahnemann S. (2000). *Organon-Synopse: Die 6 Auflagen von 1810–1842 im Überblick*. Eds. Luft B. & Wischner M. Heidelberg, Karl F. Haug.

Hall T.S. (1975). *History of General Physiology, 600 B.C. to A.D. 1900*. 2 vols. Chicago, Chicago University Press.

Haller J.S. (1984). Aconite: a case study in doctrinal conflict and the meaning of scientific medicine. *Bulletin of the New York Academy of Medicine*. 60 (9): 888–904.

Handley R. (1997). *In Search of the Later Hahnemann*. Beaconsfield, Beaconsfield Publishers.

Hanson N.R. (1958). *Patterns of Discovery: An Inquiry into the Conceptual Foundations of Science*. Cambridge, Cambridge University Press.

Harré R. (1983). *Great Scientific Experiments*. Oxford, Oxford University Press.

Harré R. (1998). *The Singular Self. An Introduction to the Psychology of Personhood*. London, Sage.

Hegel G.W.F. (1970). *Philosophy of Nature*. 3 vols. Ed. Petry M. J. London, Allen & Unwin.

Helmuth W.T. (1911). Homoeopathy. In: *Encyclopaedia Britannica*. vol. 13. 10th edn. Cambridge, Cambridge University Press.

Henderson W. (1845). *An Inquiry into the Homoeopathic Practice of Medicine*. London, Edinburgh.

Henle F.G.J. (1840). Von den Miasmen und Contagionen. In: *Pathologische Untersuchungen*. Berlin, A. Hirschwald: 1–82.

Henle F.G.J. (1846). *Handbuch der rationellen Pathologie*. 2 vols. Braunschweig, F. Vieweg.

Henshaw R.C., Naji S.A., Russell I.T., Templeton A.A. (1993). Comparison of medical abortion with surgical vacuum aspiration: women's preferences and acceptability of treatment. *British Medical Journal*. 307: 714–717.

Hentschel C., Kohnen R., Hahn E.G. (1998). Reports of complications in homeopathic treatment. In: Ernst E. & Hahn E. G., eds *Homoeopathy: A Critical Appraisal*. Oxford, Butterworth Heinemann: 136–141.

Hering C. (1879–91). *The Guiding Symptoms of our Materia Medica*. 10 vols. Philadelphia, Boericke & Tafel.

Hill C., Doyon F. (1990). Review of randomized trials of homoeopathy. *Revue d'Epidémiologie et de Santé Publique*. 38: 139–147.

Holmes O.W. (1842). *Homoeópathy and its Kindred Delusions: Two Lectures Delivered before the Boston Society for the Diffusion of Useful Knowledge*. Boston, William D. Ticknor.

Horder T. (1924). The electronic reactions of Abrams. *British Medical Journal*. 1: 179–185.

House of Commons (1854–55). *Return to an Address of the Honourable House of Commons*. Sessional Papers, no. 255. xlv: 189–226.

House of Lords (2000). *Complementary and Alternative Medicine*. Science and Technology Committee: Sixth Report. London, The Stationery Office.

Hudson R.P. (1972). Abraham Flexner in perspective: American Medical Education 1865–1910. *Bulletin of the History of Medicine*. 46: 545–561.

Hufbauer K. (1982). *The Formation of the German Chemical Community (1720–1795)*. Berkeley, University of California Press.

Hufeland C.W. (1826). Die Homöopathie. *Journal der practischen Heilkunde*. 62 (1): 3–28.

Hughes R. (1869). *On the Various Forms of Paralysis and their Treatment*. London, H. Turner.

Hughes R. (1884). *The Knowledge of the Physician*. Boston.

Hughes R. (1893). *A Manual of Pharmacodynamics*. 6th edn. London, Leath & Ross.

Hughes R., Dake J.P. (1886–91). *A Cyclopaedia of Drug Pathogenesy*. 4 vols. London, Leath & Ross.

Hunter J. (1786). *A Treatise on the Venereal Disease*. London.

Iezzoni L.I. (1996). 100 apples divided by 15 red herrings: a cautionary tale from the mid-19th century on comparing hospital mortality rates. *Annals of Internal Medicine*. 124: 1079–1085.

Inglis B. (1964). *Fringe Medicine*. London, Faber and Faber.

Irvine F.W. (1844). M. Andral's homoeopathic experiments at la Pitié. *British Journal of Homoeopathy*. 2 (1): 49–64.

Jadad A.R. (1994). *Meta-analysis of Randomized Clinical Trials* (Thesis). Oxford, Oxford University.

Jadad A.R., Moore A., Carroll D., Jenkinson C., Reynolds D.J.M., Gavaghan D.J., McQuay H.J. (1996). Assessing the quality of reports of randomized clinical trials: is blinding necessary? *Controlled Clinical Trials*. 17: 1–12.

Janet P. (1925). *Psychological Healing: A Historical and Clinical Study*. 2 vols. Transl. E & C Paul. London, Allen & Unwin.

Jardine N. (1991). *The Scenes of Inquiry. On the Reality of Questions in the Sciences*. Oxford, Clarendon Press.

Jean Paul (1826–28). *Zerstreuete Blätte*. Sämtliche Werke. Vol 2. Ed. Förster E. Berlin.

Jewson N.D. (1976). The disappearance of the sick-man from medical cosmology, 1770–1870. *Sociology*. 10: 225–244.

Johannsen (1848). Ueber den Gegenwärtigen Stand der Homöopathie in Russland. *Hygea*. 1 n.s.: 44–50.

Jonas W. (1998). Safety in homeopathy. In: Ernst E. & Hahn E. G., eds *Homoeopathy: A Critical Appraisal*. Oxford, Butterworth Heinemann: 130–135.

Jones B., Jarvis P., Lewis J.A., Ebbutt A.F. (1996). Trials to assess equivalence: the importance of rigorous methods. *British Medical Journal*. 313: 36–39.

Jones H., Hoerr N., Osol A., eds. (1949). *Blakiston's New Gould Medical Dictionary*. London, H.K. Lewis.

Juncker L.C. (1750). *Dissertatio de damno ex scabie repulsa*. Halle.

Jüni P., Witschi A., Bloch R., Egger M. (1999). The hazards of scoring the quality of clinical trials for meta-analysis. *Journal of the American Medical Association*. 282: 1054–1060.

Jütte R. (1998). The paradox of professionalisation: homeopathy and hydropathy as unorthodoxy in Germany in the 19th and early 20th century. In: Jütte R. & Risse G. B. & Woodward J., eds *Culture, Knowledge and Healing: Historical Perspectives of Homoeopathic Medicine in Europe and North America*. Sheffield, European Association for the History of Medicine and Health Publications: 65–88.

Jütte R. (1999). The historiography of nonconventional medicine in Germany: a concise overview. *Medical History*. 43: 342–358.

Jütte R., Risse G.B., Woodward J., eds. (1998). *Culture, Knowledge and Healing: Historical Perspectives of Homoeopathic Medicine in Europe and North America*. Sheffield, European Association for the History of Medicine and Health Publications.

Kant I. (1784). Beantwortung der Frage: Was ist Aufklärung? *Berlinische Monatsschrifte*. 4 (12 December): 481–494.

Kant I. (1787). *Critique of Pure Reason*. Transl. J.M.D. Meiklejohn from the 2nd German edn. London, Everyman, 1934.

Kaptchuk T.J. (1997). Early use of blind assessment in a homoeopathic scientific experiment. *British Homoeopathic Journal*. 86: 49–50.

Kaptchuk T.J. (1998a). Intentional ignorance: a history of blind assessment and placebo controls in medicine. *Bulletin of the History of Medicine*. 72: 389–433.

Kaptchuk T.J. (1998b). Powerful placebo: the dark side of the randomised controlled trial. *Lancet*. 351: 1722–1725.

Kaptchuk T.J. (2000). Debate over the history of placebos in medicine. *Alternative Therapies in Health and Medicine*. 6 (4): 18.

Kaufmann M. (1971). *Homeopathy in America, the rise and Fall of a Medical Heresy*. Baltimore, Johns Hopkins University Press.

Kelso J.S. (1995). *Dynamic Patterns: The Self-Organization of Brain and Behavior*. Cambridge, MA, MIT Press.

Kent J.T. (1885). What is homoeopathy? *St Louis Clinical Review*. 8: 425–432.

Kent J.T. (1888). The second prescription. In: Gypser K. H., ed. *Kent's Minor Writings on Homoeopathy*. Heidelberg, Haug, 1987: 232–240.

Kent J.T. (1900). *Lectures on Homoeopathic Philosophy*. Lancaster, Philadelphia.

Kent J.T. (1911). *Lectures on Homoeopathic Materia Medica*. 2nd edn. Philadelphia, Boericke & Tafel.

Kent J.T. (1912a). Classification of constitutions useless in prescribing. *The Homoeopathician*. 1: 204.

Kent J.T. (1912b). Remedies related to pathological tissue changes. *The Homoeopathician*. 2 (2): 67–68.

Kent J.T. (1912c). Severe maladies. In: Gypser K.-H., ed. *Kent's Minor Writings on Homoeopathy*. Heidelberg, Haug, 1987: 681–685.

Kent J.T. (1926). *New Remedies, Clinical Cases, Lesser Writings, Aphorisms and Precepts*. Ed. Sherwood W. W. Chicago, Ehrhart & Karl.

Kent J.T. (1945). *Repertory of the Homoeopathic Materia Medica*. 5th edn. Ed. Kent L. M. Chicago, Ehrhart & Karl.

Kienle G.S., Kiene H. (1998). The placebo effect: a scientific critique. *Complementary Therapies in Medicine*. 6: 14–24.

Kieser D.G.v. (1817–19). *System der Medizin*. Halle.

King L.S. (1958). *The Medical World of the Eighteenth Century*. Chicago, University of Chicago Press.

Kleijnen J., Knipschild P., ter Riet G. (1991). Clinical trials of homoeopathy. *British Medical Journal*. 302: 316–323.

Kleinert P.G.O. (1863). *Quellen-Nachweis der physiologischen Arzneiprüfungen*. Leipzig, Otto Purfurst.

Kollerstrom J. (1982). Basic scientific research into the 'low dose' effect. *British Homoeopathic Journal*. 71: 41–47.

Kotok A. (1999). *The History of Homeopathy in the Russian Empire until World War I, as compared with other European Countries and the USA: Similarities and Discrepancies* (Thesis). Department of the History of Medicine. Jerusalem, Hebrew University.

Kretschmer E. (1926). *Körperbau und Charakter*. 4th edn. Berlin.

Krieger E.M., Salgado H.C., Assan C.J., Greene L.L.J., Ferreira S.H. (1971). Potential screening test for detection of over-activity of the renin-angiotensin system. *Lancet*. i: 269–271.

Kuéss-Scheichelbauer (1959). *200 Jahre Freimauerei in Österreich*. Vienna, Kerry.

Kurmbahaar E.B. (1919). The blood and bone marrow in yellow gas (mustard gas) poisoning. *Journal of Medical Research*. 40: 497–507.

Lachmund J. (1998). Between scrutiny and treatment: physical diagnosis and the restructuring of 19th century medical practice. *Sociology of Health & Illness*. 20: 779–801.

Lambert J.H. (1764). *Neues Organon oder Gedanken über die Erforschung und Bezeichnüng des Wahren und dessen Unterscheidung vom Irrthum und Schein*. 2 vols. Leipzig, Johann Wendler.

Langman M. (1997). Homoeopathy trials: reasons for good ones but are they warranted? *Lancet*. 350: 825.

Last J.M., ed. (1995). *A Dictionary of Epidemiology*. 3rd edn. Oxford, Oxford University Press.

Lasveaux L. (1988). *Traitements homéopathiques du choléra dans la France du XIXe siècle*. Lyon, Boiron.

Leary B. (1987). Cholera and homoeopathy in the nineteenth century. *British Homoeopathic Journal*. 76: 190–194.

Leary B. (1994). Cholera 1854: update. *British Homoeopathic Journal*. 83: 117–121.

Leary B., Lorentzon M., Bosanquet A. (1998). It won't do any harm: practice and people at the London Homoeopathic Hospital, 1889–1923. In: Jütte R. & Risse G. B. & Woodward J., eds *Culture, Knowledge and Healing: Historical Perspectives of Homoeopathic Medicine in Europe and North America*. Sheffield, European Association for the History of Medicine and Health Publications: 251–273.

Ledermann E.K. (1945). The effect of homoeopathy and natural therapy in chronic diseases, demonstrated in a series of cases. *British Homoeopathic Journal*. 35: 52–9.

Ledermann E.K. (1949). Homoeopathy's way to recognition. *British Homoeopathic Journal*. 39 (July).

Ledermann E.K., Sutherland I., Lunt R. (1954). Homoeopathy tested against controls in surgical tuberculosis. *British Homoeopathic Journal*. 44: 83–97.

Leeser O. (1936). *Textbook of Homoeopathic Materia Medica: Inorganic Medicinal Substances*. Transl. L.J. Boyd. Philadelphia, Boericke & Tafel.

Lewis R.A. (1952). *Edwin Chadwick and the Public Health Movement 1832–1854*. London, Longmans, Green.

Light R.J., Pillemer D.B. (1984). *Summing Up: The Science of Reviewing Research*. Cambridge, MA, Harvard University Press.

Lilienfeld A. (1982). Ceteribus paribus: the evolution of the clinical trial. *Bulletin of the History of Medicine*. 56 (1): 1–18.

Lilienfeld A.M., Lilienfeld D.E. (1979). A century of case-control studies: progress? *Journal of Chronic Disease*. 32: 5–13.

Lilienfeld A.M., Lilienfeld D.E. (1980). *Foundations of Epidemiology*. 2nd edn. New York, Oxford University Press.

Linde K., Clausius N., Ramirez G., Melchart D., Eitel F., Hedges L.V., Jonas W.B. (1997). Are the effects of homoeopathy all placebo effects? A meta-analysis of randomized, placebo controlled trials. *Lancet*. 350: 834–843.

Linde K., Melchart D. (1998). Randomized controlled trials of individualized homeopathy: a state-of-the-art review. *Journal of Alternative and Complementary Medicine*. 4 (4): 371–388.

Lloyd W.E.B. (1936). *A Hundred Years of Medicine*. London, Duckworth.

Lodispoto A. (1961). *Storia dell Omeopatia in Italia*. Rome, Istituto di Storia della Medicina dell'Università di Roma.

Louis P.C.A. (1835). *Recherches sur les effets de la saignée*. Paris, Baillière.

Lully R. (1330). *The Experiments of Raymond Lully of Majorca the most learned philosopher, wherein the operations of the true Chymicall Philosophy are plainly delivered*. Transl. William Atherton, 1558, MS Ashmole 1508, Bodleian Library.

Lutze A. (1874). *Lehrbuch der Homöopathie*. 8th edn. Ed. Lutze E. A. Cöthen, Lutze'schen Klinik.

Lux J.J.W. (1833). *Isopathik der Contagionen*. Leipzig, Kollman.

MacKenzie D.A. (1981). *Statistics in Britain: The Social Construction of Scientific Knowledge, 1865–1930*. Edinburgh, Edinburgh University Press.

Malmberg H., Holopainen E., Simola M., Boss I., Lindqvist N.A. (1991). A comparison between intranasal budesonide aerosol and budesonide dry powder in the treatment of hay fever symptoms. *Rhinology*. 29: 137–141.

Marková I. (1982). *Paradigms, Thought, and Language*. Chichester, Wiley.

Marks H.M. (1997). *The Progress of Experiment: Science and Therapeutic Reform in the United States, 1900–1990*. New York, Cambridge University Press.

Martini P. (1932). *Methodenlehre der therapeutischen Untersuchung*. Berlin, Springer Verlag.

Martins M. (1835). Exposé de plusieurs expériences homéopathiques faites en Allemagne. *Revue Médicale Française et Etrangère*. 1: 205–217.

Matthews J.R. (1995). *Quantification and the Quest for Medical Certainty*. Princeton, NJ, Princeton University Press.

Maulitz R.C. (1987). *Morbid Appearances: The Anatomy of Pathology in the Early Nineteenth Century*. Cambridge, Cambridge University Press.

Mead R. (1745). *A Mechanical Account of Poisons: In Several Essays*. 3rd edn. London, J. Brindley.

Medical Council (1854–55). *Report of the Committee for Scientific Inquiries in relation to the cholera epidemic of 1854*. Parliamentary Papers, no. 1980, xxi.

Medical Research Council (2000). *A Framework for Development and Evaluation of RCTs for Complex Interventions to Improve Health*. http://www.mrc.ac.uk/complex_packages.html

Meriadec M.C. (1990). *L'Homéopathie: conception médicale à la dimension de l'homme*. Lyon, Boiron.

Meyer F.P. (1996). *Vorlesungen über Homöopathie*. Jena, Fischer.

Milcent A. (1862). Jean-Paul Tessier. *Monthly Homoeopathic Review*. 8 (6): 449–462.

Mill J.S. (1867). *Dissertations and Disquisitions*. 2 vols. London.

Mitchell G.R. (1975). *Homoeopathy: The First Authoritative Study of its Place in Medicine Today*. London, W.H. Allen.

Moher D., Fortin P., Jadad A.R., Jüni P., Klassen T., Le Lorier J., Liberati A., Linde K., Penna A. (1996). Completeness of reporting of trials published in languages other than English: implications for conduct and reporting of systematic reviews. *Lancet*. 347: 363–366.

Moher D., Jadad A.R., Nichol G., Penman M., Tugwell P., Walsh S. (1995). Assessing the quality of randomized controlled trials: an annotated bibliography of scales and checklists. *Controlled Clinical Trials*. 16: 62–73.

Moher D., Schulz K.F., Altman D.G., for the CONSORT Group (2001). The CONSORT statement: revised recommendations for improving the quality of reports of parallel-group randomised trials. *Lancet*. 357 (1191–1194).

Monro D. (1788). *A Treatise on Medical and Pharmaceutical Chemistry*. London, T. Cadell.

Morgan A.A. (1978). Bleeding gastric erosion after oral zinc sulphate. *British Medical Journal*. 1: 1283–1284.

Moskowitz R. (1992). Vaccination: a sacrament of modern medicne. *The Homoeopath*. 12 (1): 137–144.

Mössinger P. (1984). *Der praktische Arzt als Fachmann für Erfahrung und Beobachtung*. Heidelberg, Haug.

Mulrow C.D., Oxman A.D. (1997). Cochrane Collaboration Handbook. In: *The Cochrane Library [database on CDROM]*. Version 3.0. Oxford, Update Software.

Murphy M. (1993). *The Future of the Body. Explorations into the Further Evolution of Human Nature*. Los Angeles, Tarcher.

Needham J. (1974). *Science & Civilisation in China (5) Chemistry and Chemical Technology: Part 2 – Spagyrical Discovery and Invention; Magisteries of Gold and Immortality*. Cambridge, Cambridge University Press.

Newman W.R. (1991). *Summa perfectionis of Pseudo-Geber*. Leiden, Brill.

Newman W.R. (1994). Boyle's debt to corpuscular alchemy. In: Hunter M., ed. *Robert Boyle Reconsidered*. Cambridge, Cambridge University Press: 107–118.

NHS CRD (1996). *Undertaking Systematic Reviews of Research on Effectiveness*. University of York: NHS Centre for Reviews and Dissemination.

NICE (2000). *Guidance on zanamivir (Relenza) in the treatment of influenza.* http://www.nice.org.uk/docref.asp?d=12482

Nicholls P.A. (1988). *Homoeopathy and the Medical Profession.* London, Croom Helm.

Nicolson M. (1988). The metastatic theory of pathogenesis and the professional interests of the eighteenth-century physician. *Medical History.* 32: 277–300.

Noll R. (1992). *The Jung Cult: Origins of a Charismatic Movement.* London, Fontana Press.

Nurmohamed M.T., Rosendaal F.R., Buller H.R. (1992). Low-molecular-weight heparin versus standard heparin in general and orthopaedic surgery. *Lancet.* 340: 152–156.

Ober K.P. (1997). The pre-Flexnerian reports: Mark Twain's criticism of medicine in the United States. *Annals of Internal Medicine.* 126 (2): 157–163.

Oliver I. (1999). *Homoeopathy Before Hahnemann.* London, Midas Graphics.

Oosterhuis R.A.B. (1937). *Paracelsus en Hahnemann, een Renaissance der Geneeskunst.* Leiden, A. W. Sijthoff.

Osler W. (1912). *The Principles and Practice of Medicine.* 8th edn. New York, Appleton.

Osler W. (1941). Medicine in the nineteenth century. In: *Aequanimitas and Other Essays.* London, H.K. Lewis: 217–262.

Owen R.M., Ives G. (1982). The mustard gas experiments of the British Homoeopathic Society: 1941–1942. *35th Congress LMHI Sussex, UK; Papers and Summaries*: 258–269.

Oxman A.D., Cook D.J., Guyatt G.H. (1994). User's guide to the medical literature: VI. how to use an overview. *Journal of the American Medical Association.* 272: 1367–1371.

Ozanne J. (1853). Homoeopathy tested by statistics. *Homoeopathic Times.* 4 (182): 372–375.

Pagel W. (1982a). *Joan Baptista Van Helmont, Reformer of Science and Medicine.* Cambridge, Cambridge University Press.

Pagel W. (1982b). *Paracelsus: An Introduction to Philosophical Medicine in the Era of the Renaissance.* 2nd edn. Basel, Karger.

Palou J. (1966). *La Franc-Maçonnerie.* Paris, Payot.

Paterson J. (1936). Lecture demonstration showing the technique in the preparation of the non-lactose fermenting nosodes of the bowel and the clinical indications for their use. *Transactions of the 11th Congress Liga Homoeopatica Internationalis*, 24–29 August, Glasgow: 213–244.

Peirce C.S. (1935). *Collected Papers.* 6 vols. Cambridge, Mass., Harvard University Press.

Peschier G. (1835a). Mélanges. *Bibliothèque Homoeopathique*. 4: 122–126.

Peschier G. (1835b). Sur le saccharum lactis. *Bibliothèque Homoeopathique*. 4: 273–280.

Pinto G., Feldman M. (2000). *Homoeopathy for Children. A Parents' Guide to the Treatment of Common Childhood Illnesses*. 2nd edn. Saffron Walden, C.W. Daniel.

Plenciz M.A.v. (1762). *Opera medico-physica, in quatuor tractatus digesta, quorum primus contagii morborum ideam novam una cum additamento de lue bovina, anno 1761, epidemice grassante sistit. Secundus de variolis, tertius de scarlatina, quartus de terrae motu, sed praecipue illo horribili agit, qui prima Novembris anno 1755 Europam, Africam, et Americam conquassabat*. Vienna, J.T. von Trattner.

Pogue J., Yusuf S. (1998). Overcoming the limitations of current meta-analysis of randomised controlled trials. *The Lancet*. 351: 47–52.

Poitevin B. (1987). *Le devenir de l'homéopathie: éléments de théorie et de recherche*.

Porter R., ed. (1993). *Companion Encyclopaedia of the History of Medicine*. 2 vols. London, Routledge.

Porter R. (1997). *The Greatest Benefit to Mankind: A Medical History of Humanity from Antiquity to the Present*. London, HarperCollins.

Porter T.M. (1986). *The Rise of Statistical Thinking 1820–1900*. Princeton, Princeton University Press.

Principe L.M. (1998). *The Aspiring Adept: Robert Boyle and His Alchemical Quest: Including Boyle's 'Lost' 'Dialogue on the Transmutation of Metals'*. Princeton, NJ, Princeton University Press.

Quarin J.v. (1761). *Tentamen de cicuta*. Vienna.

Quin F.F., ed. (1834). *Pharmacopeia Homoeopathica*. London, S. Highley.

Rademacher J.G. (1841). *Rechtfertigung der von den Gelehrten Misskannten, Verstandes rechten Erfahrungsheillehre der alten scheidekünstigen Geheimärtze, und treue Mittheilung des Ergebnisses einen 25jährigen Erprobung dieser Lehre am Krankbette*. 2 vols. Berlin, Reimer.

Rankin G. (1988). Professional organisation and the development of medical knowledge: two interpretations of homoeopathy. In: Cooter R., ed. *Studies in the History of Alternative Medicine*. Basingstoke, Macmillan / St Antony's College, Oxford.

Rasky E., Freidl W., Haidvogl M., Stronegger W.J. (1994). Arbeits- und Lebensweise von homöopathisch tätigen Ärztinnen und Ärzten in Österreich. Eine deskriptive Studie. *Wien medizinische Wochenschrift*. 144 (17): 419–424.

Rawlins M.D. (1990). Development of a rational practice of therapeutics. *British Medical Journal*. 301: 729–733.

Reich W. (1942). *The Function of the Orgasm*, Orgone Institute.

Reilly D.T. (1996). Personal communication.

Reubi F.C. (1986). Armand Trousseau (1801–1867) et l'effet placebo. *Schweizerische Medizinische Wochenschrift*. 116 (1): 27–28.

Rickmann C. (1771). *Einfluß der Arzneiwissenschaft auf das Wohl des Staats und dem besten Mittel zur Rettung des Lebens*. Jena, Hartung.

Ricord P. (1838). *Traité pratique des maladies venériennes*. Paris, De Just Rouvier & E. Le Bouvier.

Righetti M.R. (1991). Characteristics and selected results of research in homeopathy. *Berlin Journal on Research in Homoeopathy*. 1: 195–203.

Risse G.B. (1972). Kant, Schelling, and the early search for a philosophical 'science' of medicine in Germany. *Journal of the History of Medicine and Allied Sciences*. 27 (2): 145–158.

Roberts W.H. (1986). Orthodoxy vs. homeopathy: ironic developments following the Flexner Report at the Ohio State University. *Bulletin of the History of Medicine*. 60: 73–87.

Robinson V. (1931). *The Story of Medicine*. New York, Albert & Charles Boni.

Roeschlaub A. (1799). Einige Bemerkungen ueber die Definition und Eintheilung der Medizin. *Magazin zur Vervollkommnung der theoretischen und practischen Heilkunde*. 1 (2): 279–302.

Rolf I. (1977). *Rolfing: The Integration of Human Structures*. Santa Monica, CA, Dennis-Landman.

Ronsmans C., Bennish M.L., Chakraborty J., Fauveau V. (1991). Current practices for treatment of dysentery in rural Bangladesh. *Reviews of Infectious Diseases*. 13: S351–356.

Rousseau J.J. (1796). *Handbuch für Mütter, oder Grundsätze der ersten Erziehung der Kinder*. Transl. S. Hahnemann from Principes de Jean Jacques Rousseau, sur l'éducation des enfants. Paris an 2 [1793]. Leipzig.

Routh C.H.F. (1852). *On the Fallacies of Homoeopathy and the Imperfect Statistical Inquiries on which the Results of that Practice are Estimated*. London, H.K. Lewis.

Royal College of Obstetricians and Gynaecologists (2001). *Recommendations from the study group on evidence-based ferility treatment*. www.rcog.org.uk/study/studygroup

Rückle E. (1942). Rademacher und Hahnemann. *Deutsche Zeitschrift für Homöopathie*. 58: 78–83.

Russell E. (1973). *Report on Radionics: Science of the Future*. London, Neville Spearman.

Russell I., Di Blasi Z., Lambert M., Russell D. (1998). Systematic reviews and meta-analyses: opportunities and threats. In: Templeton A. & Cooke I. & O'Brien P. M. S., eds *Evidence-based Fertility Treatment*. London, Royal College of Obstetrics and Gynaecology Press: 15–64.

Ruta D.A., Garratt A.M., Leng M., Russell I.T., MacDonald L.M. (1994). A new approach to the measurement of quality of life. *Medical Care*. 32: 1109–1126.

Sampson W., London W. (1995). Analysis of homeopathic treatment of childhood diarrhea. *Pediatrics*. 96: 961–4.

Sankaran P. (1978). *Some Recent Research and Advances in Homoeopathy*. Bombay, Homoeopathic Medical Publishers.

Schelling F.W.J.v. (1797). *Ideen zu einer Philosophie der Natur*. Leipzig, Landshut.

Schelling F.W.J.v. (1799). *Einleitung zu seinem Entwurf eines Systems der Naturphilosophie, oder ueber den Entwurf der speculativen Physik und die innere Organisation eines Systems dieser Wissenschaft*. Jena und Leipzig, Gabler.

Schenk H.G. (1966). *The Mind of the European Romantics: An Essay in Cultural History*. London, Constable.

Schier J. (1942). Die homöopathische Behandlung des Keuchhustens. *Deutsche Zeitschrift für Homöopathie*. 58: 157.

Schilsky B. (1942a). Entgegnung auf Schiers Bemerkungen. *Deutsche Zeitschrift für Homöopathie*. 58: 215.

Schilsky B. (1942b). Ueber homöopathische Behandlung des Keuchhustens. *Deutsche Zeitschrift für Homöopathie*. 58: 87–90.

Schmidt J.M. (1990). *Die philosophischen Vorstellungen Samuel Hahnemanns bei der Begründung der Homöopathie: bis zum Organon der rationellen Heilkunde, 1810*. München, Sonntag.

Schmitz A. (1942). Einige weitere Gedanken zu 'Nützt uns die Homöopathie bei der Diphtherie-Behandlung?'. *Deutsche Zeitschrift für Homöopathie*. 58: 211–213.

Schroyens F. (1993). *SYNTHESIS Repertorium homeopathicum syntheticum*. 5th edn. London, Homoeopathic Book Publishers.

Schultz C.H. (1831). *Die homöobiotische Medizin des Theophrastus Paracelsus in ihrem Gegensatz gegen die Medizin der Alten ... und als Quell der Homöopathie*. Berlin, August Hirschlaub.

Schüssler W.H. (1874). *Eine abgekürtze Therapeutik gegründet auf Histologie und Cellularpathologie*. Oldenburg.

Schwanitz H.J. (1983). *Homöopathie und Brownianismus, 1795–1844*. Stuttgart, Gustav Fischer Verlag.

Schwartzhaupt W. (1942). Nützt uns die Homöopathie bei der Diphtherie-Behandlung? *Deutsche Zeitschrift für Homöopathie*. 58: 150–153.

Schwarz D., Lellouch J. (1967). Explanatory and pragmatic attitudes in therapeutical trials. *Journal of Chronic Disease*. 20: 637–648.

Scofield A.M. (1984). Experimental research in homoeopathy – a critical review. *British Homoeopathic Journal*. 73: 161–180, 211–226.

Seemen H.v. (1926). *Kenntnis der Medizinhistorie in der deutschen Romantik*. Zurich.

Seghal M.L. (1994). Rediscovery of homoeopathy. *Homoeopathic Links* (1): 31–34.

Semmelweis I. (1861). *Die Aetiologie, Begriff, und die Prophylaxis des Kindbettfiebers*. Pest, C.A. Hartleben.

Shah I. (1964). *The Sufis*. New York, Doubleday.

Sharpe M., Hawton K., Simkin S., Surawy C., Hackmann A., Klimes I., Peto T., Warrell D., Seagroatt V. (1996). Cognitive behaviour therapy for the chronic fatigue syndrome: a randomized controlled trial. *British Medical Journal*. 312 (7022): 22–6.

Sheldon T. (1995). Please bypass the PORT. *British Medical Journal*. 309: 142–143.

Shelley J.H., Baur M.P. (1999). Paul Martini: the first clinical pharmacologist? *Lancet*. 353: 1870–1873.

Shideman D.E., Beckman H. (1958). Comments on treatment. *Wisconsin Medical Journal*. 57: 456.

Shryock R.H. (1948). *The Development of Modern Medicine: An Interpretation of the Social and Scientific Factors Involved*. 2nd edn. London, Gollancz.

Shryock R.H. (1961). The history of quantification in medical science. In: Woolf H., ed. *Quantification, a History of the Meaning of Measurement in the Natural and Social Sciences*. Indianapolis, Bobbs-Merrill, for the History of Science Society: 85–107.

Simon L. (1836). *Lettre à M. le Ministre de l'instruction publique, en réponse au jugement de l'Académie royale de Médecine, sur la doctrine médicale homoeopathique, au nom de l'Institut homoeopathique de Paris*. Paris, Baillière.

Singer C. (1928). *A Short History of Medicine*. Oxford, Clarendon Press.

Slinn J. (1995). Research and development in the UK pharmaceutical industry from the nineteenth century to the 1960s. In: Porter R. & Teich M., eds *Drugs and Narcotics in History*. Cambridge, Cambridge University Press: 168–186.

Snow J. (1849). On the pathology and mode of communication of the cholera. *London Medical Gazette*. 44: 730–732, 745–752, 923–929.

Spooner J.W. (1882). The relations of the fellows of the Massachussets Medical Society to homeopathy and homeopaths. *Boston Medical and Surgical Journal*. 107: 73–77.

Sprengel K. (1821–28). *Versuch einer pragmatischen Geschichte der Arzneikunde*. 5 vols. Vol 5, i. 3rd edn. Halle, Gebauer.

Stearns G.B. (1932). Body-reflexes as a means of selecting a remedy. *The Homoeopathic Recorder*. 47: 781.

Stearns G.B., Stark M.B. (1925). Experiments with homoeopathic potentized substances given to Drosophila melanogaster with hereditary tumors. *The Homoeopathic Recorder*. 40: 130–140.

Steiner R. (1948). *Spiritual Science and Medicine*. London, Rudolf Steiner Press.

Stiegele A. (1941). *Klinische Homöopathie. Beiträge zu ihren Grundlagen*. Stuttgart, Hippokrates-Verlag.

Stigler S.M. (1986). *The History of Statistics: The Measurement of Uncertainty before 1900*. Cambridge, MA, Harvard University Press.

Störck A. (1760). Some account of the virtues of hemlock, in curing various diseases. *The Gentleman's Magazine*. 30: 426–430.

Störck A. (1764). Some account of the use and effects of the root of meadow saffron. *The Gentleman's Magazine*. 34 (September): 426–429.

Störck A.v. (1762). *Libellus, quo demonstratur: Stramonium, Hyosciamum, Aconitum non solum tuto pose exhiberi usu interno hominibus, rerum et sea esse remedia in multis morbis maxime salutifera*. Vienna.

Suttie I. (1936). *The Origins of Love and Hate*. Harmondsworth, Penguin [1952].

Swan S. (1888). *Materia Medica Containing Provings and Clinical Verifications of Nosodes and Morbific Products*. New York, Pusey.

Swedenborg E. (1984). *The Universal Human and Soul–Body Interaction*. Ed. Dole G. F. London, SPCK.

Taylor M.A., Reilly D., Llewellyn-Jones R.H., McSharry C., Aitchison T.C. (2000). Randomised controlled trial of homoeopathy versus placebo in perennial allergic rhinitis with overview of four trial series. *British Medical Journal*. 321: 471–476.

Temkin O. (1963). The scientific approach to disease: specific entity and individual sickness. In: Crombie A. C., ed. *Scientific Change*. London, Heinemann Educational: 629–647.

Tessier J.-P. (1850). *Recherches cliniques sur le traitement de la pneumonie et du choléra suivant la méthode de Hahnemann, précédées d'une introduction sur l'abus de la statistique en médecine*. Paris, Baillière.

Tessier J.-P. (1856). On the legitimate position that homoeopathy should hold in medicine. *British Journal of Homoeopathy*. 14: 51–75.

The Lancet (1995). Quality of life and clinical trials. *Lancet*. 346: 1–2.

The Standards of Reporting Trials Group (1994). A proposal for structured reporting of randomized controlled trials. *Journal of the American Medical Association*. 272: 1926–1931.

Thomas J. (1994). Comparative study of radionics and traditionally prepared remedies. *Townsend Letter for Doctors* (May).

Torgerson D.J., Klaber-Moffett, Russell I.T. (1996). Patient preferences in randomised trials: threat or opportunity? *Journal of Health Services Research and Policy*. 1 (4): 194–197.

Tramèr M., Reynolds D., Moore R., McQuay H. (1998). When placebo controlled trials are essential and equivalence trials are inadequate. *British Medical Journal*. 317: 875–880.

Treuherz F. (1983). Heclae lava or the influence of Swedenborg on homoeopathy. *The Homoeopath*. 4 (2): 35–53.

Tröhler U. (1978). *Quantification in British Medicine and Surgery, 1750–1830* (Thesis). London, University of London.

Tromp S.W. (1949). *Psychical Physics: A Scientific Analysis of Dowsing, Radiesthesia and Kindred Divining Phenomena*. New York, Elsevier.

Trousseau A., Gouraud H. (1834). Expériences homéopathiques tentées à l'Hôtel-Dieu de Paris. *Journal des Connaissances Médico-Chirurgicales*. 8 (April): 238–241.

Tyler M. (1952). *Homoeopathic Drug Pictures*. 2nd edn. London, Homoeopathic Publishing Company.

Unschuld P.U. (1995). Plausibility or truth? An essay on medicine and world view. *Science in Context*. 8 (1): 9–30.

Unschuld P.U. (1998). *Chinese Medicine*. Transl. N. Wiseman. Brookline, Massachussets, Paradigm Publications.

Urbach P. (1985). Randomization and the design of experiments. *Philosophy of Science*. 52: 256–273.

Vakil P., King G. (1997). The homeopathic proving of two complex remedies. *Biomedical Therapy*. 15: 104–108.

Van der Steen W., Thung P. (1988). *Faces of Medicine: A Philosophical Study*. Dordrecht, Kluwer Academic.

Van Helmont J.B. (1648). Demens idea. In: *Ortus Medicinae, id est initia physicae inaudita*. Amsterdam, Elzevir.

Vandenbroucke J.P. (1997). Homoeopathy trials: going nowhere. *Lancet*. 350: 824.

Vandenbroucke J.P. (2000). Scoring the quality of clinical trials. *Journal of the American Medical Association*. 283: 1422.

Varma P.N., Indu V. (1992). *Side effects and adverse side effects of homoeopathic medicines in their lower attenuations*. New Delhi, Jain.

Vercoulen J.H., Swanink C.M., Zitman F.G., Vreden S.G., Hoofs M.P., Fennis J.F., Galama J.M., van der Meer J.W., Bleijenberg G. (1996). Randomised, double-blind, placebo-controlled study of fluoxetine in chronic fatigue syndrome. *Lancet*. 347 (9005): 858–61.

Vernois M. (1835). *Analyse complète et raisonée de la matière médicale de Samuel Hahnemann*. Paris, Baillière.

Vickers A.J. (2000). Homeopathy: analysis of a scientific debate. *Journal of Alternative and Complementary Medicine*. 6 (1): 50–58.

Vickers A.J., Smith C. (2000). Homoeopathic Oscillococcinum for preventing and treating influenza and influenza-like syndromes. In: *The Cochrane Library [database on CDROM]*. Issue 1. Oxford, Update Software.

Vithoulkas G. (1972). *Homeopathy: Medicine of the New Man*. New York, Avon.

Vithoulkas G. (1980). *The Science of Homeopathy*. New York, Grove Press.

Vithoulkas G. (1991). *A New Model for Health and Disease*. Mill Valley, CA, Health and Habitat.

Voorhoeve J.N. (1936). The 'chronic diseases' of Hahnemann considered in the light of modern constitutional theory. *Transactions of the 11th Congress Liga Homoeopatica Internationalis*, 24–29 August, Glasgow: 268–277.

Warkentin D. (1994). *ReferenceWorks*. Computer program version 1.52. Fairfax, CA, Kent Homeopathic Associates.

Waters W., Campbell M.J., Elwood P.C. (1988). Migraine headache and survival in women. *British Medical Journal*. 287 (1442–1443).

Wearden A.J., Morris R.K., Mullis R., Strickland P.L., Pearson D.J., Appleby L., Campbell I.T., Morris J.A. (1998). A randomised, double-blind, placebo-controlled treatment trial of fluoxetine and a graded exercise programme in chronic fatigue syndrome. *British Journal of Psychiatry*. 172: 485–490.

Weatherall M. (1994). Drug therapies. In: Bynum W. F. & Porter R., eds *Companion Encyclopaedia of the History of Medicine*. vol. 2. London, Routledge: 915–938.

Weatherall M.J. (1996). Making medicine scientific: empiricism, rationality, and quackery in mid-Victorian Britain. *Social History of Medicine*. 9 (2): 175–194.

Webb J. (1976). *The Occult Establishment*. La Salle, Open Court.

Wesselhoeft Jr C. (1928). Homöopathische Behandlung des Scharlachs. *Allgemeine Homöopathische Zeitung*. 176: 293–306.

Wesselhoeft Jr C. (1929). Die homöopathische Behandlung der Infektionskrankheiten. *Allgemeine Homöopathische Zeitung*. 177: 432–441.

Wessely S., Chalder T., Hirsch S., Wallace P., Wright D. (1997). The prevalence and morbidity of chronic fatigue and chronic fatigue syndrome: a prospective primary care study. *American Journal of Public Health*. 87: 1449–1455.

Whitmarsh T. (2000). More lessons from migraine. *British Homoeopathic Journal*. 89: 1–2.

Whitmont E. (1982). *Psyche and Substance. Essays on Homeopathy in the Light of Jungian Psychology*. Richmond, CA, North Atlantic Books.

Wiesenauer M., Groh P., Haussler S. (1992). Naturheilkunde als Beitrag zur Kostendampfung. Versuch einer Kostenanalyse. *Fortschritte der Medizin*. 110 (17): 311–4.

Wiesenauer M., Lüdtke R. (1996). A meta-analysis of the homeopathic treatment of pollinosis with Galphima glauca. *Forschende Komplementärmedizin*. 3: 230–234.

Wilkinson J.J.G. (1857a). *The Homoeopathic Principle Applied to Insanity. A Proposal to Treat Lunacy by Spiritualism*. London.

Wilkinson J.J.G. (1857b). *The Human Body and its Connexion with Man, Illustrated by Principal Organs*. London.

Wilkinson J.J.G. (1889). Medical specialism. *The Homoeopathic World*. 24: 390–411.

Wilkinson J.J.G. (1890). *The Soul is Form and Doth the Body Make. The Heart and the Lungs, The Will and the Understanding: Chapters in Psychology*. London, J. Speirs.

Withering W. (1785). *An Account of the Foxglove and Some of its Medical Uses*. Birmingham, G.G.J. & J. Robinson.

Wolf P. (1837). Achtzehn Thesen fuer Freunde und Feinde der Homoeopathik. *Archiv für die homöopathische Heilkunst*. 16: 1–51.

Wood M. (2000). *Vitalism: The History of Herbalism, Homeopathy, and Flower Essences*. Berkeley, California, North Atlantic Books.

Youngson A.J. (1979). *The Scientific Revolution in Victorian Medicine*. London, Croom Helm.

Zissu R. (1977–78). *Matière médicale homéopathique constitutionelle. Etudes physio-pathologique, étiologique, diathésique et clinique des remèdes*. 4 vols. 2nd edn. Paris, Librairie le François.